Prevention®

The ULTIMATE GUIDE *to*
BREAST CANCER

Prevention®

The ULTIMATE GUIDE *to*

BREAST CANCER

YOUR ESSENTIAL RESOURCE FROM DIAGNOSIS TO TREATMENT AND BEYOND

The editors of

Prevention®

**and Mary L. Gemignani, MD, MPH,
with Caren Goldman**

RODALE.

This book is intended as a reference volume only, not as a medical manual. The information given here is designed to help you make informed decisions about your health. It is not intended as a substitute for any treatment that may have been prescribed by your doctor. If you suspect that you have a medical problem, we urge you to seek competent medical help.

The information in this book is meant to supplement, not replace, proper exercise training. All forms of exercise pose some inherent risks. The editors and publisher advise readers to take full responsibility for their safety and know their limits. Before practicing the exercises in this book, be sure that your equipment is well-maintained, and do not take risks beyond your level of experience, aptitude, training, and fitness. The exercise and dietary programs in this book are not intended as a substitute for any exercise routine or dietary regimen that may have been prescribed by your doctor. As with all exercise and dietary programs, you should get your doctor's approval before beginning.

Mention of specific companies, organizations, or authorities in this book does not imply endorsement by the author or publisher, nor does mention of specific companies, organizations, or authorities imply that they endorse this book, its author, or the publisher.

Internet addresses and telephone numbers given in this book were accurate at the time it went to press.

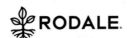

RODALE.

We inspire and enable people to improve their lives and the world around them.
rodalebooks.com

CONTENTS

Part Four: Living with Breast Cancer

Part Five: Thriving—Not Just Surviving

 Scan here or visit prevention.com/ugbcfootnotes for this book's complete footnotes.

FOREWORD

I'm a breast cancer surgeon. Every day, I see women who have recently heard the unhappy news that they have breast cancer. When they come to me, they're frightened about their future and have many questions, such as: Will they make it through the treatment process and how arduous will it be? Will they live to see their children grow up? Will they be able to enjoy the retirement plans they'd always dreamed about?

They're worried about the present, too. From dealing with health insurance to managing finances to holding on to their jobs and shuttling the kids to soccer practice–if life seemed impossibly hectic before, those four little words, "You have breast cancer," have made it seem simply impossible.

Often they are overwhelmed by the diagnosis and concerned about understanding enough to make the right decisions about treatment. All around them, family and friends are dispensing advice about the best doctors, the most up-to-date treatments, and the latest news about breast cancer research. I explain to them that it is important to understand that not everyone's breast cancer is the same, and the advice they may be receiving may not be pertinent to their diagnosis.

My first words of advice to the women who come to my office: Take a deep breath. And then take it one step at a time.

That's the advice I offer to you, too. I don't promise this will be easy, but with the information in this book, you'll learn how to manage your breast cancer journey with confidence and grace.

This book will help to answer many of the questions you already have, now that you have been told you have breast cancer. It's a primer on breast cancer—what it is, how it's diagnosed, how it's treated, how to live with it, and how to move on afterward. It will help you assemble the right medical team and work with them to choose the best treatment plan. It will discuss strategies to eat healthfully to rebuild your health and exercises to help rebuild your strength and stamina. It will give you a heads-up on important questions to ask your doctors, coping strategies for dealing with anxiety and stress, and tips on sharing the news with your family, friends, and coworkers. You'll even learn about complementary treatments that may be used to relieve some of the side effects you may experience. And you'll be inspired by the stories of women like you who have walked a path very much like yours.

As you begin your journey, I wish you health and healing, the love and support of the people you care about, and unexpected moments of joy. Knowledge really *is* power, and the information you'll find in the pages ahead can go a long way toward calming your fears, helping you make good decisions, and smoothing the road ahead.

–Dr. Mary L. Gemignani, *breast cancer surgeon,*
Memorial Sloan-Kettering Cancer Center

ACKNOWLEDGMENTS

With deep appreciation to Trisha Calvo, Nancy Fitzgerald, and Marielle Messing, our intrepid editors; to Lauren Shore-Prescott, MD, for lending her expertise; to Jess Fromm, for compiling the latest research; and to Hope Clarke, Keith Biery, Wendy Gable, and Elizabeth Krenos, for their hard work and late nights in devotion to this project.

Special thanks to the breast cancer survivors whose inspirational and informative personal stories made immeasurable contributions to this book—especially Jewell Biddle, Summer Bondurant, Crystal Brown-Tatum, Donna Deegan, Vicki Gingrich, Patricia Huxta, Elizabeth MacGregor, Lockey Maisonneuve, Meryl Marshall, Amanda Mercer, Lesley Ronson Brown, Kimberly Simanca, and Marisa Weiss, MD.

And finally, heartfelt appreciation to Gary Shiner, Ted Voorhees, and Steve Grovenburg for their considerable offerings to the process.

DEALING
with the
NEWS

Either you or someone you care deeply about has just been diagnosed with breast cancer. We know you're sad, concerned, and scared about the future. Questions are probably popping up about where to go, whom to talk to, and what to do next. And you may feel confused and frustrated because you don't have any idea where to turn for the answers.

The four chapters in Part One show you ways to begin dealing practically and creatively with your feelings, diagnosis, and prognosis; to help you assemble the best medical team you can; and to communicate effectively with your family, friends, neighbors, and coworkers.

"A journey of a thousand miles begins with a single step."

—LAO TZU

CHAPTER 1

COMING TO TERMS WITH BREAST CANCER

What happened when your doctor said, "I'm sorry to tell you that you have breast cancer"? Like so many of the women diagnosed with breast cancer each year, you probably experienced shock, denial, anger, fear, and sorrow. And in the days and weeks that followed, you most likely spent time pondering your diagnosis and, at the same time, trying to banish your worst fears. During those moments, you may have felt bewildered and frustrated as breast cancer began turning your life inside out. Chances are you started to ask some difficult questions, including a pesky, unanswerable one: "Why me?"

You undoubtedly also started searching for answers on the Internet, from friends, from magazine articles, and from books and probably discovered quite a bit to read. The Internet, in particular, can be especially overwhelming. One Google search for "breast cancer" can produce a whopping 550 million results in less than 30 seconds, not all of which are reliable.

There are two sets of statistics you've probably come across–or will–that you need to know about now.

- **You are *not* alone.** Breast cancer is the most common of all women's cancers, with the exception of skin cancer. It accounts for one in three cancers diagnosed in women. This year alone, almost one in eight

3

women of all ages will develop an invasive form of breast cancer.[1] (Men are diagnosed with breast cancer, too, although it's 100 times less common in men than in women. In July 2013, the American Cancer Society predicted that about 2,240 new cases of invasive breast cancer will be diagnosed among men.[2])

- **Breast cancer is *not* a death sentence.** Since 1991, death rates from breast cancer have declined. In fact, breast cancer has the *highest* survival rate of all cancers affecting women today.[3] There are more than 2.9 million women survivors of invasive breast cancer in the United States as of January 1, 2012.[4]

As you move through your journey, you'll be inundated with information from your own searches and from the doctors and other experts you'll be interacting with on a daily basis. You'll also, no doubt, be receiving advice and information from well-meaning family, friends, coworkers, and other acquaintances. Deciphering all this (and figuring out what makes sense for *you*) is where this essential *Prevention* guide comes in. In the pages that follow, you'll find information about breast cancer that's trustworthy and all in one place. It comes from knowledgeable sources: our lead doctor, top-notch research institutions and medical journals, and respected breast cancer organizations. We've also defined the medical language that you'll be hearing throughout your treatment and recovery to make it user-friendly and to reduce some of the stress and anxiety you're probably feeling. And wherever possible, we've included healing wisdom that you can take with you on your journey from diagnosis to recovery.

WHAT DOES BREAST CANCER MEAN TO YOU?

Longtime survivors say they're encouraged by efforts worldwide to find a cure and by the long-term survival statistics. But they also report that when they received the news that they had breast cancer, the numbers took on new meaning: "I know what my diagnosis says," so many women told us. "It says I have breast cancer. I know what the statistics are–that I have more of a chance of surviving this disease than ever before. But what does breast cancer *really* mean for me?"

a look at the numbers

As of January 2012, it was estimated that more than 2.9 million women were living in the United States with a history of invasive breast cancer and an additional 226,870 women who would be diagnosed that year. The median age of those learning they had invasive breast cancer was 61.[5]

There is no simple answer to this question. Consider just a few of the countless meanings of breast cancer that may come to mind. First, there are the technical meanings in medical dictionaries. These are straightforward, and that's good, because your doctors need precise definitions in order to understand your case and plan your treatment. You want members of your medical team to be clear with you and with each other about the meanings of tumors, the stages of cancer, lesions, metastasis or the development of secondary malignant growths, and so on.

But there are many other meanings of breast cancer in terms of how it affects you emotionally, physically, socially, and financially. These meanings first show up in the form of questions such as: *What quality of life will I have? Will my family and friends be there to help me? Will I have to give up my job? Will I still be lovable? Why does this scare me so much? What will happen to my family/my children if I die?*

These are the toughest questions, and they don't have concrete answers. Even if you seek help and advice from others, only *you* will be able to answer them. So remember, although your desire for immediate answers is understandable, try to be patient. In the end, surprising answers will come your way when you least expect them. Some will spontaneously show up when you're pondering them alone in the middle of the night or while you're talking to someone about something else. And others will only come through experience and by riding out your new learning curve.

start a journal

One of the best things about keeping a journal is that you can express yourself vividly and honestly. In one study about journaling, early breast cancer patients wrote about their illness, breast cancer trauma, and facts related to breast cancer for 20 minutes a day over 4 days. The study concluded that the practice significantly improved quality-of-life outcomes. The researchers recommended using journaling for early breast cancer patients because it's practical and easy.[6]

GETTING STARTED

Journals can be anything you want them to be. You can buy a special blank book or a lined notebook with a cover that grabs your attention. Or you can journal on your computer—by just writing up documents and attaching pictures or by using a journaling app like:

Capture 365 Journal PRO by Sockii (for iPhone and iPad; sockii .com/portfolio/capture-365-journal/). Keeps track of your journal entries and photos in a calendar-like format.

Day One by Bloom Built (for Mac computers, iPhone, and iPad; dayoneapp.com). Allows you to include text, pictures, locations, routines, medicine you are taking/took—and so much more—to visually catalog your entire journey from diagnosis through recovery.

FINDING WAYS TO TALK ABOUT YOUR BREAST CANCER

Early on, many women don't talk about the medical side of their breast cancer. Instead they use symbolic words to express and explore what they feel is happening to them physically, emotionally, and spiritually. They find that words borrowed from things like novels, nature, and video games help them "see" what they feel.

Diaro Personal Diary by Pixel Crater (for Android and Mac; diaroapp.com). Keep a journal of your experiences—and sync across all devices you use. This app also has a search option to help you find previous entries based on key words you used.

Private DIARY (for Android; privatediaryonline.com developed by Mihalich DS Group). This password-protected daily journal allows you to keep track of events, emotions, and pictures throughout your journey. There's also a free version.

Besides traditional ways of journaling, you may want to go public with your reflections. You can blog online or have a dedicated Facebook page about living with breast cancer. Many women enjoy using art materials to express themselves. One woman did a musical journal online. Daily she listened to one piece of music that expressed her feelings about her breast cancer, then made a journal entry about what the music "said" to her. Scrapbooking is another popular way of journaling.

When it comes to keeping a journal, anything goes!

Don't get anxious about the days you don't feel like writing. This practice shouldn't be a source of stress in your life, but just one way to record your thoughts, questions, and emotions throughout your healing journey. And remember: Unless you decide to share it, no one has to read the journal but you.

Susan Carter is a licensed professional clinical counselor who works with breast cancer patients at the University of Toledo Medical Center Eleanor N. Dana Cancer Center in Ohio. When asked about the words her clients use to describe their breast cancer, Carter reported that an older woman called her tumor "a squatter" that took up residence in her breast. "And who or what gave it the right to do that?" the woman demanded. Another woman named her cancer Kudzu, Carter added, because it was like the rapidly spreading vine that grew fast and took root in places it wasn't supposed to. One young patient kept calling hers Frank. When asked why, she replied, "Frankly, my breast cancer doesn't give a damn about me. So I call it Frank and keep reminding him that his days are numbered." One woman even used the word *iceberg*. "I found my lump myself," she explained. "It was like a tiny piece of an iceberg near the surface. Little did I know how much stuff was hidden below."[7]

Many women with breast cancer recall powerful images that struck them once they started talking about their breast cancer. Of course, it's no surprise that some women used unrestrained profanity when their doctor said *breast cancer*. "It added some good color to our conversation," said one survivor. "Of course, the doctor also said sympathetically that I wasn't the first one to react that way."[8]

How you describe your illness is up to you. You may not feel comfortable calling it a name other than what it is–"breast cancer" or "my breast cancer"–and that's perfectly okay. What matters is that you become comfortable talking about it, as this will come in handy in the chapter on telling others, on page 48.

POINTS TO PONDER

Begin thinking about how breast cancer might affect your quality of life in the future. Here are some tips.

Don't Spend Energy Wondering *If* You'll Be a Survivor Someday

Instead, try saying "I am a survivor" out loud, or just picture these words in your mind's eye. Now believe and embrace them wholeheartedly. If you still feel doubtful, consider these other ways of describing the word *survive*: to continue, endure, live, persist, carry on, and go on. In other words, in their own way, each of these words already describes the most important survivor in the world–*you*.

Why Do This?

You need to focus on the positive right now. Researchers have found that optimism and positive thinking can lower rates of depression, lower levels of distress, increase feelings of well-being, and allow you to cope better with stressful situations. This in turn can reduce the harmful effects of stress on your body, which is important to your healing.

Don't Try to Push Your Breast Cancer Out of Your Mind

There will be so many times you'll want to forget about your illness. That's completely normal. But we do recommend that you be aware of the ways that you are either dealing with it or choosing not to. So try not to permanently store your thoughts and feelings about your diagnosis in a locked box or a dark corner. Find ways to express (and respect) your feelings by joining a support group, journaling, or even volunteering for a breast cancer cause.

Why Do This?

Coming to grips with the news that you have breast cancer is not a one-time thing. Getting the news is just your first step as a survivor. But processing the impact of your diagnosis on your life takes lots of time–days, weeks, months, and even years–which is why understanding how you want to deal with it now could impact the course of your entire journey.

Accept That There Will Be Steps on Your Journey Only *You* Can Take

Breast cancer can feel lonely and isolating at times, particularly during surgery, chemotherapy, and radiation. This might make it seem hard to move forward. But know that you will never travel the entire length of your healing path alone. You have your medical team, your spouse or partner, your family, friends, coworkers, neighbors, and even other survivors who will be helping you and encouraging you every step of the way.

Why Do This?

Loneliness is isolating and can lead to feelings of sadness and depression, which can negatively affect your healing. Understanding up front that there *will* be isolating times during your journey can help you to anticipate them and better cope with them. But knowing, too, that you have a community of supporters whom you can reach out to is comforting as well.

CREATING A CARING CIRCLE

Your medical team will be among your most constant companions now and in the future. In Chapter 3, you'll learn how to surround yourself with the most dedicated and skillful experts available to you. Of course, you know other core groups of caring people who may want invitations to join your team and help you reach your goalpost, too. This includes your spouse or partner; your family, relatives, neighbors, friends, coworkers; and members of breast cancer organizations, faith communities, and social organizations. Likewise, support groups, therapists, complementary healing practitioners, and, without a doubt, other survivors will be there for you as well. Never forget that these other survivors are some of your most caring comrades, wise mentors, cheerleading role models, fierce fund-raisers, and sisters and brothers in "the cause," because each of them has walked many, many miles in shoes like yours.

And finally, remember to take this *Prevention* guide along with you, too. See it as a constant companion that's always ready to offer you:

 BETWEEN THE LINES

step back before moving forward

As you read this, stop for a moment and flip back to the Contents pages. Consider that your user-friendly road map, and refer to it as necessary while you go through every part of your healing journey. Take a few minutes to let your eyes scan the chapter titles and point you wherever you want, or need, to go right now. Maybe you'll continue in this chapter, but if not, that's perfectly okay. You may find yourself going to Chapter 4, where you'll learn how to break your news to others. Or you might wind up in a different section altogether. Wherever you find yourself going, trust your reasons for being there. We want you to become engaged with the information you're reading and not race through it. Remember: You can always double back to this chapter or any others as needed.

- Solid medical and scientific information about breast cancer that comes from leading experts in all related fields

- User-friendly definitions and explanations of the different types of breast cancer and the most current procedures, treatments, therapies, clinical trials, and other protocols being used

- Words of practical wisdom from breast cancer researchers, physicians, and other specialists in pursuit of cutting-edge treatments and a cure

- Road maps to navigate a mountain of information about the causes of your illness, treatments, finances, emotions, health insurance, patient's rights, and obligations to yourself and others

- Clear answers to wide-ranging and baffling questions you may struggle with

- Profiles in courage and reflections on everyday survivorship skills from women who once felt as you do now

- Information about lifestyle factors that can help improve your quality of life and minimize the risk of a recurrence

- Updates about safe complementary/alternative medicine, backed by research and recommended to alleviate symptoms and side effects and help heal your body, ease your mind, and uplift your spirits

- Suggestions, tools, and resources to assess nutritional needs and bolster your diet during treatments, plus ways to incorporate dietary modifications and delicious recipes into your daily life

- Tips to understand the benefits of exercise while you're a patient and ways to use exercise to fortify your physical and psychological well-being

- Steps that relatives—mothers, daughters, sisters, aunts, and cousins—can take to prevent breast cancer or detect it early

- Advice on how to live life to the fullest in the present moment and plan for the future

Channeling Hope

Amanda Mercer was in peak physical condition in the winter of 2012. A former collegiate swimmer, the then 43-year-old attorney had been training for nearly 2 years to swim across the English Channel and back later that summer. She was part of a relay team of six determined women who'd set out to not only break the world record but also to raise money for ALS (amyotrophic lateral sclerosis, also known as Lou Gehrig's disease) research.

She felt a lump in her breast, and tests revealed that she had stage II malignant ductal carcinoma. "It's a crushing thing to hear you have cancer," she says. "But I was most upset about possibly not being able to do this swim."

She underwent a lumpectomy, 16 weeks of chemotherapy, and 6 weeks of daily radiation. And swimming the English Channel? That happened 16 days after her final chemo infusion. "I'm a goal-oriented person," she says, "so having something else to focus on helped me get through the low points of treatment."

The women broke the world record, finishing in 18 hours 55 minutes. The film *Swimming Towards a Cure: A Documentary about Raising Hope* details their efforts to raise awareness for ALS.

After the swim, Amanda began her daily radiation therapy and set about rebuilding her life postcancer, posttraining, and then coping with surgery to treat a brain aneurysm.

One year later, Amanda is back to her normal life again. She's set aside her law practice for the time being and is working on a book about her recent experiences.

She'd like women who've been diagnosed to know . . . *it's going to be hard, but you will make it through. Find something else to focus on—don't make your life all about your cancer.*

Breast cancer is . . . *beatable.*

Tomorrow will . . . *be better.*

*"Nothing in life is to be feared.
It is only to be understood."*

—MARIE CURIE

CHAPTER 2

DEALING WITH DIAGNOSIS AND PROGNOSIS

di · ag · no · sis (noun) \dī ig 'nō səs\

1. The identifying of an illness, such as cancer, in a patient through physical examination, medical tests, or other procedures

2. The identifying of the nature or cause of something, especially a problem or fault

3. A decision or conclusion reached by medical or other circumstances

That's what the dictionary has to say about diagnosis. Here's what goes into understanding what a breast cancer diagnosis means to you medically and personally.

THE TESTS

According to the Centers for Disease Control and Prevention, there are multiple steps in the diagnosis of breast cancer. Most fall within four categories, and a positive cancer diagnosis may be made at any one of the steps.[1]

Breast exams can be done by you at home or by a health practitioner. Self-exams can find palpable tumors, but they're not effective for finding early lesions (pathologic changes in the tissue). Clinical exams are often part of routine gynecological checkups, and they sometimes uncover palpable tumors.

Screening imaging (mammogram) is done when a patient has neither symptoms nor palpable lumps. A mammogram finds tumors before they're palpable and still easily treatable. A radiologist's report uses phases to indicate that there is a worrisome lesion. For example, the words "suspicious for malignancy," "suspicious for tumor," "suspicious findings," "suspicious nodes," or "suspicious mass" mean that you will proceed from your screening mammogram to further diagnostic evaluation.

Diagnostic imaging is used when cancer may be present and for further evaluation of findings on your screening mammograms. They are done for women with symptoms, a history of breast masses, and/or abnormal results from a mammogram. Diagnostic imaging helps to differentiate benign lesions from malignant ones. Here are some examples of diagnostic imaging:[2]

- *Diagnostic mammograms* are more thorough than screening mammograms and may include multiple additional pictures of the breast. A radiologist will report his interpretation of your findings by using a BI-RADS score, which runs on a scale from 0 to 5:

  0: Additional testing is necessary.

  1–2: Nothing suspicious was found.

  3: There is a less than 2 percent chance that you have cancer, but you will need to follow up with another mammogram in 6 months.

  4: With a BI-RADS score of 4, the radiologist can't ascertain that what he sees is benign and will request a biopsy to be sure.

  5: This is almost certainly cancer, highly suspicious, and a biopsy is necessary.

- *Ultrasound* is usually used after a screening mammogram shows a mass, or if breast tissue is dense and obscures the mammogram, to help determine if it is solid or cystic (liquid filled).

- *MRI, or magnetic resonance imaging,* uses radio waves and a powerful magnet linked to a computer to create detailed pictures of the breasts. It can be used as a screening tool in women who are considered high risk for developing breast cancer.

- *Bone scans* require injecting a radioactive agent to detect whether cancer has spread to bone tissue.

- **PET (positron-emission tomography) scans** light up areas of metabolic activity. Breast cancers are more active than the benign tissue and produce strongly lighted areas.

Biopsies. When you are sent for a breast biopsy, it does not always mean your doctor knows you have cancer. A biopsy is an effective way of diagnosing the cancer but is also helpful in knowing which lesions can be left alone. There are a few types of biopsies.

- **Fine-needle aspiration** can be performed if you have a lump in your breast. This is performed by your doctor, utilizing a needle and syringe (like when you have blood drawn), and a few of the cells are suctioned out of the lump for examination.

- **Core-needle biopsy** requires a hollow needle to extract small pieces of breast tissue. A *stereotactic core-needle biopsy* uses x-rays and a computer to determine where the needle will be placed. A *vacuum-assisted core biopsy* is guided by ultrasound or MRI and can take more tissue for testing than a standard core biopsy.[3]

  You can read more about these procedures on page 85.

THE PATHOLOGY REPORT

Once the tests your doctor ordered are complete, several factors determine whether or not you get the "good" news you've been hoping for. It all gets under way in the pathology lab. Pathologists are physicians who identify diseases by studying cells and tissues. After you have your tests and a biopsy, the specimens are sent to a laboratory where a pathologist examines them under a microscope. Afterward, the pathologist writes up the findings in your pathology report. It includes information about your general health, descriptions of how your cells look under the microscope, and your diagnosis. The report is sent to the surgeon who performed the biopsy or to an oncologist who ordered the tests. This doctor then reviews your pathology report, along with other information about your health and medical history, to consider options for your treatment and prognosis. We'll discuss what goes into a prognosis beginning on page 18.

Unless you feel that you need to discuss something in your report with the pathologist, you probably won't talk to her.

THE WAIT

You already know that diagnostic tests and procedures set off alarm bells: "Do I?" or "Don't I?" Whenever we have important and urgent medical tests, it's difficult for most of us to get through the troublesome waiting period to learn the results. Some women call whatever news they get their "verdict" because it feels like they've been waiting for a jury to make a decision. Here's what one survivor journaled about waiting: "Getting my results has become a game I now call 'hurry up and wait.' Hurry up to get this test or that test done ASAP. Then wait for what feels like an eternity for the results."

Have you already finished playing that game? Or are you still playing it? Most patients find that when it comes to getting a breast cancer diagnosis and then going through their treatment, they don't play it just once but several times.

As annoying and frightening as the waiting game can be, it's also a time when all undiagnosed patients hope that they will be one of the people beating the odds. It's also when they experience and learn about their doubts and many of their deepest fears in new ways. If you're still

 BETWEEN THE LINES

asking for information

Your doctor may call you personally to give you information about your pathology report and then have a nurse schedule an appointment to discuss it further. If he is not straightforward and you want to know for sure whether or not you have breast cancer, never be too scared, shy, or polite to ask for more details. If you don't ask and later feel unsettled, give yourself permission to call back and ask to speak to the doctor. If the doctor isn't available, leave times that you are available for a return call.

waiting or have just gotten your diagnosis, try to be aware of *all* your hopes, fears, and doubts by acknowledging them. Try using your journal as a helpmate that can give voice to each of them. Think of it as a trusted friend who's giving you a precious gift at a most distressing time–the gift of listening and never judging anything you have to say.

THE APPOINTMENT

If you're still waiting for your test results as you read this, make sure that you take someone you trust with you to your appointment. It's always helpful to have a caring hand to hold and an extra set of ears to rely upon if you receive disappointing and frightening news. Not only can this person write down what the doctor says, she can ask additional questions that may be in *your* best interest. You may also want to plan ahead to record your conversation, but be sure to ask permission beforehand because some cancer centers have a policy about recordings.

The following are sample questions that patients ask their doctors when they get their diagnosis. The information comes from renowned breast cancer organizations that support and advocate for the cause. If you feel that it's premature to ask any of them at this appointment–or maybe you're not emotionally ready to hear certain answers–that's okay. When you *are* ready to learn the answers to these questions, you can refer to them in this book and call your doctor's office to discuss them.

What kind of breast cancer do I have?

- Is it invasive or noninvasive?
- How advanced is it?
- Do you know if it is aggressive?
- What is the size of the tumor?

What surgery is recommended for my cancer?

- A lumpectomy (surgery that removes the tumor and a small amount of normal tissue around it)?
- A mastectomy to remove part or all of my breast?
- A sentinel node biopsy to determine if my cancer has spread? A sentinel lymph node is the first lymph node(s) to which cancer cells are most likely to spread from a primary tumor.[4]

Will I need tests before my surgery to see if the cancer has spread to any other organs, such as my liver, lungs, or bones?

- When and where will the tests be done?
- How soon will I get the results?

After my surgery, will I need radiation or chemotherapy–or both?

- When do these treatments get started and for how long?

What are the chances that my cancer will come back or that I'll develop another type of cancer?

Where can I find a support group?

YOUR PROGNOSIS

prog · no · sis (noun) \präg ˈnō səs\

1. The likely outcome or course of a disease; the chance of recovery or recurrence
2. Forecast; prognostication

stage (noun) \stāj\

1. The classification of the severity of a disease on the basis of established symptomatic criteria to plan treatment and assess prognosis

grade (noun) \grād\

1. A degree of severity of a disease, such as breast cancer, or an abnormal condition, determined by assessing the structure and growth pattern of cells, to determine how quickly the disease/condition is likely to grow and spread[5]

What Exactly Is It?

During the appointment with the doctor who gives you your diagnosis, you'll also have the opportunity to receive your prognosis. According to the National Cancer Institute (NCI) at the National Institutes of Health, lots of information is factored into a prognosis. But most important to you will be the type and location of your cancer, the stage of the disease, and the cancer's grade. You'll also learn about your treatment options and any additional health problems you may have that could affect the course of the disease or its treatment.

When estimating your prognosis, your doctor will use statistics. These are numerical data that are collected, organized, analyzed, interpreted, and then presented. Breast cancer statistics are not personal guesstimates, but rather, they are conclusions about patients that are gathered over a period of time.

However, it's important to remember that your case is unique. You're not merely a statistic, stage, or type. So your doctors can't estimate with absolute certainty what course your breast cancer will take. Additionally, they can't be conclusive about your outcome, either. Throughout your treatment, your body, mind, and spirit will influence how you navigate your particular road to healing. So if you don't have your prognosis yet–and are still trying to decide whether or not you want it–seriously consider your reasons both for and against getting it.

First, keep in mind some encouraging news. Today, numerous statistics conclude there are more breast cancer treatments and higher cure rates than ever before. Add to that the fact that the numbers of women who die from breast cancer are declining.

Deciding in favor of getting your prognosis will satisfy your curiosity about the outlook for your type and stage of cancer, which in turn can help you to better cope and make plans for yourself and others. This can be especially empowering at a time when so many important aspects of your life feel as though they're spinning out of control.

Or you may be one of the many women who decide they're better off without this information. Ira R. Byock, MD, director of palliative medicine at Dartmouth-Hitchcock Medical Center in Lebanon, New Hampshire, and a member of Cancer.Net's Psychosocial Oncology Advisory Panel, puts it this way:

> Not everyone wants to know their chances of being cured or how long they can expect to live. Some people feel that knowing their prognosis is depressing or bad luck. In some cultures, people believe that talking about dying is unwise and can sometimes cause a person to die. In fact, many of us have some tendency to feel that talking about dying can somehow invite misfortune. We shush our ill mother or father if they bring up the possibility that they might not get better–"Don't talk like that!" we say, as if talking about it will make it come true.

It is okay not to want to know your prognosis, but living with cancer certainly highlights the fact that life is precious and that every one of us will die one day.[6]

Does that describe your attitude? Then the option of immediately having access to details about the future can be frightening rather than helpful. So instead of taking the risk of feeling more vulnerable or fearing that negative feelings could lead to depression or a self-fulfilling prophecy, you might opt to put your prognosis on a shelf for the time being–or forever.

Elizabeth Glasson, a blogger and author of *A Glass Half Full: A Breast Cancer Blog Revisited*, was one of those patients. In 2007, she was diagnosed with a grade 3, stage III tumor in her left breast. In a brief statement about why she didn't want her prognosis, she wrote: "Every case is entirely different and treatment is tailored to the individual. All I know is that statistically I'd be happier not having it than having it–but other than that–the future seems to me to lie between a hearty combination of faith, medicine, and most of all, luck."[7]

Whether you get your prognosis or not, whatever the report says is always open to the most important interpretation in the world–yours. If you see that information as a "glass half full" that motivates you, go for it. But if you choose not to get your prognosis, it will be important for you (or someone you bring with you to your appointment) to inform your doctor and members of your medical team not to give it to you. You can always change your mind later. Most doctors will accommodate your wishes and focus on giving you the information you want, when you want it.

BASIC SURVIVAL SKILLS

Remember: You're a survivor right from day one. To get a better understanding of what that means, let's consider what the American Cancer Society has to say.

sur · viv · al (noun) \sər ˈvī vəl\
There are at least three distinct phases associated with cancer survival, including the time from diagnosis to the end of initial treatment, the transition from treatment to extended survival, and long-term survival. In practice, however, the concept of

weighing the pros and cons

Puzzling over the pros and cons of having your prognosis and wondering how it might affect you? This exercise is a simple way to help you make your decision. You'll also find it useful when you have to make decisions concerning your treatments, your family, your finances, and many other things.

Step 1: Ask yourself two questions. Even if they seem obvious, try saying them aloud. It can be helpful and a powerful way to hear them anew. "Is it helpful for me to know my prognosis?" "Am I better off not knowing?" If either is easy for you to answer with conviction, then go no further. But if you find yourself wondering or engaged in a hard tug-of-war of *Should I or Shouldn't I,* continue on.

Step 2: Divide a piece of paper into quarters. Label the first one at the top: "Pros of getting my prognosis." Label the other one at the top: "Cons of getting my prognosis." The two on the bottom are: "Pros of *not* getting my prognosis" and "Cons of *not* getting my prognosis." Other words for *pros* and *cons* can be *benefits* and *costs, upsides* and *downsides, positives* and *negatives,* or *costs* and *promises.*

Step 3: Fill in each column—and don't rush to finish. Some reasons for doing one or the other will come quickly. Others may take time. Be patient. When you're ready, tally the results in each quarter to get an overall picture of the importance of getting or *not* getting your prognosis.

survivorship is often associated with the period after active treatment ends. It encompasses a range of cancer experiences and trajectories, including:

- Living cancer-free for the remainder of life
- Living cancer-free for many years but experiencing one or more serious, late complications of treatment

- Living cancer-free for many years, but dying after a late recurrence

- Living cancer-free after the first cancer is treated, but developing a second cancer

- Living with intermittent periods of active disease requiring treatment

- Living with cancer continuously without a disease-free period[8]

Naturally, even though you're already a survivor, it can be upsetting every time you find yourself asking: *Will I be here next year? Five years from now? Ten years? Much longer than that?* The questions may scare you. Plus, you've probably heard all kinds of sound bites in the news about how long people survive breast cancer, but now you can't recall any that may apply to you.

Use Statistics and Other Information with Care

You may find yourself turning to the Internet–the place where you can get most of the statistical information you want or need. But be careful about statistics and studies.

While we encourage you to be resourceful and informed, we also advise you to be cautious as you look for information about breast cancer online. This is a vulnerable time for you. Remember that both the positive and the negative numbers you see and hear about surviving breast cancer are conclusions drawn at the end of lengthy and complicated studies. Unless you're an expert, those numbers can be misleading, confusing, and very troublesome. So be careful about trying to figure out how the latest statistics apply to you. Studies can take a long time–sometimes a decade or more. Therefore, it's helpful to know how long a study that interests you took. One reason is that over a long period of time, the study may include data based on the experiences of women treated with older therapies, so the analysis of the data may not reflect recent advances in breast cancer detection and treatment that may be available to you now.

Additionally, there will always be important information in the studies that the media doesn't include. That's why they call most of the news reports we read and listen to "sound bites." For example, one gold standard resource for the media is the renowned *New England Journal of*

Medicine. In 2005, it reported the results of a new study showing that survival rates for women with breast cancer are rising. During the early 1960s, the 5-year relative survival rate was 63 percent. Today it's 90 percent. And women who are diagnosed with localized breast cancer now have a 99 percent survival rate.[9] According to the study, the two most important factors for the rise are improvements in treatments and the use of widespread mammography screening.[10]

Of course, that's very exciting and hopeful news, especially because in 2012, more than 60 percent of breast cancers were diagnosed in this stage.[11] However, many of the sound bites in the media never reported that survival rates still drop when breast cancer has spread (metastasized) to nearby lymph nodes and drop even further if distant lymph nodes or other organs are involved.[12]

So if you have your diagnosis and choose to get your prognosis, it's especially important to consider how many small bits of information you're getting from a much longer scientific article. When it comes to your long-term outlook, it's never wrong to ask questions that help clarify what you read, see, and hear.

One of your first, and most heartfelt, questions for your doctor is likely to be: "How bad is this exactly?" One way he may answer that question is to explain the stage of your cancer.

ARM YOURSELF WITH KNOWLEDGE

Remember: When it comes to cancer, ignorance is hardly bliss. Here is a primer to help you understand the nuts and bolts of staging tumors and how this will help your doctor determine your prognosis.

Staging Your Tumor

First things first. You've probably heard about cancer stages dozens of times, from friends and relatives and from interviews with survivors. Staging is important when doctors make a prognosis. To help ensure it's accurate, your doctor needs to know where your cancer got started and how far it may or may not have spread. That ranges from stage 0, when your cancer is "in situ" (limited to one specific place), to stage IV, when it has spread to distant organs.

Most cancer centers, research institutions, hospitals, and organizations use a basic format to stage all types of cancer. What varies may be the type of cancer or the system used. Some systems, such as the following one that's used by the Cleveland Clinic, incorporate additional information. You'll notice that, in this case, the stages are subdivided. When you get your prognosis, you'll probably get basic information. Don't hesitate to ask about subdivisions if you want to know more.

Stage 0: Disease localized to the milk ducts (carcinoma in situ)

Stage I: Cancer that's smaller than 2 centimeters (about an inch) across and has not spread

Stage II: A tumor less than 2 centimeters across that has spread to the underarm lymph nodes (IIA); or a tumor between 2 and 5 centimeters (with or without spread to the lymph nodes); or a tumor larger than 5 centimeters that has not spread to the lymph nodes under the arm (both IIB)

Stage III: Also called locally advanced breast cancer, involves a tumor larger than 5 centimeters that has spread to the lymph nodes under the arm, or a tumor that's any size with cancerous lymph nodes that adhere to one another or to surrounding tissue (IIIA). Stage IIIB breast cancer is a tumor of any size that has spread to the skin, chest wall, or internal mammary lymph nodes (located beneath the breast and inside the chest).

Stage IV: Any tumor, regardless of size, that has spread to areas away from the breast and lymph nodes under the arm, such as the bones, lungs, or liver.[13] For more information on staging, see Chapter 5.

Getting More Information

Your doctor may also order additional imaging tests, such as a chest x-ray, mammograms of both breasts, bone scans, computed tomography (CT) scans, MRIs, and/or PET scans. Blood tests may also be done to evaluate your overall health and because, sometimes, they indicate whether or not the cancer has spread to certain organs.[14]

And then there are still other pieces of the puzzle. To work up the best treatment plan possible, tailor-made for you, your doctor will also take these things into consideration:

- The size of the breast cancer
- Whether the cancer is invasive or in situ
- The stage of the breast cancer (whether it is only in the breast or has spread to the lymph nodes or other places in the body)
- The type of breast cancer

- The rate of cell growth
- How likely the cancer is to come back (recurrence)
- Whether the cancer has just been diagnosed or is a recurrence
- Your age
- Your menopausal status
- Your general health

ASKING THE BIG QUESTION

The one persistent question that every patient struggles with is "Will I die from this?" No one can know for sure. Every day, people who learn they have breast cancer get a prognosis that seems to ensure them a cancer-free life beyond their treatment. But because each of us is unique, there are no guarantees. For example, there could be a recurrence of the breast cancer, a new type of cancer, or some unrelated condition or disease that causes someone to die sooner than imagined. And on the flip side, every day, someone who gets a disheartening prognosis miraculously lives beyond all expectations.

One of the editors of this guide found a high school classmate on the Internet and called to reconnect. He was delighted, but sadly his biggest news was that he had stage IV breast cancer. It was a recurrence 10 years after his first bout. "There is no stage V," he said. "And this time it's every-where and very aggressive." As they continued to talk about the past and then the present, his positive attitude surprised her. He said that, for a long time, his mantra was to always live life joyfully. He loved his work teaching junior high school social studies. "I decided to keep teaching through my treatment because it gave me so much joy," he said.

The day after his doctors said they had exhausted all possibilities for new treatments, he retired. His plan was to travel and do other things on his bucket list. He went as far as the Great Wall of China and to dozens of other places. When he came home for good, he mentored students and lived for another 3 years. Shortly before he died, he sent an e-mail saying "No regrets. I've been true to myself. I've lived joyfully and cancer has been part of the joyride." You just never know.

Earlier we quoted Dr. Byock's thoughts about getting your prognosis. Here are his thoughts about the enormous question of life expectancy:

A person's prognosis is always an estimate, and multiple studies have shown that it is often a *rough* estimate. . . . The statement "No two people are exactly alike" certainly applies to people living with cancer.

Some studies have shown that doctors tend to overestimate their patients' life expectancies. This may be because specialist physicians tend to think mostly about the diagnosis they are treating, while a patient may die from a complication caused by a separate condition. It may also be true that doctors' hopes for their patients cause them to believe that the people they care for—and care about—will live longer than "average patients."[15]

IT'S TIME TO MOVE ONWARD

Today, thanks to new procedures, collaborative research, medical teamwork, and new ways to address patient care holistically, you are the beneficiary of a worldwide campaign to treat breast cancer, heal patients

crossing the threshold

This practice uses the power of imagination to visualize a story in your mind's eye, so go someplace where you can sit or lie quietly.

Take a step back in time to reflect on the day you got your diagnosis. See yourself in your doctor's office hearing *"You have breast cancer"* for the first time. Notice how you're reacting to those words.

When you're ready, visualize yourself leaving your doctor's office, and go to a familiar place with a threshold (a place with a gate or door, literally or figuratively). It can be a place that's part of your life now or one from the past—perhaps the front door of your current home or a childhood one. It can also be a line in the sand at a beautiful beach or a thin, ribbonlike stream separating one bank from another. Once at the threshold, stand before it for as long as you need as you try to come to terms with your diagnosis.

Whenever you're ready, visualize yourself taking a step to straddle the threshold. Take a deep breath, looking back in the direction of the world you knew before your diagnosis. There's no rush. Look back for as long as you need to.

Look toward the other side of the threshold. Though many things ahead are invisible, begin to see the healing path you'll travel. Try to look farther ahead. Notice the guideposts along the way that lead to reassurance, recovery, inner peace, and other milestones.

As you continue to stand in this place—still looking to the future— take a moment to ask yourself if there's anything you might want to leave behind. It may be something that you don't find helpful or no longer need—a worry, fear, attitude, or daily routine. If there's something you want to shed, see yourself taking it off or out of a bag of woes and leaving it on the ground.

When you're ready, see yourself taking a step to completely cross over the threshold. Take another step away from it and another, and feel your body and mind—and your invincible spirit—moving you bravely forward on your journey to healing and wholeness.

innovatively, and find a cure for your disease. Not only is this campaign global, it's growing exponentially, too. Yet as reassuring as that may be, coming to terms with breast cancer is not a once-and-for-all kind of process. Each new phase of your healing journey may mean finding new strength to move forward courageously all over again.

Remember the earlier discussion about using symbolic words and images to describe and deal with breast cancer? In her book *Wellness Wisdom*, survivor Alice McCall reflects on her journey: "Images have enormous power, and images freed from deep within ourselves can change us profoundly."[16]

So now that you have your diagnosis and possibly your prognosis, try the Personal Practice on page 27 before moving on to the chapters that follow. It's designed to bring up images that can help you see where you've been before breast cancer and then help you cross over and navigate your healing path more positively and confidently.

As you begin to gather your medical team and caring circle and then begin treatment, you'll travel to new, challenging, and mysterious places. You may never have planned to go there, but now you must stop to visit these places on your healing journey. Remember to carry this guide with you every step of the way. You'll come to know it as a dependable companion designed to point you in the right directions. The goal isn't to read and absorb every word or to go through the chapters in order–unless you want to. As we suggested earlier, feel free to browse. You're sure to discover that you have reliable information at your fingertips that can help you find answers to your questions, seek reassurance, develop confidence, and live every bit of your remarkable life to the fullest from this moment on.

Reaching the Finish Line

Donna Deegan, a former television news anchor, is no longer tethered to her desk at northeast Florida's leading news station. Instead, the 52-year-old mother of two is on a tireless mission across the country and back to her native Jacksonville, raising funds for underserved women with breast cancer and for research and patient care.

She founded two organizations in her hometown: the National Marathon to Finish Breast Cancer and the Donna Foundation. Together they've raised more than $5 million and served more than 6,500 women.

Donna was diagnosed for the first time in 1999 when she was 38. She had a lumpectomy, then chemotherapy and radiation, but in 2002, a PET scan revealed breast cancer in a deep lymph node. And in 2007, breast cancer came around one more time.

Despite painful surgery and a round of chemotherapy, she still ran the organization's first marathon. "It was my way of saying that where there's a positive will, there *will* be a way to finish breast cancer.

"You may feel that you have to run a 'marathon' to survive," says Donna. "And once you begin, it may seem like it's impossible to finish. But with the support of thousands of others cheering you on, it encourages you physically, emotionally, and spiritually to get there."

She'd like women who've been diagnosed to know . . . *it can be life-changing in a positive way.*

Breast cancer is . . . *going to be cured.*

Tomorrow will . . . *be better than today.*

"Some patients, though conscious that their condition is perilous, recover their health simply through their contentment with the goodness of the physician."

—HIPPOCRATES

CHAPTER 3

ASSEMBLING THE RIGHT MEDICAL TEAM

About every 3 minutes a woman somewhere in the United States learns she has breast cancer,[1] and it turns her life upside down. For you and each of them, one of the most pressing items on the agenda is finding a doctor you can trust to take you through this process. This cancer doctor, also called an oncologist, who'll be with you throughout your entire breast cancer journey, is the person you literally trust with your life. This chapter will help guide you through the process of finding a team of experts in whom you can have confidence to make the decisions necessary for your treatment and recovery.

FINDING THE RIGHT DOCTOR—FOR YOU

You want the best doctors in the world to treat you. And that's completely understandable. But you've got to put the time in to find them (and that's how this chapter can help). One national survey of 7,600 American adults found, surprisingly, that "Americans spend more time researching a refrigerator than they do choosing a doctor or hospital."[2] So put yourself in charge by following these steps.

Step 1: Start with Your Primary Care Doctor or Gynecologist

Chances are this is the doctor who found your cancer, so this is a good place to start. The American Cancer Society recommends asking her this question: "If you found out that you or someone you love had this cancer, which doctor would you go to for treatment?"[3] Ask for two or three names and find out, if possible, what cancer treatment center your doctor is affiliated with.

It's natural to have questions and doubts as you move through this process, but communicating your thoughts at every stage is the key to getting the right information for you. When the coauthor of this guide heard her trusted gynecologist's recommendation for a breast cancer surgeon, she initially told him, "No." (She had her mind set on a doctor at a well-known medical school 2 hours away.) Her doctor listened to all her reasons and then said, "I'm recommending this doctor because he is the surgeon I would send my wife, mother, or sister to." That's all it took to convince her that she didn't have to travel far for the right doctor.[4]

Why Do This?

You've trusted your primary care doctor or gynecologist with your care thus far, so it's worth starting your process with a frank discussion with her about the best possible options for a cancer doctor.

Step 2: Get Recommendations from Survivors

Start gathering information from survivors who are friends and relatives. Think of them as trusted leaders who have "been there/done that." They'll give you their honest opinions of doctors and may even turn you on to other experts they've heard about.

Why Do This?

Not only will you get recommendations for doctors, hospitals, and other experts, you'll start to build a support network to call on throughout your treatment and recovery process. Chances are they'll give you other personal advice as they discuss doctors and hospitals with you—and this is invaluable. Be sure to jot everything down in your journal.

finding a doctor I can trust

Whenever we put our lives in another person's hands, trust becomes a major issue. Although your reasons for trusting or not trusting someone may be based on facts, the conclusions you draw about them are precolored by your first impression. According to a study conducted at New York University, researchers found that we make 11 major decisions about one another in the first 7 seconds of meeting. Some of the qualities we assess so quickly include whether or not someone is trustworthy, competent, likeable, and confident.[5] (That's why meeting with a doctor before selecting him or her as your health-care provider is critical.)

With that in mind, reflect on people—including doctors—you trust. Next, finish the sentence below.

When I say "I trust someone," I mean that person is . . .

After making your personal statement about trust, use the following exercise to figure out the qualities you want in doctors and others on your team.

Don't worry about whether your answers are "right." This isn't a test. For example, look at the first question in the list that follows: "Which of my doctors do I trust the most—and why?" For you, the right answer may be your family doctor or gynecologist. But someone else's may include their dentist or their beloved pet's vet.

Step 3: Conduct a Web Search—Carefully

The first place to start is at cancercenters.cancer.gov, the official Web site for the National Cancer Institute. When you click on Cancer Centers on the top bar, you'll be taken to an index of the top cancer treatment centers throughout the country. Find a center near you and call; all of these centers have dedicated patient access lines so you'll be able to speak to

In your journal, write your answers to these questions. Give yourself permission to write whatever you want.

- Which of my doctors do I trust the most—and why?
- Are there other doctors I trust who have treated relatives and friends?
- Why is it that I never trusted Dr. X?
- If I were to name one or two qualities that I want most in my doctors—like a degree from a prestigious university or a warm bedside manner—what would they be?

Take a look at your responses. Then, in order of their importance, prioritize your list. Spend time thinking about what this exercise says about the kind of doctors you want. Then ask yourself two new questions: *Which of the qualities/attributes I chose are of the utmost importance to me now? Are these hopes and expectations for my doctors realistic?*

You'll be getting a lot of unsolicited advice. Don't take someone else's advice and recommendations too seriously unless they're actually qualified to give it. Your goal is to make the best choices in the best ways you can. By doing this, you'll not only trust your doctors, but you'll also trust the most important person in the world—you!

someone about top doctors there, the ease of getting an appointment, and additional resources to contact.

The American Board of Medical Specialties (ABMS), which publishes the *Official ABMS Directory of Board Certified Medical Specialists*, is another good source. Their guide lists specialists, their field of specialization, and their education. The directory is available online at abms.org.

While numerous online sites rate doctors, it's better to skip them altogether. As tempting as it may be to see how these sites rate a doctor you're considering, we don't recommend it because the ratings have come from unverified patients. Some may have used the doctor you're researching while others have not.

Why Do This?

You can find helpful information online from reputable cancer centers like the National Cancer Institute, the American Cancer Society, the National Breast Cancer Foundation, Susan G. Komen for the Cure, People Living Through Cancer, and the Cancer Information Service. You should never start your search online, but you should make it one part of your selection process.

Step 4: Make Sure the Doctors—And the Hospitals They're Affiliated With—Are Accredited

To fine-tune your list of possible candidates (and hospitals), call the doctors' offices or do a Web search to answer these questions.

Is the doctor board-certified? Board certification is a trusted sign that the doctor is highly trained in his field. Keep in mind, though, that some cancer specialties don't have board certification. For example, breast cancer surgery doesn't have board certification, but these doctors can be board-certified in general surgery or surgical specialties.

Is the hospital accredited? The Joint Commission sets standards for, evaluates, and accredits health-care organizations in the United States. The Commission on Cancer of the American College of Surgeons also accredits facilities that provide the best in cancer diagnosis and treatment and comply with established standards. These facilities also have access to clinical trials that you may want to take part in.

Is the doctor affiliated with an accredited mammography facility? You will need posttreatment mammograms to track your healing, so be sure that the mammography facility your potential doctor is affiliated with is accredited by the American College of Radiology's Mammography Accreditation Program. This accreditation provides facilities with review by other doctors and critical feedback on staff qualifications, equipment, quality control, image quality, and radiation doses. It also ensures that the facility is certified and inspected regularly by the US Department of Health and Human Services.

Why Do This?

To ensure you get the best possible care from the doctor and hospital or cancer center you'll be working with. It will also ease your mind to know you're working with the best of the best.

Step 5: Interview Your Top Choices

Once you've narrowed your list to two or three doctors, book informational appointments with them. Many doctors encourage this practice. Bring your list of questions. And be sure to ask the doctor how much experience she has treating your type of cancer and how many cases like yours she has treated in the last year and the last 5 years.

You'll also want to get a feel for the doctor's demeanor: Is she compassionate and understanding and, most importantly, does she listen to your concerns and what you have to say? You want an expert partner in the process, not someone who dictates without taking time to listen.

Why Do This?

First, the response you receive when you call to set up an informational interview tells you something about the doctor or the practice's willingness to work with you. Second, you wouldn't hire somebody to work for you without conducting an interview first. So it makes sense to interview your doctor, who is probably the single most important person in your life right now (besides you!). She will be working side by side with you throughout the entire healing process. Plus, you might discover that the doctor whom all your friends admire doesn't pass your "sniff test."

Step 6: Ask about a Patient Portal

You've narrowed down your choices; this last step can help you make your decision. Ask if the doctor's practice offers you a patient portal. These are secure sites on the Internet where all your visits to this doctor (and others in the practice) are posted, along with procedures and test results. Some portals are linked with other doctors and hospitals, too. (If a patient portal is available, and you decide to go with this doctor, you'll need to ask for an account and PIN.)

Not all physicians are up to speed with this technology, but it can make doctor visits and results much easier for you to coordinate. Plus, you'll be able to easily share the information with loved ones who are sure to ask many questions throughout the process. The only downside: If you see different doctors from different practices, you may have to set up separate accounts for each of your doctors, but it may be worth the effort.

Why Do This?

It allows your records to be available to you 24/7. In most cases, these records can even be downloaded, so you can print out copies for other doctors or medical professionals.

WHO'S WHO ON YOUR BREAST CANCER TEAM

You've gotten the information you need to choose a doctor to guide you through your treatment and recovery. But you'll need others to be part of your breast cancer team, too. The following information is a primer to help you navigate who's who.

Your Team of Experts

Foremost on your team will be doctors specializing in breast cancer. They include general and oncology surgeons, medical oncologists, plastic surgeons, and medical and radiation oncologists. Today, it's customary to find these doctors all working together in private practices and in hospitals. They form teams that go by several names, such as a multidisciplinary team, tumor board, or tumor conference. In many medical centers, team members meet weekly to review their patients' progress, discuss new patients, and make collaborative recommendations. Here's what each member of your team specializes in.

Breast surgeons are doctors who specialize in surgically removing breast tumors and conserving as much of the breast as possible. They usually complete additional training in breast surgical oncology. They also perform surgery to diagnose or treat cancer.

Medical oncologists are doctors who practice oncology, the branch of medical science dealing with tumors, including the origin, development, diagnosis, and treatment of malignant neoplasms (tumors).[6] Whenever someone has breast cancer or some other form of cancer, the leader of her medical team is usually an oncologist. These doctors specialize in the medical treatment of cancer. All oncologists have a thorough knowledge of the ways that cancers behave and grow, and their training allows them to determine the risk of a recurrence of your breast cancer and the need for and benefits of additional (adjuvant) therapies, such as chemotherapy, hormonal therapy, and radiation therapy.

Plastic surgeons are doctors with training in breast reconstructive techniques.

Radiation oncologists are specialists with additional/advanced training in cancer treatment using radiation therapy.

Radiologists are doctors who interpret x-rays or other forms of imaging, such as an ultrasound or MRI. Some centers have specific breast imaging specialists who concentrate on mammography, ultrasonography, and MRI of the breast.

Surgical oncologists are doctors who perform biopsies and other surgical procedures on the breast or the axillary lymph nodes (near the underarm area). They complete their general surgery residency and then go on to receive additional training in surgical oncology.

Your Support Team

Your breast cancer physicians aren't the only ones who may be involved in your treatment. There will be others—both medical and nonmedical—who make up your team.

Home health aides assist patients who need help moving around, bathing, cooking, or doing household chores.

Hospice care providers work in homes or dedicated centers with terminal breast cancer patients and their loved ones. They focus on providing comfort, controlling pain and other physical symptoms, and offering emotional support.

Nurses/nurse practitioners are health-care professionals with wide-ranging skills and degrees. Registered nurses assigned to breast cancer patients often serve as their case managers.

Nutritionists help patients choose foods that provide enough calories and nutrients to help them feel better when suffering from nausea, heartburn, or fatigue related to chemotherapy and other treatments. They can

navigating breast cancer

Breast cancer professionals recognize how overwhelming the health-care system can be for patients. That's why many routinely provide a patient navigator to guide you (and your loved ones) through it.

These trained professionals (and sometimes laypeople) are your "go-to" advocates. Though programs differ, all of them strive to enhance your quality of life and help you:

- Get answers to wide-ranging questions and concerns
- Understand complicated medical information or provide missing information
- Figure out health insurance or deal with having none
- Find resources for managing stressful issues such as transportation, financial problems, and child care
- Locate support for emotional issues
- Overcome language and cultural difficulties as well as biases based on age, race, religion, nationality, sexual orientation, etc.

If your medical team or health-care facility doesn't have a breast cancer navigator on staff, check out Chapter 12. Many of the resources listed there can help you get services you need.

You can also check the Internet. Search Google for "patient navigation services." First look at the results for nonprofit organizations that specialize in breast cancer, such as the American Cancer Society (cancer.org) or the Livestrong Foundation (livestrong. org). You'll also see results for private for-profit services. Be sure to look at credentials and consumer reviews carefully before signing up.

also provide information about the foods that can help nourish you post-treatment.

Oncology social workers are professionals trained to counsel people affected by cancer and help them access practical assistance.

Patient navigators can either be medical professionals or people from other fields. They provide services and support that help patients and their families navigate the intricacies within the health-care and insurance systems.

Psychiatrists are medical doctors who specialize in helping people who are depressed and/or anxious. They can prescribe medications, such as antidepressants, that help improve the quality of life for some breast cancer patients.

Psychologists have a PhD or other degree rather than a medical degree; they counsel patients who feel depressed, anxious, or sad about treatment side effects.

Radiation physicists perform diagnostic tests and plan and administer radiation dosage.

Radiation technologists help place you in the correct treatment position so that the proper dose of radiation is delivered to the proper site.

Spiritual counselors and clergy help patients deal with questions from a religious and/or spiritual perspective and find ways to help

start a breast cancer file box

You'll be receiving lots of pathology reports and other information. Start a file box (you can find inexpensive plastic ones at your local drugstore), and create sections to keep all the information organized. Remember: Always order hard copies of your pathology report and other medical records from your doctor's office. (You can also download and print information from a patient portal, if your doctor's office uses this service.) You may also consider getting copies of your "films"–screening and diagnostic mammograms or other images. This way, you can take records with you to visits and not have to wait for them to be ordered.

patients face fears, concerns, and treatment and look forward to the future.

THE POWER OF CLEAR COMMUNICATION

Unless you decide you want to be told what to do and when to do it in the months ahead, you'll be looking for doctors who engage you in conversations and listen respectfully to what you contribute.

This means that you have to make your medical concerns and questions known to your doctors. Though we'd all like to believe our highly trained specialists are mind readers, they aren't. You must learn to be a careful communicator, so keeping track of your questions throughout the process is important.

It will be very hard to listen carefully to everything your doctors say during such a stressful time. Following these tips will ensure that clear communication flows between you and your doctor.

Avoid Making Assumptions

Be forthright. Tell your doctor when information sounds confusing and speak up if you need clarification. Does your mind wander when your doctor explains something technical? This can happen easily during such a stressful time. If it does, simply ask the doctor to repeat the information.

Bring a Scribe

Take along a friend or relative who can serve as a note taker and an extra pair of ears. If you have something to say privately to your doctor, wait until the end of the appointment so you can speak to the doctor alone, and ask your scribe to meet you in the waiting room.

Use Questions to Communicate

Don't dismiss the stream of questions that pop into your head. Instead, remind yourself that rather than being silly or unimportant, well-communicated questions can help express your concerns. If the answers you get aren't satisfactory, try restating your questions. Here are a few tips for asking clear and appropriate questions.

Listen. The old saying goes "You can hear a lot just by listening." That's particularly true when it comes to listening for answers to your medical questions.

Don't interrupt. If you believe that what you have to say is important at that particular moment, then by all means break in, but do so politely (it sounds obvious, we know, but it's easy to forget niceties when you're anxious). If your doctor asks you to "hold on," don't get angry. Just wait. The answer to your question may be in the next sentence. If it's not, you can ask the question afterward. Also, it's easy to get ahead of what the doctor is telling you and mentally complete her thought. Try to not let this happen and, instead, stay focused on the conversation at hand.

Try asking a couple of short, to-the-point questions instead of a long, complicated, or vague one. This will help to ensure clear answers that are helpful and easier to remember.

Avoid asking leading questions (those that try to influence the answer and persuade the other person to agree with you). During stressful and scary times, we all want certainty that everything will be okay. But since no one can predict the future, your doctor can't honestly say yes to the question "If I do everything you tell me, I'll be cured, right?"

Be clear in your questions. Open with a statement that tells the person you heard what he or she was saying. For example, you might say something like this: "If I heard you correctly, you said that I may not need chemotherapy if my breast cancer hasn't spread to my lymph nodes. Can you tell me more about my lymph nodes and why that's the case?"

Of course, you'll always have questions that you don't need to discuss with your doctors or anyone else. These are the deeply personal ones in your heart that facts, figures, and other data can't really answer. Only you can. They can be the hardest, because sometimes it takes patience for those answers to come.

WHEN TO SEEK A SECOND OPINION

Once you've found the right cancer doctor and team, you may find yourself needing or wanting a second opinion. This is completely normal; it doesn't mean that you're being indecisive. Seeking an impartial second opinion means asking other breast cancer specialists for their unique perspectives. Think of it as a way to do additional research and provide an extra measure of confidence and peace of mind when you finalize your medical team and treatment. These are reasons why and when you should seek out a second opinion.

There's uncertainty about the type or extent of the breast cancer you have. It's hard to feel confident about your treatment options when there are doubts about your breast cancer.

You've been given several treatment options and find it hard to choose. Another set of eyes, ears, and experience can help make your choice easier.

It's difficult to communicate with your doctor. This is an anxious time for you and if, for whatever reason, the communication isn't clear, a second opinion may help you sort things out.

You've been told you have a less common or rare cancer. This is a good time to get a second opinion from a doctor who specializes in your form of breast cancer.

Your intuition tells you to get a second opinion. There's no doubt you have breast cancer, but you do have some doubts about doctors, treatments, and other options. A second opinion will help you calm the uneasiness that your doubts may generate.

Your health insurance requires a second opinion. This may be a surprise, but there it is–a built-in reason to get one.

Your doctor says, "Go for it." Many doctors welcome second opinions as a way to ensure that you're getting the best possible treatment plan.

Recent research from the University of Michigan Comprehensive Cancer Center in Ann Arbor suggests that it is worthwhile to opt for a second opinion, particularly if you're getting the second opinion from someone on a multidisciplinary tumor board (made up of surgeons, medical oncologists, radiation oncologists, radiologists, and pathologists).

In the study of 149 breast cancer patients, 77 of the participants (52 percent) were advised, on the second opinion, to change their original treatment plans. The study authors found the initial treatment recommendations often did not consider new surgery techniques, such as delivering chemotherapy before surgery to make breast conservation possible or sentinel lymph node biopsy, a technique to determine whether cancer has spread beyond the breast. The researchers also found that radiologists–during a second opinion–reinterpreted imaging results in 45 percent of patients, in some cases identifying previously undiagnosed second cancers. More than a quarter of the patients were recommended to undergo another biopsy.[7]

Furthermore, pathologists had a different interpretation of tests–including the stage of the cancer–for 43 patients.[8] The latter was particularly important, since the process of staging assesses the aggressiveness of a malignant tumor, which in turn guides treatment.

Before You Get a Second Opinion

You've found the doctor you want to meet with for a second opinion. Before you book your appointment, though, consider these important points.

Check with your health-insurance provider. This way, you'll know if second opinions are covered (sometimes they aren't–and if that's the case, you'll need to decide if you want to pay out of pocket). If your insurance will pay all or part of the costs of getting a second opinion, nail down *exactly* what will come out of your pocket. You may be required to pay something more than your usual co-pay at the time of your first office visit. (For more information about the financial side of breast cancer, go to Chapter 8.) Also check with your health-insurance provider to find out if the doctor is "in" or "out" of network. You can often do this online at the Web site for your insurance company and then just call for more information.

Make sure you have copies of all your medical records to take with you.

Ask someone you trust to go with you and be your second set of eyes and ears. If someone accompanied you to get your diagnosis and prognosis, ask that person to go with you this time, too.

what doctors think about second opinions

One doctor who doesn't need to be convinced of the value of second opinions is Marisa Weiss, MD, president and founder of Breastcancer.org and a breast cancer survivor. (Read her survivor story on page 73.) In an article explaining the value of second opinions, she writes:

> Because of my unique diagnosis and complex family history, there were a number of complex decisions to be made where there was no right answer. My medical oncologist encouraged me to seek a second opinion and was very open to getting input from other medical oncologists on the best solutions moving forward.[9]

What to Expect from a Second Opinion

To provide a second opinion, a doctor will review your medical reports and test results and then consider your diagnosis and possibilities for treatment. On one hand, a second opinion may confirm everything your physician has already told you, which can provide a real sense of relief. On the other hand, it may also point out new options based on additional observations about the type and stage of your breast cancer. In turn, this may result in a recommendation for a different course of action or treatment facility. Ultimately, you can expect a second opinion to give you:

- A way to eliminate doubts that keep you from being able to make a choice

- Another lens through which to view and review your diagnosis, prognosis, and options for treatment

- The peace of mind that comes when you feel confident that *you* are making the right choice rather than having someone else make it for you

how do you react to anxiety?

From the moment you received your diagnosis, did the news cause certain things the doctor was saying to slip right by you? That's completely natural during stressful times. The primary reason: anxiety. Anxiety makes it difficult to focus, hear what others are saying, and understand options.

When we *react* to something, it's usually a result of our built-in fight-or-flight response warning us to take one of two actions: to *fight* what threatens our life or take *flight* and run away from it.

When we *respond* to something that causes anxiety, we override that automatic and emotional "gut instinct" to fight or flee. Instead, we stop and begin thinking about our options. We use the part of our brain that helps us figure things out and make choices.

Use this exercise to learn how you deal with making decisions in anxious times. In your journal, write down what happened when you learned you had breast cancer. For example:

- "I felt sick to my stomach."
- "My ears started ringing and I couldn't hear anything."
- "I fought back tears."

Next, ask if there's anything you might do differently in the future now that you know that emotional reactions to bad news are not just instinctive but normal.

Learn to cope with anxiety by asking yourself these questions:

- As I build a medical team, what can I expect to push my buttons?
- What are the healthiest ways to manage my anxiety about this?
- What do I need to think about, write down, and have handy when I speak to my new doctors, nurses, and others?
- Who can I ask to come with me to my appointments to help me manage everything?

Keep in mind that the doctor who gives you a second opinion may give you better, more optimistic news than the first doctor did. Or you might like the bedside manner of the second doctor better. The bottom line: Don't assume that the second doctor is necessarily correct.

If the second opinion is drastically different from the first, you may even want to seek out a third opinion–and that's okay (it's commonly done, so you wouldn't be the first to do this). If you do decide to take this route, go about finding one exactly the way you found your main doctor and even your second-opinion doctor.

If the second opinion is very close to what your original doctor recommended, ask the doctors to discuss your treatment options. If they seem hesitant to do this, explain that it's very important to you to get the best treatment possible, and doing this would help make that happen. Be persistent.

In the end, you may decide to work with a different doctor based on what you learned from your second (and even third) opinions. Don't feel bad about switching; you must be 100 percent confident in your doctor and the treatment plan you're pursuing. Seeking out different opinions is a good strategy for doing this.

WRAPPING UP YOUR SEARCH

As you start to make headway with your team, take a deep breath. You don't need to have every detail in place right after getting your diagnosis unless your doctor advises otherwise. This means you have time to:

- Begin to thoughtfully process what's happened to you physically and emotionally since you learned you might have breast cancer
- Get a second (or third) opinion if you want one

Fit for Life

Today, Lockey Maisonneuve, 47, is the founder of MovingOn, an exercise program for breast cancer survivors and a blogger for the Web site Positively Positive. But the road that took her there was tough. It began in 2006 and included a mastectomy, chemotherapy, and radiation, a preventive mastectomy, breast reconstruction, and finally saline implants.

Once her last surgery healed, Lockey found a new calling. "I no longer felt comfortable at my gym and other places. One day, I talked to a nurse about the importance of exercise for women who had just finished their treatments. After listening, she suggested that I start a program there."

Lockey is passionate about her new niche. From firsthand experience, she knows that when you're no longer a patient, you feel that your life should get back to normal. But how exactly are you supposed to do that after everything you've been through?

Because exercise can be about much more than just physical rehabilitation, she began to see it as a way for women to begin the transition to their post–breast cancer lives as they learn to gain control over their bodies holistically. "I believe that whenever I can help a patient or a survivor to gain a little more strength and flexibility in their bodies, they also gain the strength they need in their souls to continue on and be well."

"I know it will always be about so much more than the exercise," she says. "I see the women come to know the real survivor in their body, mind, and spirit. They begin to look inward and touch the survivor who's there now and the one they want to be in the future. And I do, too."

She'd like women who've been diagnosed to know . . . *to use the challenge of breast cancer as an opportunity to learn, grow, and be true to yourself.*

Breast cancer is . . . *not something I would wish on anyone.*

Tomorrow will . . . *provide another opportunity for growth, healing, and inspiration.*

*"Do not protect yourself by a fence,
but rather by your friends."*

—Czech Proverb

CHAPTER 4

BREAKING THE NEWS TO FAMILY, FRIENDS, AND COWORKERS

When you learned that you had breast cancer, did you want to tell some people about it right away but weren't sure if you should? Or did you wish the world would go away so you could hunker down and not say anything to anyone? Perhaps you've already done one or the other. Talking about your diagnosis and prognosis with other people is not easy. Indeed, it's difficult, uncomfortable, and scary at times, especially since you're still trying to come to terms with the news yourself. With that in mind, we hope you'll refer to this chapter often for advice on delivering your news to others and keeping the lines of communication open throughout your entire journey.

Whether or not you've started telling people about your breast cancer, at some point, the news is going to get out to an even wider audience. Here are some things to think about (all will be addressed in this chapter):

- Who needs to know about your breast cancer right now and who can wait?

- How do I communicate what I want to say about breast cancer to different people—my spouse, children, parents, siblings, employer, and those I don't know well?

- How can I prepare myself to deliver my news without getting emotional (and is it okay if I do)?

- What obstacles will I run into when I tell people?

- How do I keep the lines of communication open and healthy–particularly with my spouse and/or my family and friends–throughout my journey to recovery?

- How do I talk about sensitive issues like sex (with my spouse), cancer (with my kids), and more?

Throughout this chapter, you'll also find tips for managing your reactions and responses to what others may say or do when they get the news.

BEING TRUE TO YOURSELF

During your journey from diagnosis to recovery, you may experience strong urges pulling you in opposite directions. One urge, for example, might be a desire to share your news with lots of people. A conflicting impulse might be to clam up and keep it all to yourself. How you react to this internal tug-of-war usually depends on inborn tendencies to either want to be alone (this suggests that you're introverted) or to spend time with other people (a sign you may be extroverted). All of us fall somewhere along a continuum of introverted and extroverted, and that can change during our lifetime, particularly during periods like this when stress is common.

Knowing something about your personality type can be helpful when you tell others about your breast cancer. Introverts, for example, often feel emotionally exhausted after explaining what's happened whether the conversation went well or poorly. And once it's over, they often feel drained and want to be alone to recharge their batteries. Extroverts may react just the opposite and feel as though they've gotten a positive boost that makes them want to keep going. This knowledge can also be used throughout your treatment and recovery when you need to deliver news of your progress.

Are You an Introvert?

If you're an introvert, your friends, relatives, coworkers, and neighbors may say that you're shy, withdrawn, and aloof (though a better way to describe you may be to say that you're reserved). This doesn't mean that you don't like and care about people. It's just that you're not fond of spending time in crowds.

You might be an introvert if you prefer a quiet evening alone or with another person instead of going to a party or even just spending time with others. Or you may just prefer to focus inwardly instead of seeking input from others, especially when it's time to figure out personal issues.

If you're an introvert, then plan to get ready to report your news "live" by first spending time alone. Try going someplace where you won't be disturbed to figure out what you want to say. This doesn't necessarily mean packing your bags and leaving town for a few days. More practical ways can be writing in your journal, going for a long walk in a park, or driving somewhere that feels safe and comforting. You can also get "away" by listening to music you love, practicing yoga, meditating, or pouring yourself a soothing cup of coffee or tea.

Are You an Extrovert?

If you have an extroverted personality, you feel energized by outside stimuli, such as people, events, and community happenings. Also your family and friends are apt to describe you as outgoing, a people person, ambitious, and the life of the party. Crowds, social gatherings, and family reunions invigorate you mentally, physically, and spiritually, too. If you haven't had contact with others for a long time, you start to feel exhausted, and even a little depressed. You prefer to act rather than spend time thinking about things.

As soon as you got your diagnosis, you may have wanted to break your news to lots of people right away. If you haven't done that yet, try this instead: Tell just one or two people, observe their reactions, and learn what they think about the news. Think of this as a trial run. Afterward, you can use their feedback to help you organize your thoughts for telling a much larger audience.

CONTROLLING THE MESSAGE

Sharing bad news with people you love and care about can be tough. Though you don't want your news to distress people, you know that inevitably it will. In some cases, you might even feel disappointed after conversations. "It could have gone better," you may tell yourself. Or "Why did

I allow my brother to push the same old buttons and make me angry? I wish I had never said anything."

In every situation, though, it's always helpful to remember these key points about delivering your news:

- You *can* control the content of the news you choose to share.

- You *cannot* control another person's reactions and responses to your news.

To accomplish all this, you need to focus on building up your confidence. No matter how much confidence you typically have, learning that you have breast cancer can make you fearful and uncertain about a lot of things, including how to talk to others about your diagnosis. After all, you're stepping out the door to tell people about a deeply personal event in your life. To become more self-assured about your news and how to deliver it, follow these steps.

Step 1: Plan Ahead

Begin smoothing the way for this big step by doing some prep work.

Why Do This?

Professional speakers know how to monitor and maximize their comfort level when they talk to people. This way, they can seamlessly manage their discomfort level when they encounter unexpected glitches, such as forgetting what they were saying or becoming distracted by someone interrupting. To prepare yourself to talk about your breast cancer confidently, it will be helpful for you to anticipate and address concerns, questions, or even a look on someone's face that may startle or fluster you or even cause you to cry.

Step 2: Keep Lists—Lots of Them

Ever since your diagnosis, you've been bombarded with details pulling you in different directions. Not only can many of these details throw you off course, but they can also set you into intellectual and emotional overload. And that can diminish your ability to stay focused, maximize your brainpower, and make difficult decisions. But if you make lists (you may even want to keep them in your journal so you don't lose them), you have guides to keep you on track. Here's how to get started.

what questions do you have about breast cancer?

Begin by pondering the following questions, and write the answers and your feelings in your journal as a way to help you figure out what and how to communicate with everyone in your life. Start by asking yourself: *What do I know for sure about my diagnosis, prognosis, and about breast cancer in general? And what do I need to learn more about? What can I talk about easily? What will be the hardest things for me to talk about? What do I not want to talk about at least for now?*

Now take your self-talk deeper by answering these questions.

What do I fear or dread most about telling others? Everything? Saying "I have breast cancer" out loud? Being emotional? Being labeled? What people will think of me? Am I worried about the looks of pity on their faces? What about unsolicited advice; how will I handle that? Am I concerned about not having the right answers or all the answers? How am I going to handle unexpected outbursts of crying?

What happens to me when I talk about the private parts of my body publicly? Is it easy for me to say the word *breast* or does it embarrass me? Do I use *breast* like any other word, or do I use slang such as *boob* instead? Does my word choice depend on whether I'm talking to a man or a woman or a relative, friend, or doctor? Do I look right at the person I'm talking to or do I avoid eye contact? Do I mumble the words or use body language that diminishes or distracts from what I'm trying to say?

When people ask me questions that are too personal, do I tell them I'm not going there, or do I try to answer those questions anyhow? How good am I at maintaining my boundaries even when someone doesn't respect them? Am I quiet when someone's behavior toward me is not acceptable, or do I respond by telling them so?

If my prognosis is discouraging, what will I say or do if someone asks me if I'm going to die?

List the people you have already told about your diagnosis. Usually, these are your spouse or partner, your parents or adult children, and perhaps your closest friend.

Write up an "ASAP" list. Include other family members and friends, your employer, and possibly a therapist or clergyperson. Next to each name note how you want to make contact. Will you talk to them one-on-one or in a small group (e.g., your coworkers)? Or will you phone some people individually? Is handwriting a letter a better way for you to deliver the news to some?

Create a "hold" list. These are the people whom you're less close to personally and/or geographically. Of course, there's a practical side to doing this: You will have fewer people to tell. The downside is that the time lag allows your news to get out anyhow. So don't be surprised when someone who's been put on hold reaches out to you first. When that happens, be ready to tweak the (possibly inaccurate) information that's being passed around. You may want to temporarily exclude young children, as they need special attention (something we'll discuss later in this chapter). An aging parent who is ill might be another person to put on hold.

It's okay to create a "difficult-to-deal-with" list. Reasons can range from an intuitive dread to a still-simmering feud to past negative communication experiences. You can always move people off this list later. Just know that right now it's better to trust your instincts.

Why Do This?

Lists can help you gain mental control of your situation so you feel more confident about how you'll cope with telling others. Lists can also help you efficiently organize and prioritize your thoughts.

Step 3: Be Timely

You don't have to tell everyone your news immediately, but know that timely and accurate information helps to calm people's anxiety and prevent the spread of rumors. You already know that when your doctor told you that you have breast cancer, your anxiety shot up. So it's not a stretch to imagine those closest to you having heightened anxiety about it, too.

Why Do This?

You want to be the one to take your story into the public arena. This allows you to control the message and prevent people from possibly spreading inaccurate information. It will also give you a chance to let people know that you don't really feel comfortable with them talking to others about it right now.

UNDERSTANDING WHY YOUR WORRIES RUN WILD—AND HOW TO GET THEM UNDER CONTROL

Before you even say anything to anyone, human nature will cause you to imagine people reacting to your news. The scenarios you picture in your mind's eye may have some people looking sad and concerned. You'll imagine them offering comforting words, compassionate hugs, unconditional love, and helpful resources. But in your imagination, others may appear to react negatively, looking as though they're annoyed, angry, disinterested, or disappointed in you. Perhaps you'll hear them telling you what to do or challenging what your doctor says is best.

Once you've told someone about your breast cancer, it's also easy to imagine that they're thinking something different from what they're saying or that their response could have been better than it was. This is normal, particularly during times of stress. But remember, you can't second-guess someone else's anxiety about your breast cancer. The only anxiety you can try to manage is your own. Understanding *why* your mind thinks this way during stressful times (also called cognitive distortions) will help you realize that many of your worries about telling people your news or about your illness are simply unfounded.

As you read through this list, jot down in your journal what type of thinking you most often engage in and what's a more positive way of looking at the situation.

All-or-nothing thinking means you tend to look at things in black or white, with no middle ground, such as, "That conversation was a total failure."

Catastrophizing is expecting the worst-case scenario to happen. For example, "I'm going to die" or "They're going to burst out crying, and I'm not going to be able to handle the situation."

Diminishing the positive means you come up with reasons why positive things (news from your doctor, reactions from others) don't matter. "My doctor told me that the outcome is likely to be positive, but he didn't really mean that." Or "She seemed to be genuinely concerned about me, but I know she doesn't really care."

Emotional reasoning is believing that the way you are feeling right now about your situation is reality. For example, "I just know that things are not going to go well."

Jumping to conclusions is just what it means: You're making negative interpretations about a situation (and worrying about it) before it even happens. For example, "I just *know* she's going to start offering me all sorts of advice about what I should be doing."

Labeling is how you see yourself based on your own perceived (and usually nonexistent) shortcomings. "I don't handle sickness well." Or "I didn't deliver that news well; I'm no good at communicating stuff like this."

Overgeneralization is taking a single negative response from someone and assuming that everyone's response will be like that. "Well, that didn't go over like I expected. I just can't do this."

Personalization is when you take responsibility for things that are outside your control (like your breast cancer). For example, "It's my fault that I got this breast cancer. I should have never . . . (fill in the blank)."

"Shoulds" and "should-nots" involve holding yourself to a rigid list of what you should and shouldn't do when it comes to telling others about your breast cancer and then beating yourself up if you don't follow these "rules" to a tee. For example, "I should have never gotten into that discussion about taking a long-term leave from work."

Mental filtering is when you focus on the negative responses to your news while filtering out all the positive ones. For example, "Nobody seems to care" (when actually people *do*).

SHARING THE NEWS WITH THOSE CLOSEST TO YOU

We wish there was a one-story-fits-all way to break your news to those who are most important to you. Having one handy would certainly make this tough task a lot easier. But because your husband or partner, children, parents, dearest friend, and employer are important to you in similar yet very different ways, that's not an option.

Telling Your Husband/Partner

The fact that your husband or partner has probably known from the beginning doesn't diminish the emotional impact of your diagnosis. At times, you may feel that breast cancer is an intrusive third party in your relationship. It's this aspect of breast cancer that can take your relationship on unexpected emotional roller-coaster rides if you don't plan ahead to talk about what's happening for each of you. That's why it's very important to keep the lines of communication between you timely, open, honest, and ever-flowing. Since this chapter covers the most important aspects of sustaining healthy communication, offer to share it with your husband or partner.

Naturally, obvious issues such as child care and household tasks will be relatively easy to bring up and discuss even if they've become more complicated since your diagnosis. But others, such as finances, sexual intimacy, and changes in emotional needs, can become touchy. To keep these concerns from having a negative impact on your relationship, it's important to begin talking about them as soon as possible rather than allowing your anxieties about them to take on a life of their own. The best way is to formally sit down without distractions (hire a babysitter if you need to keep children occupied, and turn off your phones and the TV so you're not interrupted). If you need to set a formal time to have this talk, then do it, but just make sure you sit down in a quiet place. And don't just casually talk while you're doing other things (such as cooking dinner or doing the dishes); you need to be focused and deliberate in the topics you cover. Here are some tips to get you started.

Talk—And Listen

When you get anxious, it's easy to nervously talk (and talk), without giving the other person time to respond. That's completely normal, but allow time for your partner to talk, too. If your partner doesn't say much, it doesn't mean he doesn't care. Your partner may just need time to process everything and reflect.

Make It Clear That You Want
Your Partner to Respond

Sometimes your spouse or partner may not think you want someone else to talk and may remain quiet throughout your conversation, not knowing what to say. Reassure your partner that you *do* want to hear his or her thoughts and that it's important that you deal with this *together*.

Prepare a List of Questions

Use this section as a guide. It contains a few of the topics you should begin discussing (issues you probably never planned to confront in your relationship). Of course, there's no way to answer many of these questions until later. However, right now, finding answers is less important than opening the doors to communication and making sure they stay open. Now is the time to look ahead and anticipate what will be coming down the road so you can face it together.

What toll is breast cancer going to take on the family finances? Are there savings or other resources to fill in the voids created by your taking medical leave? What about the unforeseen medical expenses that are sure to come up? Money is already a source of marital discord in everyday life, and it can become a source of serious concern unless you talk about this throughout your entire journey.

How do you both feel about the potential physical changes, such as hair loss and/or noticeable weight gain or loss, which could result over the course of your treatment? What about the ways that surgery and postoperative treatments may change your appearance? Know that feelings of poor self-esteem and unattractiveness could develop throughout the process, particularly if you have chemotherapy. A recent study from the nonprofit Cleveland Clinic Foundation found that fewer than 20 percent of the women studied reported poor body image following partial mastectomy and breast reconstruction, but those who had chemotherapy had a hard time with it because of the fatigue, nausea, mouth sores, diarrhea, and hair loss that can accompany treatment.[1] (This is something to anticipate and discuss with your partner if your doctor tells you that you need chemotherapy.)

If you have a mastectomy, your breast will be removed. What about that possibility makes you and your partner apprehensive or fearful? Is reconstructive surgery important to both of you, neither of you, or just one of you? How important is physical sensation in the breasts for you and your partner? (Once you discuss this, be sure to speak to your doctor about it and write it down in your list of questions.)

How are you going to deal with the inevitable changes to sex and your libido? Breast cancer affects the sexual desires of women differently. This is especially true for premenopausal women because breast cancer treatments can jump-start menopause. If that happens, it's not a stretch to imagine that you'll be physically exhausted and that your libido will be diminished. Some breast cancer treatments can cause decreased estrogen and vaginal dryness and, as a result, painful intercourse. This is the time to bring these topics up with your spouse or partner.

The journey may also take its toll on you (or your partner) in the form of depression or extreme anxiety, which may have to be treated with medication. This medication may also reduce your libido and/or affect sexual function.

Your partner may also be the one who is worn out, lacks desire, develops depression, or becomes impotent. How are you both going to cope with this?

All are issues that you need to address now with your partner and over the course of your treatment and recovery. Again, neither of you will probably have many of the answers to these questions, but bringing them out in the open now paves the way for honest and frank conversation as you both move through the process of treatment and recovery.

Know when to call in help. If you or your partner is having a hard time communicating and is feeling angry, anxious, or scared, you may have to book an appointment with a family therapist or counselor. Know that this is normal and many couples do it; it doesn't mean your relationship is flawed or destined for separation or divorce. Coping with the ups and downs of marriage is challenging enough every day; adding a serious illness like cancer to the mix is hard for any couple to work through on their own.

Some organizations that can help you locate a therapist or counselor near you include the American Psychological Association Help Center (apa.org/helpcenter/), the American Association for Marriage and Family Therapy (aamft.org), Cancer Support Community (cancersupportcommunity.org), and the National Register of Health

Service Providers in Psychology (findapsychologist.org). And if you're having trouble discussing sexual issues, a marriage therapist can help. Also, there are sexual health counselors available to you at cancer treatment centers. Be sure to ask your doctor about them.

Telling Your Children

The root meaning of the word *compassion* is "to suffer with." If the love and compassion you feel for your children puts you at a loss for the right words to tell them you have breast cancer, you're not alone. Be reassured that we're here to help you find those words so you can address your children's questions, concerns, and fears truthfully and compassionately.

The key: Don't procrastinate. Kids are very intuitive and sensitive. Before you've said a word, they may have already sensed something is going on but been afraid to ask. And if you wait too long, their fears can escalate. Remember that your first goal is to tell your children and then keep the lines of communication open throughout your journey to recovery. After all, they're passengers on your journey, too.

There are lots of ways to prepare yourself to be calm and fully present for your children when you break the news. For example, many women find that getting professional advice beforehand from a therapist, social worker, school guidance counselor, or clergyperson helps. So does the been-there-done-that wisdom of other breast cancer survivors.

Of course, recommendations for telling your children about breast cancer are readily available online, too. Professionals who work for nonprofit breast cancer organizations usually write trustworthy articles with helpful advice and practical tips. However, it takes time to cull the numerous Web sites for the most reliable information–and this can be a distraction. That's why we point you to the most helpful advice here. Think of this as a checklist for a special mission.

Build your confidence beforehand so you come across as calmly as possible. Children will sense your peacefulness and presence. This, in turn, will help them freely express their feelings, thoughts, and questions.

Talk to your partner (or to your child's biological father) about whether or not you want to make this a team effort. If your partner is available and comfortable doing so, the show of solidarity may help reassure your child that this is a family affair. It will also enable you to see them and hear their concerns through an extra pair of eyes and ears.

Pick a place and time that will be free of disruptions and distractions. This isn't a good time for phone calls, ringing doorbells, or an impatient dog to get in the way.

Speak to each child individually. It will be a special one-on-one time for you to be fully present to each other. This can open up opportunities for you to really focus on each child's reactions and talk about breast cancer in language she can understand. This approach also gives your children permission to talk to you in ways they might not with a sibling around.

Start out slowly, and don't overload young children (under 8 years old) with too much information at once. Preteens and teens can be given more.

Assure, and reassure, your child that he or she is loved and, that no matter what happens, will be cared for and safe.

Use age-appropriate language. You want to communicate honestly what is happening, but be sure to use language that won't overwhelm or confuse your child. For example, for a preschool-age child, you might say: "There is something in Mommy's body that isn't supposed to be there. It can make Mommy very sick." For a school-age child (and older), it's okay to say the name of your disease, how you learned about it, where it's located, and what your medical team will do to take care of you. For example, "I am going to have to stay in the hospital so the doctors can give me some medicine to help me get well again. It takes a long time to get well when someone has breast cancer." Also explain that things at home may feel, look, or be different. Include changes in your appearance (for example, possible hair loss) and availability, as well as less obvious ones, like your stamina and who will be doing routine tasks around the house.

Pay attention to children's body language for helpful feedback about their thoughts, feelings, and worries. Ask questions that invite them to talk about their concerns.

Read one or more of the books written for children about cancer to get a better understanding of your child's concerns and questions. Because children love repetition, the books written for their age group can also keep communication going when you're unavailable. When possible, you can read aloud with young children, ask them to read to you, and do any suggested projects together. Although older children are apt to look up information on the Internet, they may still find that reading a book that captures their feelings and fears will reinforce what you've said in ways that the Web can't. A book may also spark ideas for future conversations.

Look for books with four- or five-star ratings and positive reviews like these three that have the American Cancer Society seal of approval:[2]

- *Because . . . Someone I Love Has Cancer: Kids' Activity Book* by the American Cancer Society. This spiral-bound book for kids ages 6 and up comes with five self-sharpening crayons and offers activities to discover inner strengths and enhance self-esteem. It also has a 16-page removable guide for caregivers with family and group activities.

- *Nana, What's Cancer?* by Beverlye Hyman Fead and Tessa Mae Hamermesh. This is a story geared for children 5 and up that centers around Tessa, a 10-year-old girl who wants to understand the confusing world of cancer. She asks her nana, who explains the facts in a comforting way that eases fears.

- *Our Mom Has Cancer* by Abigail Ackermann and Adrienne Ackermann. Written and illustrated by sisters Abigail and Adrienne, this picture book for children 4 to 8 is an honest account of what it's like to have a mom going through cancer.

Telling Your Employer and Coworkers

As soon as you get your diagnosis, or shortly thereafter, it's important to discuss with your doctor how your breast cancer might affect your job performance. We say *might*, because every patient is unique. No two people with a similar diagnosis react to either their breast cancer treatments or their work responsibilities exactly the same way. Once you have spoken with your doctor, follow these guidelines.

Call to make an appointment to speak, in person (if possible), with the appropriate person where you work. This can be your employer, a supervisor, and/or a human resources officer. If you're asked why you want the appointment, you can say that you have breast cancer or that you want to discuss a recent medical diagnosis privately before letting

dealing with kids' questions and concerns

When it comes to having concerns, every parent knows that their child will have troubling ones about breast cancer. Here are some of the questions that children of all ages (yes, adult children, too) may ask and how you can respond.

"Did someone cause you to get breast cancer?" Think of this question in terms of, "Did I say or do something that caused you to get sick?" Explain to them that breast cancer is not someone else's fault—and particularly not their fault.

"Can I catch cancer from you?" Tell them that cancer is not like a cold or flu; it can't be caught from other people. And because you can't give it to them or anyone else, they can touch, hug, and kiss you, and you can do the same.

"Will you still be able to . . . ?" Reassure them that everyone in the family is going to be working together to keep things running smoothly and ensure everyone is cared for.

"Can I help you, Mom?" The answer is "Yes!" When you provide opportunities for children to pitch in, it affirms their desire to try to make you well. Plan to ask if they can take on certain chores or be available at certain times. If they enjoy drawing, ask them to make you cards when they have time. If they love to sing or play an instrument, tell them how much you would enjoy listening to them before dinner or at bedtime. There are lots of opportunities disguised as chores or requests. It may be as simple yet profound as asking a busy teenager for a nightly hug, kiss, or prayer.

---

others at work know about it. Or you can just say that you need to discuss a personal concern. Say whatever you feel comfortable with. Remember to also ask that the reason for the appointment be kept private until after you get together. Keep in mind that giving your news is better done face-to-face, if possible, than over a phone call; it's more personal, and it may even be more reassuring to you to be able to read and interpret the emotions and body language of the person you speak with.

Be well prepared for the meeting, no matter what the size of your company or your relationship to your employer. Take a list of important questions with you, including ones about medical leave (and whether or not you'll be able to return to work after your surgery or during treatments), as well as compensation during medical leave. If you were given an employee handbook when you were hired, go through it carefully before your meeting. Search for answers to your questions and, if you can't find them, make sure they're on your list of things to discuss.

Figure out when you want your coworkers to know before your meeting. You may say something the same day, but that will depend on what you learn from the meeting and how you feel after that meeting. You may have already planned to meet privately with some coworkers who are friends or survivors. Depending on what's comfortable for you, plan to talk to others in person when and where it's best for you.

PREPARING TO SHARE THE NEWS

Disclosing heartfelt and devastating news to those we love can be tough. To make it easier, try writing down what you want to say beforehand.

Begin with a rough draft. Read all the way through this chapter first. Then start writing a rough draft of your "speech." Think of it as a trial run that you can return to as often as you need to. Here are some tips.

Say thank you. Your appreciation can be for coming to hear your news, for friendship, or for any other reason you want to give.

Set the stage. Ease into your "discussion" with a personal anecdote. For example: "We've all known women who have had breast cancer. Honestly, I never thought I'd be one of them. But now I am, and I'd like to tell you about what that means to me and to you."

Stick to the most important details. Not everyone you're talking to needs to know everything about your diagnosis and prognosis. Consider handing out a basic information sheet about your type of breast cancer. You can get this from your doctor's office or the Internet. You can use it as a point-by-point "cheat sheet" when you're talking; and afterward, others can refer to it.

Finish your rough draft. Write about minor details that you may or may not end up using. If you decide they're just not right for a particular audience or they make your discussion run too long, keep them in your journal or file them away under "Future Questions to Bring Up."

Practice. Try standing in front of a mirror while reading the rough draft to boost your confidence.

Once you get going with this exercise, don't be surprised if you feel like you're writing a book. Remember this is a *rough* draft. So if it feels cathartic to let it all out, go for it. You can edit and polish it later.

COMMUNICATING THROUGH CHANGE

Breaking the news to people about your cancer is only the first step. How you deal with and interact with people from this point on will change, and knowing what to expect will help prevent possible anger, confusion, anxiety, and even feelings of uneasiness. Here are some examples of changes that will occur.

People will want to know how you're doing. Expect ongoing requests for the latest news about your progress, treatments, and how you are doing overall. This will be especially true at home or work where routine questions like "How are you doing?" or "What's new?" will take on a new and important meaning. Where in the past people may not have paid much attention to your answers, now they will. You'll need to figure out how you want to respond to questions like this and how much you want to let people know as you move through your treatment.

Your cancer may become the "elephant in the room"–something that everyone sees and knows about, but no one wants to talk about. Ask yourself if you're okay with this. You don't need to discuss your cancer all the time, but if it's making you and others feel uneasy or act strange, then you need to bring it up. You could give people a chance to open up to you with, "Is there something you want to talk to me about?" or even "Are you okay with everything that's been going on?"

Your family dynamics will change. To prevent communication from breaking down, talk to your partner about the situations that are worrying you. Consider having a family meeting. You may want to invite close extended family members, too. Call it "Comments, Concerns, Complaints, and Questions."

- **Let people know you want to talk about the ways breast cancer may be causing change in your family.** Explain that you're interested in hearing their comments, concerns, complaints, and questions about the changes.

- **Open the meeting with a statement about a positive personal change that's directly related to your breast cancer.** It may be hard at first to think of one, but your work in your journal can help you determine some things you could say. It could be something like: "I'd like to begin by saying that ever since I got my diagnosis, I've felt more supported and loved than I can ever remember. I am so grateful for that because breast cancer is changing everything for me. Sometimes it makes me realize how much I've taken for granted before it happened. Thank you for being there in so many ways as we learn how to go through this together."

- **Mention a change that's concerning you.** It could simply be, "I'm concerned about the television being on during dinner. We never kept it on before I got breast cancer, so why is this happening now?" Or you can use the same example and then take it to a deeper level: "Is the television staying on because it's hard to talk or there's nothing to say?"

- **Ask people to share their concerns.** If it seems like there is prolonged discussion about one particular concern, ask to schedule another meeting–possibly the next day or week–to discuss that one issue. Remind your family that the purpose of the meeting is to get everyone's comments, concerns, complaints, and questions on the table, and prolonged discussions about any one of them can prevent that from happening.

- **Prepare yourself for complaints and other negative comments and concerns.** If you feel your buttons being pushed, remember you're not alone–others may be experiencing that same feeling. Keep yourself from reacting negatively by taking a moment–and a deep breath. Even calling a meeting break can help defuse the situation. After the break, people might be calmer and less anxious. Keep in mind that the objective of the meeting is to address the unease so you can move on to a healthier place on your journey.

It's okay *not* to have cancer be the center of all conversations. Once someone is diagnosed with cancer, it's hard for the focus to shift back to the general news of the family (accomplishments at work for a partner, school news and sporting events for children, and even just the daily business of living) or even random discussions with friends and/or

a simple script: what to say

You may be finding it hard to use the right words to tell people your news. Or you've shared your news with those closest to you and just don't know how to tell your coworkers or acquaintances. While there is no one-size-fits-all script, we created this basic script for you to use as a starting point. Change, or add, whatever you want to make this yours. Begin by saying:

It's really important to me that you listen to everything I have to tell you. I know you'll have questions, so if you could wait to ask them until after I'm done, that would mean a lot to me. I know you'll understand once you hear what I have to say.

Know that this is very hard for me, so if I'm silent for a few minutes as I'm talking, understand that I may not be finished yet. I may need these moments to gather my thoughts.

I know that once I say what I need to say, you'll want to help me with advice. Thank you so much for this. But right now, I'm getting a lot of information from a lot of people, which is a little overwhelming for me. So if you could not share advice with me right now, I would really appreciate that.

I have breast cancer. "I just found out . . ." (include when you were told). "It's stage . . ." (if you want to share this). "I start my treatments . . ." (include when, if you want to share this information).

Please be sensitive to the fact that there are things that I want to know—and don't want to know—about my illness right now. There's some stuff I'm just not ready to deal with yet. It's not that I'm in denial. I'm just trying to take things one step at a time. So if I don't want to talk about something, please respect that.

Thank you so much for being here for me and listening to my news. It means so much to me to have you in my life and as I'm going through this journey to healing.

coworkers. Know that it's important for you, as well as for everyone else, to take their mind off your illness. It's okay to take a break from treatment discussions, prognosis, and breast cancer and just go to lunch, catch up on work gossip, see a movie or a play . . . whatever works for you. What you'll find is that everyone, including yourself, will become less anxious.

COMMUNICATING YOUR EXPECTATIONS

What do you expect of others while you're on your journey to recovery? It might be that you're hoping family members will take over your everyday tasks while you're away for surgery or treatments. Or maybe you'd like your husband or a dear friend to spend more time with you. Naturally, you can't assume that others will meet your needs unless you communicate them clearly. But doing so can be tricky.

Perhaps you think you're being selfish if you tell people what you'd like them to do, or perhaps you just assume your needs are so obvious they'll know. But since no one can read your mind, you can never assume anyone knows what you think or hope unless you talk about those desires with them. To better understand what *your* expectations are:

- **Write down exactly what you expect from others.** Doing this can help clarify what you need and why you need it. This is also a good way to avoid asking for something that's come to mind on the fly and you haven't thought through carefully. For example, you may have already assumed that it would be your husband or partner who will drive you to chemo treatments (the side effects of chemotherapy treatments may prevent you from being able to drive afterward). But this may not have even crossed your partner's mind. Another example, which may be awkward to bring up, might be wanting sex (or even just more comforting "snuggle time") with your husband or partner but not knowing how to ask for it, particularly during times when you may not feel that you're attractive. Or it might just be that you want someone to *not* say anything to others about your breast cancer or to keep you in their thoughts and prayers when you have surgery.

- **Plan ahead about who you will ask to do what.** Once you have your list, figure out who can best fulfill the expectations on it.

- **Prioritize each expectation.** You may need certain people, like your partner or spouse, to do more than one thing. But you may find that because they're satisfying one expectation, they don't have the time or energy for another. Prioritizing will help you and them to figure out what they should be focusing their energy on.

how do you respond to offers of help?

Is "No, thanks" your standard response when unexpected offers of help come your way? If so, why is it? Perhaps it's because you were raised not to accept help, or taught that if you do, you have an obligation to repay that debt someday. It could be because you think that accepting help makes you look weak. Or maybe you're just someone who feels as though you're imposing or you're just too embarrassed, proud, or stubborn to ask for, or accept, help.

If any of these reasons describe why you might reject sincere offers of help or never ask for it, you're not alone. But in order to fortify yourself physically, psychologically, and emotionally, you may need to change your attitude about accepting help. According to the American Psychological Association, getting help when you need it is a crucial step in building your resilience and facing challenges during adverse times.[3] So to reap the benefits of help, try reframing negative thoughts about accepting help and look at it through a positive lens instead.

Think about how people help one another and strangers after natural disasters. Recall watching the news and empathizing with those who suffered and those who generously gave gifts of their compassion, time, and other resources. You probably teared up at times because the recipients were so grateful for the kindness of

- **Communicate your expectations considerately and appropriately.** We suggested that you take the lead when you talk about your expectations, but also remember that there are good and bad ways of doing this. Even when dealing with difficult people, try to be polite and appreciative, not pushy or insistent. It seems obvious, but it's easy to start demanding things from others when you've been through so much.

others. But so often the helpers expressed their gratitude, too, especially for the immeasurable gifts of appreciation and learning what a real difference they have made in another's life.

To get started:

Write in your journal about instances in your life when someone's help (no matter how small) surprised you. It could be something as simple as someone allowing you to cut in line after seeing you were rushed. It could be a coworker offering to pitch in with a last-minute project you were stressing about. Whatever comes to mind, write it down in your journal. List the emotions that you felt at that time, too.

Now write about instances in your life when you had the opportunity to help someone else and how it made you feel. What you'll probably discover is how good helping others made you feel, and you'll understand why people are reaching out to you now.

So when someone offers to help you, say "Yes." Don't automatically deprive yourself of the special gift you are being offered. Instead, accept needed help and think of it in terms of a gift exchange. And finally, don't forget to also ask how you might help them. This is one time when a regifted gift is the perfect one.

dealing with employment discrimination

Not all employers are compassionate and accommodating when it comes to how your treatments affect your job performance. Sometimes their reaction to your illness may result in job discrimination.

So it's important right from the start to talk to your employer about accommodations for your illness. That's because you may need to:

- Take leave for doctors' appointments, to find doctors or treatment centers, or to recuperate from treatment
- Schedule breaks or have a private place to rest or take medications
- Make adjustments to your work routine, such as working at home, adjusting the temperature in the office, using the phone or computer to contact doctors, or passing minor tasks to another employee
- Request reassignment to another, more manageable job

As a woman with breast cancer in the workplace, you need to know about your rights under the Americans with Disabilities Act (ADA).

The ADA is a federal law that prohibits most employers from discriminating against employees because of or during an illness. If you work for a company with 15 or more employees, the ADA

Also be sure to ask others about *their* expectations. You can't know what others expect of you unless you ask. And sometimes people don't even realize they're putting expectations on you. For example, your mother might make a statement like "Of course you'll be well enough to come for Thanksgiving." In this situation, it's best to be forthright. For example: "I really hope that can happen. Everyone who will be there can help protect you when you apply for a job, after you've been offered one, and as an employee during your illness.

Complementing the ADA is the Family and Medical Leave Act (FMLA) and antidiscrimination legislation on the state level. For more information about the federal laws and job discrimination in the workplace, go to the US Equal Employment Opportunity Commission's Web site: eeoc.gov/facts/cancer.html.

But what if you don't fall under the ADA guidelines and you feel discriminated against by a supervisor at your place of employment? First talk to your human resources department and/or the head of your department. If applicable, keep going up the chain of command.

If that doesn't work and you feel your employer may be at fault, Barbara Hoffman, JD, an expert for Breastcancer.org, recommends the following:

- Contact your local bar association for advice.

- Check out the National Employment Lawyers Association (nela.org) for information about attorneys specializing in employment discrimination.

- Contact cancer advocacy organizations like the National Coalition for Cancer Survivorship (canceradvocacy.org) and the Patient Advocate Foundation (patientadvocate.org).

knows I have to go through surgery, chemotherapy, and radiation, and I should be finished by then. But right now, I don't know for sure how long that will take or how I'll feel afterward. I hope I can come. I know we'll both be disappointed if I can't. So let's see what happens over the next 6 months." Keeping the door open for honest conversation and communication is critical.

MOVING ON

As you move forward, remember to go wherever you need to in this guide. Continue to refer to the resources in these four chapters whenever you need them to help you sustain the journey ahead. Sidestepping, jumping ahead, and backtracking are all positive ways to get where you need to be in the most positive and healing ways possible. Safe travels.

Agent of Change

Breast cancer doctor Marisa Weiss was an acclaimed radiation oncologist for more than 20 years. The author of four books of advice for breast cancer patients, she thought she had all the answers.

But in 2010, when she was diagnosed with early-stage breast cancer, questions answered countless times for others became her own: *Where do I go from here? What are my treatment options? How do I tell my children?*

Marisa, 51 at the time of her diagnosis, had lots of practical and personal answers handy. But even so, the Philadelphia-based physician says, "The unexpected shock and uncertainty comes over you like a tsunami." Storms like that leave you feeling vulnerable and disoriented, so it's important to pull together an action plan. "You start by working with the best people you can to come up with a strategy."

More than a decade before her own diagnosis, Marisa founded Breastcancer.org as a way to get medically reviewed, user-friendly information to millions of women anywhere, anytime. She knew how little time doctors have to spend with their patients and believed all of that had to change. Convinced that it was imperative for her to become an agent of that change, Breastcancer.org was born.

Today, her vision has created a Web site that's had a huge impact. In a world where breaking news about breast cancer can be complicated, it's hard for patients to understand data that their lives may depend on. Breastcancer.org gives women and their loved ones authoritative, up-to-the-minute information that helps them make vitally important choices.

She'd like women who've been diagnosed to know . . . *many brave women have blazed the trail for you—don't try to do it alone!*

Breast cancer is . . . *the most common cancer to affect women.*

Tomorrow will . . . *bring us closer to preventing this disease and, for those women still diagnosed, closer to the cure.*

PART TWO

DECIPHERING
the DIAGNOSIS

In the following pages, we'll introduce you to the latest science and research regarding breast cancer, homing in on what you need to know to understand your diagnosis and make informed decisions.

We'll provide an introduction to the causes and genesis of breast cancer, as well as give you an up-to-date look at recent research into the molecular basis of tumors, which has led to the development of new, highly effective medications. We'll also explain how to read your pathology report.

The good news is that medical research has progressed considerably in recent decades and is improving all the time. You have options when it comes to treatment. In the following pages, we'll guide you through what you need to know to make the best decisions for your situation and diagnosis.

"When you get into a tight place and everything goes against you, till it seems as though you could not hang on a minute longer, never give up then, for that is just the place and time that the tide will turn."

—HARRIET BEECHER STOWE

CHAPTER 5

WHAT IS BREAST CANCER?

B y now, you've had time to think a bit about your diagnosis, and the questions that probably keep coming to mind are "How did I get this cancer?" and "Was it because of something I did, I ate, or I didn't do?" Understanding exactly what breast cancer is will help you answer these questions and give you an idea of why and how medical treatment can help.

First off, it's important to understand your cells and how they work. Healthy cells go about their everyday business signaled by directions from DNA–the so-called genetic "recipe" found in every cell–and then they die a natural death, called apoptosis. But mutations in DNA can make this process go awry. And in many types of cancer, the cells don't receive their usual signal to stop dividing, so they keep producing new growth. This leads to out-of-control cell division and, eventually, a tumor, which can be benign (meaning it's usually non-cancerous, slow-growing, and doesn't metastasize, or spread to other parts of the body) or malignant. Malignant tumors, which grow at greatly varying speeds, can metastasize to other parts of the body (and organs) and interfere with healthy functioning.

When a tumor develops in the breast, it often begins in the milk ducts. But it can also occur in lobules (the glands that produce milk) and sometimes in fatty tissue (see the illustration on page 79). The most common breast cancers are named based on where they arise and whether they've invaded surrounding tissue. For example, ductal carcinoma in situ is cancer that hasn't spread beyond the ducts (*in situ* is Latin for "in position," meaning the cancer hasn't spread beyond its original location).

WHAT CAUSES BREAST CANCER?

This is what scientists and doctors like to call a loaded question. The truth is that no one really knows definitively what causes breast cancer—or, for that matter, any type of cancer. In fact, a Google search for the "answer" will bring you 63 billion results in about 0.3 second (that's always a good indication no one really knows the answer, although everyone likes to offer an opinion about it). And speaking of opinions, you're sure to get a lot from well-meaning family members, friends, coworkers, and acquaintances about what may have caused your breast cancer. By all means, listen politely, and then go ahead dealing with your health-care team for information that applies to your cancer (and that includes how they think it might have developed).

Genetics do play a part, but not as much as people think. In fact, only 5 to 10 percent of breast cancers are hereditary,[1] meaning the disease was passed on from family members. Scientists and researchers are trying to understand the reasons why the rest of breast cancer cases occur. Let's just say that much research still needs to be done.

Top 10 Risk Factors for Breast Cancer

Some risk factors you can't control—and some you can. Here's a look at both.

Risk Factors You Can't Control

These risk factors, like age and heredity, put you at higher risk.

Sex. Sixty percent of women who develop breast cancer don't have a major risk factor other than being a woman. Men *can* develop breast cancer, but it's about 100 times less common in men: Just 2,240 American men will be diagnosed with the disease in 2013.[2]

Age. The older you are, the higher your risk. Eighty percent of new cancers are diagnosed in people over 55,[3] more than half of new breast cancers occur in women over 60, and more than one-third occur in women over 75.[4] Also, breast cancer is more common later in life—after menopause—in Europe and the United States than in other parts of the

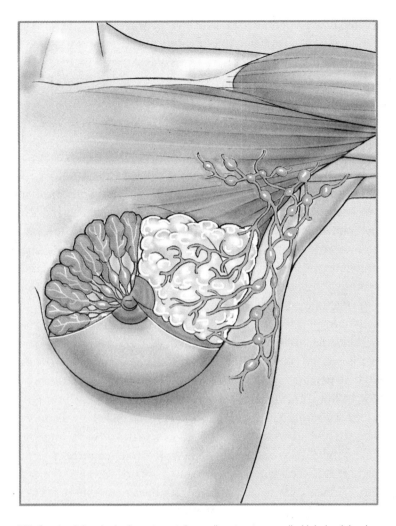

Milk-forming lobes in the breast contain smaller structures called lobules (glands that produce milk) and bulbs that express milk. The breast is also made up of blood and lymph vessels, ducts connecting the milk-producing lobes to the nipple, and stroma, a fatty connective tissue.

world, such as Japan or Africa, but scientists haven't figured out why.[5]

Race and ethnicity. According to the American Cancer Society, white women are slightly more likely to develop breast cancer than African American women, but African American women are more likely to die of this cancer. But in women under 45, breast cancer is more common in African Americans. Asian, Hispanic, and Native American women all have a lower risk of developing and dying from breast cancer.[6]

Exposure to hormones. If you got your period early in life–also called early menarche–and/or went into menopause late, you've been exposed to the female reproductive hormones estrogen and progesterone for a long time. (These hormones are what regulate your periods.) This long-term exposure puts you at higher risk of breast cancer. According to the American Cancer Society, studies have found that women using oral contraceptives (birth control pills) have a slightly greater risk of breast cancer than women who have never used them, though the Pill has been shown to reduce risk of endometrial and ovarian cancers.[7]

Genetics. In the early 1990s, scientists discovered a genetic disposition to breast cancer in mutations of the genes BRCA1 and BRCA2 (named for BReast CAncer). These tumor suppressor genes flew into the spotlight in mid-2013 when the actress Angelina Jolie revealed she had undergone a preventive double mastectomy. Jolie fit the profile for highest risk: Not only was she a carrier of the BRCA1 mutation, but her mother died of ovarian cancer and an aunt of breast cancer.[8] Doctors estimated her lifetime chance of developing breast cancer at 87 percent.[9] Risk associated with these two mutations differs, however, and is calculated based on a number of highly individual factors–it can be as low as about 45 percent.[10]

Not all women will make a choice similar to Angelina Jolie's, but preventive mastectomy is an option for BRCA carriers. For a woman with a first-degree relative who's had breast cancer, getting tested can provide a measure of relief from anxiety, and a more informed sense of the risks for you or your children. Still, the genetic causes of breast cancer are largely a mystery. Only about 40 percent of hereditary breast cancer is linked to these two genes,[11] and only 5 to 10 percent of breast cancers are hereditary.[12]

Risk Factors You *Can* Control

Researchers estimate that 50 to 75 percent of cancers are the result of modifiable risk factors. Researchers have also determined that certain lifestyle choices have been linked to breast cancer.

Exposure to carcinogens. No matter what you read–or what anyone else tells you–some environmental risk factors *do* seem to exist. In fact, so-called endocrine-disrupting chemicals and carcinogens (which may increase breast cancer risk) are present in many working environments. For example, one study found that women who worked in certain jobs, such as plastics manufacturing and food canning, had more than *twice* the risk of developing premenopausal breast cancer compared to women who did not work in these environments.[13]

Pesticides in food and chemicals in household cleaning products and other everyday substances may also cause cancer. Unfortunately, though, not enough studies to date have focused on environmental causes like these. In fact, a 2013 government report criticized the lack of funding for such efforts.[14]

Smoking (and secondhand cigarette smoke) exposes you to carcinogens as well, which is why smoking is considered a risk factor for many cancers, including breast cancer.

Diet. Studies are conflicting as to whether eating certain foods can increase or decrease your breast cancer risk. But what has been proven: High-fat diets can lead to being overweight or obese, which is a breast cancer risk factor. (See more on diet in Chapter 9.)

Alcohol intake. When it comes to alcohol, those who have two to five drinks daily have about $1\frac{1}{2}$ times the risk of women who don't drink.[15]

Obesity. Fat cells make estrogen. And when breast cells are exposed to extra estrogen over time, the risk of developing breast cancer is higher.[16] One 2006 study found that women who gained about 55 pounds or more after the age of 18 had a 45 percent increased risk of developing breast cancer compared with those who maintained their weight. Gaining weight after menopause can also increase a woman's risk. That same study found that putting on 22 pounds after menopause increased the risk of developing breast cancer by 18 percent.[17]

Lack of exercise. Exercise is key to preventing breast cancer because it controls blood sugar and limits blood levels of something called insulin growth factor, a hormone that can affect how breast cells grow and behave. Exercising also helps you maintain a healthy weight (see Chapter 10).

HOW BREAST CANCER IS DETECTED

Perhaps you had a routine mammogram that returned suspicious results, or you or your doctor discovered a lump in your breast, as is often the case.[18] Either way, you most likely got a definitive diagnosis after imaging tests and a tissue sample, or biopsy. In this section, we'll explore the various imaging techniques and explain how to understand the results of a biopsy.

The Latest Imaging Techniques

Various imaging techniques are used to detect cancer. Chances are you'll recognize the one (or more) you had done. But keep in mind that you'll most likely need additional imaging as you move through your treatment and healing process. These imaging techniques are detailed in the following pages.

Mammography is an imaging tool that uses x-rays to look inside the breast and detect tumors as small as 5 to 10 millimeters, and sometimes as small as 1 millimeter (keep in mind that an inch is 25 millimeters, so this is extremely small).[19] Usually, two views of the breast are taken: craneocaudal (CC) and mediolateral oblique (MLO). Mammography is considered the gold standard of breast imaging, but it has certain disadvantages, particularly for women with dense breast tissue. For example, it can't detect cancer outside the fatty area of the breast, such as near the underarm (one reason why physical exams are still important).[20] It also can't reliably differentiate between problematic growths and dense tissue, which can lead to false negatives for women with dense breasts.[21] Also, breast implants can obscure mammogram images.

When choosing where to have a mammogram done, be sure to select a facility that is FDA certified and that does a lot of mammograms. Chances are, if you had a screening mammogram that raised red flags, you've already gone for (or are scheduled to go for) a diagnostic mammogram. A diagnostic mammogram is still an x-ray of the breast, but it's done to study more closely the area of concern. Note that it's important to either get all of your mammograms done at the same facility or have your old films available so the radiologist can compare them.

Digital mammography is increasingly available, but it hasn't been shown to improve identification over traditional film mammography. But just like pictures taken with your digital camera, it does make it easier for your doctor to examine your images (the original pictures can be magnified and looked at in many different ways on the computer screen) and to send them to other specialists if necessary.

Ultrasound imaging uses sound waves to create images. It can help distinguish a benign cyst from a solid mass, which could be a tumor. Plus, it's useful in imaging breasts with dense tissue or implants, which can be hard to read on a mammogram. It's also harmless, since it's not invasive, uses no radiation, and has no side effects associated with the sound waves.[22]

But why–if you've already been diagnosed with breast cancer–would you need an additional ultrasound? You might have one if your doctor suspects that your cancer may have spread to your lymph nodes in your underarm area (this is called an axillary ultrasound). You might also have an ultrasound to measure a tumor and determine exactly where it's located prior to neoadjuvant chemotherapy (this is treatment given before primary therapy; for example, chemotherapy to shrink a tumor before it can be removed surgically).

PET (positron-emission tomography) scanning is another imaging technique, but it works very differently than a mammogram. First, it's

 BETWEEN THE LINES

can mammography radiation cause breast cancer?

Chances are, like many survivors, you've had more than just a few mammograms in the years prior to your diagnosis. And like so many other survivors, you may be thinking that the radiation from this imaging technique might be one of the reasons you got breast cancer in the first place. It's a valid thought, but both digital and film mammography use a very small amount of radiation, which isn't dangerous at recommended screening levels.

The American Cancer Society puts it in perspective this way: If you have yearly mammograms starting at age 40 and continue until you're 90, you'll get a total of 20 to 40 rads (a measure of radiation dose). To put it another way, flying from New York to California on a commercial jet exposes a woman to roughly the same amount of radiation as one mammogram.[23] Also, as one researcher puts it, your chances of developing breast cancer from the radiation in a digital mammogram is 1 in 1,000, and of dying from it, 1 in 10,000. Yet the lifetime risk of breast cancer is 1 in 8 or 9.[24]

not used to diagnose cancer (as a mammogram or ultrasound does) because it doesn't detect very small tumors well. It's used after someone has already been diagnosed with breast cancer in order to determine if the cancer has spread to the lymph nodes or other areas of the body and to assess if metastatic breast cancer is responding to treatment.

With a PET, you're injected with a substance that contains a small amount of radioactive material (which emits less radiation than a standard x-ray) mixed with sugar. More radioactive material accumulates in areas that have increased levels of chemical activity (this shows up as a brighter spot on the scan). Since cancer cells are more active than normal cells, they show up brighter on the scan.

If you're pregnant, this radioactive material could potentially harm the fetus. And if you're breastfeeding, the radioactive material could contaminate the breast milk. In either case, talk to your doctor about the risk/benefits of having a PET scan done.

Be sure to ask your doctor whether another test that doesn't use radiation could work just as well. One 2012 study calculated that PET scans can raise breast cancer risk by as much as 20 percent, particularly in younger women who receive several scans.[25]

Magnetic resonance imaging, or MRI, uses a powerful magnet and radio waves to create very detailed images. The radio waves bounce back off breast tissue, and a magnetized coil surrounding each breast measures the intensity of the echoes.[26] There are benefits to this type of imaging: It doesn't use radiation, it doesn't involve the breast being flattened (which many women know can be extremely painful), and it's unhindered by dense breast tissue or implants. But because it is so detailed, it can lead to more false-positive results (which means it can find something suspicious that very often turns out not to be cancer) and result in unnecessary biopsies. This is why an MRI isn't typically recommended as a screening tool for women who are at average risk of developing breast cancer. It's also expensive, adding more than $1,000 to your bill.[27] Plus, the approximately 1-hour procedure, which is done in an MRI machine, can make a patient feel extremely claustrophobic.

An MRI, however, can be useful as an adjunct to mammography and ultrasound imaging for women at higher-than-average risk of developing breast cancer. In fact, the American Cancer Society recommends that high-risk women–from the age of 30–have both a breast MRI and a mammogram every year. This includes those who have a strong family history of breast cancer and those with the BRCA1 or BRCA2 mutation.

An MRI can also be done if you're diagnosed with cancer in one breast. A breast MRI–used in conjunction with mammography–can offer a more detailed look at the opposite breast (and has a better chance of finding the cancer, in this situation, than just a mammogram alone).[28]

An MRI is also usually recommended prior to surgery and as a follow-up diagnostic therapy once your treatments are finished. But a recent review of data from breast cancer studies conducted by Memorial Sloan-Kettering Cancer Center in New York found that women who had an MRI prior to surgery to determine the extent and severity of their tumor ended up having their entire breast removed (a mastectomy) instead of having breast-conserving surgery. Researchers theorized that an MRI, which is so detailed in its imaging, might make a cancer look worse than it actually is.[29] If you're concerned about having an MRI, discuss possible alternatives with your doctor.

BIOPSY PROCEDURES

When your physical exam–combined with mammography, ultrasound, or other imaging tests–turned up suspicious results, a tissue biopsy was most likely the next step. Several days before any biopsy, you're usually asked to stop taking aspirin or other blood thinners, as they can interfere with blood clotting and healing. There are three different types of biopsy procedures.

Fine-needle biopsy is used most often for lumps that can be felt on a physical exam. During this 10-minute outpatient procedure, the breast area is first injected with a numbing medication. Then a very thin needle attached to a syringe is inserted (sometimes guided by an ultrasound) into the lump to take a sample of cells, which are then examined in the lab. You may have some swelling, soreness, and pain afterward.[30]

Stereotactic core biopsy is typically done in a radiology suite for lesions that are not palpable. You either lie facedown on a table or are seated in a chair while your breast is placed between imaging plates and a mammogram is taken. Your breast is numbed with local anesthesia, and the radiologist makes a tiny nick and then inserts a slightly larger needle than what's used in fine-needle aspiration. The radiologist then takes samples of suspicious tissue revealed in imaging (usually an abnormality called microcalcifications, which are white specks of calcium in the breast tissue). Usually, 5 or 10 "cores" are taken to ensure a complete sampling of the area.[31] Occasionally, biopsies are guided by MRI or ultrasound, or performed as a surgical procedure, depending on the location of the suspicious tissue.[32]

Afterward, a tiny titanium "clip" (about the size of a sesame seed) is inserted in the breast to mark the biopsy site; it remains in the breast permanently so anyone reading future mammograms knows that this area has already been evaluated. It's also a way for doctors to tell exactly where the tissue–if cancerous–has been removed. (If you have concerns about having clips inserted in your breast, discuss this with your radiologist; if you speak up, you may not need to have them inserted.) Temporary bruising and pain are typical side effects.

HOW TO READ YOUR PATHOLOGY REPORT

After your biopsy is analyzed, the lab will send a pathology report to your doctor. You will have a chance to review the report with your doctor at your follow-up or postoperative visit. If she doesn't offer, be sure to ask your doctor to review it with you, and ask for a copy of it so you can write notes and review it later.

The pathology report is comprised of several components. The first is identifying information about you, including your name, date of birth, medical record, and your doctor's name, date of procedure, and date of pathology report. The second is a clinical information section that gives the history of how your cancer was identified. This is written by your surgeon and helps the pathologist know the details about you. The gross description section provides information on what your tissues looked like before they were examined under the microscope; it also includes measurements of the tissue that was removed.

The diagnosis section gives all of the pertinent information regarding what your cells look like under the microscope and discusses the type of cancer, tumor size, grade, lymph node status (whether lymph nodes have tumor cells in them and, if so, how many nodes). It will also give molecular information such as ER, PR and HER2 status. In this part, the pathologist will report on your margins. The final diagnosis section gives a summary of the information presented, and it is this information that your doctor will use to determine your stage.

Staging

Staging is a word used to describe how doctors evaluate the size of a tumor and the extent of cancer in a biopsied tissue sample or following surgery. The tumor-node-metastasis (TNM) system is commonly used for staging.[33] (A newer method of characterizing tumors, based on molecular characteristics of cancer cells, is explored later in this chapter in "How 'Molecular Analysis' Is Changing Breast Cancer Treatment–For the Better" on page 92.) You'll find the terms used here are the same as those used by your medical team, so it's helpful to become familiar with them.

In the TNM system, the number following each letter refers to the size of the tumor or the cancer's spread through the body.

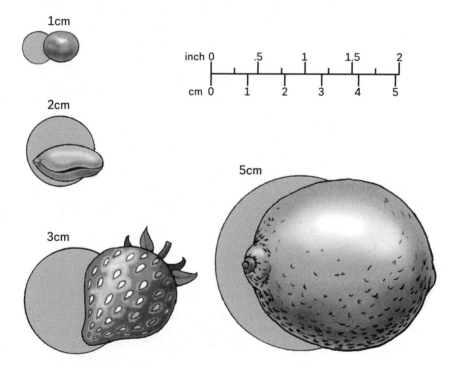

A T1 tumor is less than 2 cm across, the size of an unshelled peanut, or smaller, such as a 1-cm-wide pea. T2 tumors run from 2 to 5 cm across, about the size of a strawberry. T3 tumors are 5 cm wide, or roughly the size of a lime.

CANCER STAGING GUIDE: TUMOR-NODE-METASTASIS

Below you'll find the terms used on a pathology report written with the TNM system. Tissue will be graded on location of a primary tumor, whether it has spread to the lymph nodes, and whether it has spread beyond the lymph nodes. These factors add up to the stage.

PRIMARY TUMOR (T)

TX	Primary tumor cannot be evaluated
T0	No evidence of primary tumor
Tis	Carcinoma in situ (early cancer that has not spread to neighboring tissue)
T1, T2, T3, T4	Size and/or extent of the primary tumor

REGIONAL LYMPH NODES (N)

NX	Regional lymph nodes cannot be evaluated
N0	No regional lymph node involvement (no cancer found in the lymph nodes)
N1, N2, N3	Involvement of regional lymph nodes (number and/or extent of spread)

DISTANT METASTASIS (M)

MX	Distant metastasis cannot be evaluated
M0	No distant metastasis (cancer has not spread to other parts of the body)
M1	Distant metastasis (cancer has spread to distant parts of the body)

STAGE	DEFINITION
Stage 0	Carcinoma in situ (early cancer present only in the layer of cells in which it began)
Stage I, II, and III	Higher numbers indicate more extensive disease: greater tumor size and/or spread of the cancer to nearby lymph nodes and/or organs adjacent to the primary tumor
Stage IV	The cancer has spread to another organ

Sources: National Comprehensive Cancer Network Cancer Staging Guide 2013 and National Cancer Institute

You may also find several other categories in your pathology report.

In situ means early-stage cancer is present only in the cells in which it began.

Localized means the cancer is limited to the organ in which it began, without evidence of spread.

Regional means the cancer has spread beyond the original (primary) site to nearby lymph nodes or organs and tissues.

Distant means the cancer has spread from the primary site to distant organs or distant lymph nodes.

Unknown is occasionally used to indicate there's not enough information available to indicate a stage.

THE DIFFERENT TYPES OF BREAST CANCER

Researchers are discovering that there's not just one breast cancer, but many. Here's a guide to the major types.

Lobular Carcinoma in Situ (LCIS)

Lobular carcinoma in situ, or LCIS, is an abnormal growth in the lobules of milk glands. It's technically not considered a cancer and has long been regarded as simply a risk factor for breast cancer. Women with a history of LCIS have a risk of about 1 percent per year, or 20 to 25 percent over a lifetime, of developing breast cancer.[34] Women diagnosed with this condition have several options. Watchful waiting involves at least yearly mammograms and regular clinical and self-guided breast exams. Tamoxifen (Nolvadex), which is approved by the FDA for all women, and raloxifene (Evista), which is approved for postmenopausal women, block the effects of estrogen in the body and reduce the risk of breast cancer in women with LCIS by 56 percent.[35] Lumpectomy may be considered;[36] a more drastic option is double, or bilateral, mastectomy, which decreases the chance of breast cancer by 97 percent.[37] LCIS increases the risk of cancer in both breasts, no matter where it first occurred, so if mastectomy is chosen, both breasts must be removed for the procedure to be effective.

Ductal Carcinoma in Situ (DCIS)

If lobular carcinoma in situ is an indication of possible later cancer, ductal carcinoma in situ (DCIS) is generally considered an early stage of cancer itself–in fact, it's categorized as "stage 0." However, highly effective treatments are available, and survival rates for this condition are close to 100 percent.[38] One in five breast cancers diagnosed each year are DCIS, which often shows up as calcium deposits, called microcalcifications, in

better understanding your cancer

Knowledge is power; and when it comes to your breast cancer, this old saying becomes even more applicable. When you understand what kind of cancer you have and how it's being discussed among your medical team, you'll feel more empowered to ask questions. Plus, you'll know how to target your research to learn about the cancer and the treatments that can help.

So, with that in mind, after having read this chapter, take a moment to go through your pathology reports. You should have copies of every report that's issued in your medical file (see "Start a Breast Cancer File Box" on page 39). If you don't, don't worry. Just call your doctor's office and ask that they be sent to you. You can always pick up this journal exercise afterward.

Once you have your pathology reports, write down in your journal the type of cancer you have, as well as the way it's being described medically. Then, using the information in this chapter, jot down notes about your cancer (try to include as many characteristics as you can), as well as any questions you still have. Be sure to bring your journal with you to every doctor's appointment so you can take notes and so you don't forget what questions to ask.

Use this journal entry as your guide throughout your journey, whether you're in your doctor's office, in the treatment center, or just sitting down at your computer doing research. Think of this exercise as owning your cancer, so you know exactly how to kiss it good-bye for good!

isolated locations or spread throughout the breast. Though the "in situ" means it occurs in only one place, there's a higher chance than with LCIS that DCIS will morph into invasive cancer down the road. As a result, DCIS is often treated similarly to invasive cancer—lumpectomy and radiation or mastectomy and possibly tamoxifen. The risk of DCIS progressing to invasive cancer after lumpectomy alone is 20 percent; combined with radiation, the risk drops to 11 percent.[39]

Invasive Cancer

Invasive cancers, just like in situ growths, can arise in the milk ducts, or lobules, and are named accordingly. Invasive (or infiltrating) ductal carcinomas make up 80 percent of breast cancers,[40] while invasive (or infiltrating) lobular carcinoma is found in 10 percent of all breast cancers.[41] However, both these forms have spread beyond the confines of the milk glands and, left unchecked, have the potential to spread to the lymph nodes, bones, and the rest of the body in a process called metastasis. Both have similar progressions—one is not worse than the other—though invasive lobular cancer can usually be treated with hormone-blocking drugs (see "How 'Molecular Analysis' Is Changing Breast Cancer Treatment—For the Better" on page 92).[42]

Rare Forms of Breast Cancer

Rare forms of breast cancer make up about 10 percent of invasive ductal carcinomas. These include:

Medullary begins in the milk ducts and is a soft, fleshy mass that resembles a part of the brain called the medulla. It's more common in women who have a BRCA1 mutation.

Mucinous (or colloid carcinoma) begins in the milk duct and is made up of tumors that "float" in pools of mucin, an ingredient found in mucus. This cancer tends to affect women after they've gone through menopause.

Tubular tumors begin in the milk ducts and are small (about 1 centimeter) and made up of tube-shaped structures called tubules. This type of cancer isn't likely to spread outside the breast.

Papillary cancer also begins in the milk ducts and consists of finger-like projections, or papules. It accounts for less than 1 percent of all breast cancers and isn't likely to spread to the lymph nodes.[43]

Paget's disease, which occurs in the nipple and surrounding areola, involves an additional tumor inside the breast in about half of all cases,[44] may be invasive or noninvasive, and makes up less than 3 percent of all cancers.[45] It's often mistaken for dermatitis or eczema on the nipple because it causes flaking, crusty or thickened skin, along with possible yellowish or bloody discharge from the nipple.

Inflammatory breast cancer also typically begins in the milk ducts and causes breasts to become red, swollen, tender, and warm to the touch. While it occurs in 1 to 3 percent of all breast cancers,[46] it spreads rapidly and is usually diagnosed when it's either stage III or stage IV.

How "Molecular Analysis" Is Changing Breast Cancer Treatment—For the Better

Not all cancer cells are the same (not even all breast cancer cells). Each different type of cancer, in each different type of person, acts differently and has a genetic "on-off" switch. Finding that switch–and figuring out which treatment (or combination of treatments) turns it off–is what's dominating cancer research now and is why administering a one-size-fits-all treatment for breast cancer is quickly becoming obsolete.

Scientists have found that different breast cancers respond to different hormones and proteins in the body (this is described as the molecular characteristics of cancer, or biomarkers). It's this discovery that has allowed the development of revolutionary new drugs that inhibit cancer growth.

Your pathology report should indicate whether the biopsy or surgery found a biomarker-responsive tumor. Below, we review the most important information you need to know about each type.[47] Understanding this language is the key to better understanding your medical team when they're discussing your cancer and the treatment protocol they select for you.

Luminal A comprises 45 to 60 percent of all breast cancers. It's slow-growing, as well as:

- Estrogen receptor positive (ER+)
- Progesterone receptor positive (PR+)

Luminal B comprises 10 to 15 percent of all breast cancers. It's faster-growing than luminal A and is:

- Estrogen receptor positive (ER+)

- Human epidermal growth factor receptor 2 positive (HER2+)
- Either progesterone receptor positive (PR+) or progesterone receptor negative (PR−)

HER2 includes 10 percent of breast cancers. It's:

- Estrogen receptor negative (ER−)
- Progesterone receptor negative (PR−)
- Human epidermal growth factor receptor 2 positive (HER2+)

Triple negative, also known as "basal-like," makes up 10 to 15 percent of all breast cancers. It's fast-growing and called triple negative because all its biomarkers are negatives.

- Estrogen receptor negative (ER−)
- Progesterone receptor negative (PR−)
- Human epidermal growth factor receptor 2 negative (HER2−)

While triple negative has traditionally been considered to have the worst prognosis since it's fast-growing and no drugs are available to treat it, researchers recently discovered that this type of cancer, too, has a genetic "on-off" switch–a regulator called miR-708.[48] So drugs that make use of this pathway may not be far off. Triple negative breast cancer also is more responsive to chemotherapy than hormone-sensitive cancers, and if women with this type of cancer make it past the 5-year mark, they're not likely to experience a recurrence.

Making Choices

Vicki Gingrich knows the importance of making thoughtful choices. At age 37, Vicki was diagnosed with stage III, ER-/PR+, six positive node invasive ductal carcinoma. "When it comes to cancer, every patient needs to consider the ramifications of saying 'yes' or 'no' too quickly," says this 23-year survivor.

A friend who was diagnosed at 37 prompted Vicki to have a lump in her breast checked. "While our kids went trick-or-treating, we talked about her experience." The next day, Vicki called her doctor.

A mammogram and biopsy revealed a tumor the size of a Ping-Pong ball and six positive lymph nodes. "Driving home, I went nuts," she recalls. "But before I got there, I pulled myself together. My sons were only 8 and 10 years old. I was scared, but I had to be there for them."

After her mastectomy, Vicki entered a clinical trial. For 6 months, she received intravenous Adriamycin and 5FU on Day 1 and Day 8 and, simultaneously, 2 weeks of oral Cytoxan. Two weeks without drugs followed. She also received tamoxifen and Zoladex for 5 years. Eventually, the Zoladex caused a premature prolapse of her uterus and led to a total hysterectomy, ending her participation in the trial. So she and her doctor chose a 10-year regimen of tamoxifen instead of the usual 5.

During this time, Vicki coauthored the book *Show Me: A Photo Collection of Breast Cancer Survivors' Lumpectomies, Mastectomies, Breast Reconstructions and Thoughts on Body Image*. "Finally," says Vicki, "a woman could actually see results of real women who made choices that best suited their lives."

She'd like women who've been diagnosed to know . . . *be your own advocate, ask questions, seek help and support!*

Breast cancer is . . . *so much more than just a kind of cancer. It's scary, hopeful, and life-changing in the same breath.*

Tomorrow will . . . *wait . . . live and enjoy today!*

PART THREE

FINDING *the* RIGHT TREATMENT

Now it's time to consider which treatments to pursue. Treatments for breast cancer have traditionally included lumpectomy or mastectomy, lymph node removal, radiation, and chemotherapy. But standards for treatment are moving in an increasingly personalized direction, and much depends on your diagnosis and prognosis. Consider your values, preferences, and lifestyle when pondering your options, along with the information presented in this chapter and the advice of your medical team, and take the time you need to be comfortable with your decisions.

"I am not afraid of storms,
for I am learning
how to sail my ship."

—LOUISA MAY ALCOTT

CHAPTER 6

SURGERY AND RADIATION

By now, you've probably received your treatment plan from your doctor. You may have even begun treatment. Wherever you are in your healing journey, this chapter will guide you through surgery and radiation and give you everything you need to know so you understand what's happening to your body and why.

First, it's important to understand that breast cancer treatment falls into two general categories: The first is local (also called locoregional) and the second is systemic (also known as adjuvant therapy). Local treatment involves surgery with or without radiation. Systemic therapy addresses the whole body. In the next chapter, you'll get information about systemic treatments, which include chemotherapy, immunotherapy, and hormone therapy.

Clinical staging takes into account your medical history, physical examination, and testing you have had. It is what your surgeon uses to help advise treatment courses. Your clinical stage differs from your true pathologic stage, which is usually determined after surgery is complete and your doctor knows the tumor size and status of your lymph nodes.

Local treatment decisions depend on a number of factors including your tumor stage, but they hinge on the often-difficult choice between lumpectomy and mastectomy, as well as lymph node biopsy or removal. In the following sections, you'll find descriptions of surgical options as well as recommendations and outcomes. If you don't know your tumor characteristics and staging, check your pathology report (see page 86 for tips on how to read it).

CHOOSING A SURGERY

The type of surgery you undergo–lumpectomy or mastectomy–depends on the type of tumor you have, how big it is, and where it has spread.

Lumpectomy

Also known as breast-conserving surgery, only the tumor and a small rim (or area) around it are removed with a lumpectomy. Your surgeon may also call it a partial or segmental mastectomy, wide excision, wedge resection, or even quadrantectomy (a word that technically means one-quarter of the breast is removed, though some surgeons use it interchangeably with lumpectomy).

Whatever the term, techniques from plastic surgery now commonly help make the end result aesthetically pleasing, so your breast looks as close as possible to how it did before surgery. During this surgery, it's typical that the general shape of the breast as well as the nipple are kept. Because some tissue is removed, you'll have a scar and your breast may be smaller and firmer. You may also experience some numbness. Be sure to talk with your doctor about how much breast tissue she will be removing and what your breast will look like after the surgery (ask your doctor to show you pictures of what your breast might look like afterward). If you don't feel comfortable with your doctor's response, it's not too late to get a second opinion or even find another doctor.[1] Some surgeons are more experienced in breast conservation techniques than are others.

When it's recommended: Lumpectomy may be a good choice if your tumor is small or you have stage I or II breast cancer. It has proved to be most effective when followed by radiation, as it reduces the risk cancer will return in the treated breast, but radiation has its own risks. Generally, radiation therapy is part of breast conservation therapy, but you should discuss with your doctor whether you may be a candidate for skipping radiation.[2] Women with stage I breast cancers that have the following factors are considered potential candidates, but age is also a huge

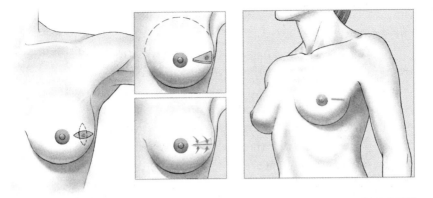

During a lumpectomy, only the tumor and some surrounding tissue are removed, leaving a small surgical scar but preserving the breast.

factor (the younger you are at diagnosis, the more likely the radiation is necessary to protect you from the risk of recurrence).

- **Your tumor is less than 2 centimeters across** and has been removed with "clear" margins (see "What Are Tissue Margins?" on page 102).

- **Your tumor is hormone (estrogen or progesterone) receptor positive,** and you're taking a hormone-blocking medication such as tamoxifen.

- **No cancer cells were found in your sentinel lymph nodes.**

But discuss this with your doctor and your health-care team to determine what will give you the best outcome.

What to expect: If your tumor can't be felt, you'll need another mammogram or ultrasound at the hospital on the day of surgery. When a tumor is not felt, it needs to be localized with a wire prior to surgery. This is called a needle localization, and it helps your surgeon find the area that needs to be removed as part of the lumpectomy. Newer techniques such as radioactive seed localization also assist your surgeon to find the specific area to be removed. You'll either have local anesthetic to numb just the surgery area, intravenous sedation, or general anesthesia. Be sure to talk to your doctor about your options prior to surgery.

Most surgeons use a scalpel to make an incision in the skin of the breast and an electrocautery knife, which uses thermal energy to minimize bleeding while removing the tumor tissue from the breast. Most of these incisions are curved, like a smile or frown, to follow the natural curve of the breast.

A separate incision is made in the area of the armpit called the axilla for your surgeon to remove the sentinel nodes (see "Sentinel Node Biopsy" on page 106). If an axillary node dissection is perfomed–which means removal of multiple lymph nodes in the axilla–a rubber tube called a drain is inserted into your armpit to collect excess fluid that can accumulate in the space where the lymph nodes were. The drain is connected to a plastic bulb that creates suction to help remove fluid. Finally, your surgeon will stitch the incision closed and dress the wound. The entire surgery usually takes anywhere from 15 to 40 minutes. You typically don't need to stay in the hospital overnight, though sometimes you do if you're having your lymph nodes removed.

If you had a drain inserted, it usually stays in place for 1 to 2 weeks after the surgery. If you are going home with the drain, be sure to get instructions from your doctor or a nurse about how to care for it. The detachable drain bulb (which is where the fluid collects) needs to be drained several times a day, and the amount of fluid drained needs to be recorded. Make sure to bring your drain log booklet to your follow-up appointment. The log will help your doctor or nurse know when the drain is ready to be removed.

Recurrence after lumpectomy: If your lymph nodes test positive for cancer cells (see "Sentinel Node Biopsy" on page 106), the chance of a local recurrence–that is, cancer in the same breast–is 11 percent within 5 years. If the lymph nodes are negative, the risk is reduced to about 7 percent within 5 years.[3] The addition of radiation can help, too: Only about 6 percent of women will experience a recurrence of cancer in the same breast with a combination of lumpectomy and radiation.[4] Without radiation, women have a 15 to 35 percent chance cancer will recur in the same breast.[5] Systemic therapies such as chemotherapy, addressed in the next chapter, can lower your chances of recurrence further.

Mastectomy

This procedure removes the tissue of the entire breast, dramatically reducing the risk of cancer recurrence in that breast; however, this does not affect the possibility of cancer occurring in the opposite breast (or

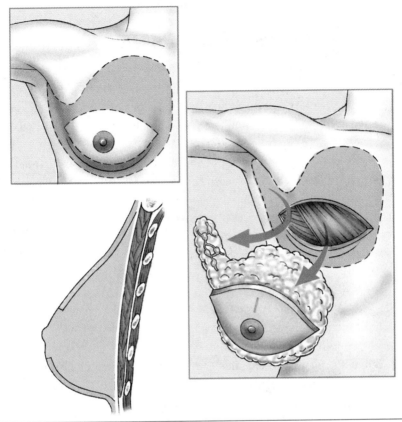

A modified radical mastectomy removes the tissue of the entire breast and axillary lymph nodes, indicated by the shaded area. Modern procedures leave most of the breast skin intact, which is essential to reconstructing a natural-looking breast.

elsewhere in the body). In a *total (or simple) mastectomy*, all of the breast tissue–which lies between the collarbone and ribs, from the side of the body to the breastbone in the center–is removed. In a *modified radical mastectomy*, in addition to removing the breast, an axillary node dissection is also performed, which involves removing multiple lymph nodes. A simple mastectomy can be converted to a modified radical mastectomy if the sentinel lymph nodes are positive and your surgeon proceeds with removing multiple lymph nodes in the axilla (armpit). A *radical mastectomy*, in which the breast, muscles in the chest wall, and numerous lymph nodes are removed, was once common but is no longer necessary in most cases.[6]

what are tissue margins?

When a surgeon excises a tumor—not just a breast cancer tumor—a pathologist will check the edges, or margins, of the tissue for cancer cells. If none are found, the excision is considered to have clean or negative margins, which is a good indication the surgery was successful in removing the cancer.

If, however, the edges are positive, it means cancer cells lined the edge of the excised tissue. In this case, a second surgery (called a re-excision) or even mastectomy may be necessary, since the most important goal of surgery is to remove all existing cancer tissue.

Once the pathologist examines the margins, the information will appear on your pathology report. Be sure to ask your doctor whether your tumor had positive or negative margins, then discuss with her your next steps.

When it's recommended: Mastectomy is usually chosen over lumpectomy as a treatment choice if:

- **Your tumor is larger than 5 centimeters** (2 inches) across.

- **Your tumor is large relative to your breast** or you have multiple tumors in different areas of the breast.

- **Your mammogram showed broadly scattered microcalcifications** (calcium deposits that are associated with DCIS).[7]

What to expect: At the hospital, your surgeon (or a nurse) may mark with a felt-tip pen exactly where the incisions will be made. This procedure is usually done if you're having immediate reconstruction and is performed while you're sitting up, allowing your doctor to see where the natural curves of your breast are. Since you'll be given general anesthesia for this procedure, you'll have a needle with a long intravenous tube connected into your arm and taped into place.

During surgery, your doctor will make an incision (usually in the shape of an oval around the nipple and running across the width of the breast). If you're having a *skin-saving mastectomy*, your surgeon will make a smaller incision, usually around the areola area of the nipple. He will then separate the breast tissue from the overlying skin and from the chest wall muscle underneath and remove all of the breast tissue (including the cancerous tissue) through that incision, leaving most of the breast skin intact. This is important if you're planning on having reconstructive surgery, because the implant goes under the muscle and skin, creating a natural-looking breast. Otherwise, if you're not having a skin-saving mastectomy with reconstruction, your doctor will remove the excess tissue and the skin.

Once the tissue is removed, the doctor closes the incision with stitches that dissolve over time so they don't need to be removed. (In some cases, surgical staples are used; these do need to be removed, usually on the first follow-up visit after surgery.) This procedure takes anywhere from 2 to 3 hours. If you're having immediate reconstructive surgery, it will take place following tissue removal.

After the tissue is removed, surgical drains that collect excess fluid will be inserted. You will have a surgical bra placed after surgery that has a fastener for the drain tubes. Generally, you will keep using this bra until the drains are removed. You'll usually stay at the hospital for 1 or 2 nights.

Keep in mind that if you haven't had reconstructive surgery, you won't be able to wear a prosthesis or be fitted for the bra that holds the prosthesis just yet. Your body needs to heal for a while before that can happen, but each person is different, so talk to your doctor about timing. There are boutiques, often associated with your medical center, that can help fit you for a prosthesis.

Also, some women experience something called phantom pain, which could be a feeling of pressure, itching, or physical pain even though the breast is no longer there. This same feeling is experienced by people who've had a limb amputated. The brain continues to send signals to nerves in the breast area that were cut during surgery, even though the breast is no longer there. Typically, acetaminophen or ibuprofen can address this pain.

Reconstructive surgery: Breast reconstructive surgery that takes place immediately after a mastectomy is called *immediate reconstruction*. *Delayed reconstruction* is the term used if you want reconstructive surgery to be done months or even years later.

If you are having reconstructive surgery right away, you'll have what's called a tissue expander put in place under the skin and muscles of the chest wall. This is essentially a balloon device with a tiny bit of saline in it. Three to 4 weeks postsurgery, you'll go in for weekly office visits with your surgeon to have a small amount of saline added through a small needle inserted in the skin. This allows the skin and chest muscle to gently stretch to accommodate the implant. And then, once the expander is the desired size, you'll wait 4 to 6 weeks before the next stage of surgery. (If you're having chemotherapy, though, you'll need to wait until chemotherapy is completed to start this second stage of surgery. If you're having radiation, discuss with your doctor whether you should be getting reconstruction now or delay it.) During the second surgery, you'll go under general anesthesia again, and the tissue expander will be removed and replaced with implants of the same size. (These implants are usually made of silicone gel or saline.) You won't need to stay in the hospital overnight for this surgery. It's important to note that, while reconstructive surgery restores the shape of the breast, sensation to the breast doesn't always return.

The entire process—from mastectomy to reconstructive surgery—takes anywhere from 3 to 6 months.

The question of whether to have breast reconstructive surgery is an important one for many women. Some women find that reconstruction allows them to move on from a mastectomy more easily; others are content with prosthetics. The choice to have the procedure or not is entirely personal. If you're considering it, you should know that insurance companies that cover breast cancer treatment are required by federal laws to also cover breast reconstructive surgery or prostheses following mastectomy. But many women aren't aware it's an option. In one recent study, 70 percent of women weren't informed by their health-care team that reconstruction was available.[8] So be sure to talk to your insurance company before surgery about exactly what's covered—and what's not.

Keep in mind that it's not necessary to schedule reconstructive surgery at the same time as your mastectomy. Indeed, it may be wiser to wait. Some studies have found that reconstruction may have fewer complications if it isn't performed along with a mastectomy.[9] While the reconstructed breast and nipple (if you're able to save it) will have no sensation, you may feel better knowing that implants are now much safer than they were a decade or two ago, and studies have shown implants will not increase your chance of a breast cancer recurrence after a mastectomy.[10]

what's a tissue flap procedure?

Tissue flap surgery (also called autologous tissue reconstruction) is a way to rebuild the breast after a mastectomy that uses skin, fat, and muscle from another part of your body. It's performed by a plastic surgeon. The two most common types of tissue flap procedures are the *TRAM flap* (or *transverse rectus abdominis muscle flap*), which uses tissue from the lower tummy area (and results in a "tummy tuck"), and the *latissimus dorsi flap*, which uses tissue from the upper back.

There are upsides and downsides to this type of surgery. The advantages include using your own tissue, which behaves like your own tissue (for example, as you gain or lose weight, your breasts will enlarge or shrink accordingly). There's also no need to worry about replacement of implants or potential rupture. Also, many women opt for this type of reconstructive surgery because they're not putting anything "foreign" (such as silicone or saline implants) into their body.

On the downside: The operations will leave two scars—one where the tissue was taken and one on the reconstructed breast. While the scars fade over time, they never go away completely. Also, the breasts may not be completely even (in size and shape) on both sides. And because healthy blood vessels are needed for the tissue's blood supply, this type of reconstructive procedure is usually not an option for women with diabetes, those with connective tissue or vascular disease, or smokers. Last, recovery from this type of procedure is longer than with implant-type reconstructions.

If you decide—along with your doctor—that this might be a good option for you, be sure to ask to see pictures of how it will look (best- and worst-case scenarios), so you can make the best, most informed decision about what's right for you.

Also, it's important to know your options for nipple reconstruction and discuss them with your plastic surgeon. For example, you might want to consider 3-D nipple tattooing, which re-creates an almost real-looking nipple and is typically covered by insurance. (For more information, watch this video about the procedure: tinyurl.com/ons3bqt.)

Mastectomy and radiation: While radiation isn't always recommended after a mastectomy, it may be considered under certain high-risk circumstances, such as if:

- **Your tumor is larger than 5 centimeters** (whether in one mass or spread in several places throughout the breast).

- **The excised breast tissue has positive margins** (that is, cancer cells are found at its edge; see "What Are Tissue Margins?" on page 102).

- **Cancer is found in four or more lymph nodes** (or sometimes fewer, if you have more risk factors).

- **Cancer has spread to the skin.**[11]

Recurrence after mastectomy: While a mastectomy significantly reduces the chance of cancer returning, it does not eliminate it completely. Women who have had a breast removed have a 5 to 10 percent chance of recurrence in the same breast. Radiation therapy can reduce this to 3 to 5 percent, but radiation also carries risks (see page 111) that may not be worth the small associated benefit.[12]

If your lymph nodes are negative for the spread of cancer, the risk of cancer recurring in the same breast within 5 years is 6 percent. If one to three lymph nodes contain cancerous cells, the risk is 16 percent, which can be lowered to just 2 percent by adding follow-up radiation therapy. If four or more lymph nodes contain cancer, the risk of recurrence is 26 percent within 5 years, while radiation reduces this risk to 6 percent.[13]

Sentinel Node Biopsy

Lymph nodes are part of the body's lymphatic system, which plays a role in eliminating waste and is an important first defense against immune intruders such as bacteria and cancerous cells. The sentinel lymph nodes, which are found at the underarm, are the first stop in cancer's spread through the body. As a result, these lymph nodes are routinely checked in lumpectomy or mastectomy procedures.

During a sentinel node biopsy, a radioactive substance or blue dye is

lumpectomy or mastectomy?

Outcomes for lumpectomy with radiation and mastectomy have been compared head-to-head in a number of trials. Survival rates for both methods are consistently nearly identical.[14] Still, the decision whether to have a lumpectomy alone, lumpectomy with radiation, or mastectomy may not be easy. Here are a few questions to consider as you evaluate options:

- **How do you approach your health?** Do you prefer to do everything you can to be healthy, or are you usually content with less aggressive or possibly risky measures?

- **Are you a worrier?** Some women would rather opt for a mastectomy, knowing they'll have less cause to worry about recurrence. Others are comfortable with some uncertainty.

- **Will losing a breast bother you?** Some women report feelings of loss and grief after a mastectomy, even when they thought they were comfortable with their decision.

- **How do you feel about reconstructive surgery?** While reconstructed breasts won't experience sensation, they can help you move on from treatment because your breasts will look similar to the way they looked before.

- **Will the daily routine of radiation be difficult for you?** Most courses of radiation last for 3 to 6 weeks and require being at a facility once a day, 5 days a week, beginning about a month after surgery. (However, many facilities are offering with shorter courses.[15])

- **Do you have risk factors for a recurrence,** such as family history or a mutation in the BRCA genes that will increase your risk for developing another breast cancer either in the same breast or the other breast.

- **Which choice are you likely to regret the least?** Some women find it helpful to consider how it would feel to live with each option, and then choose the one they're least likely to regret over time.

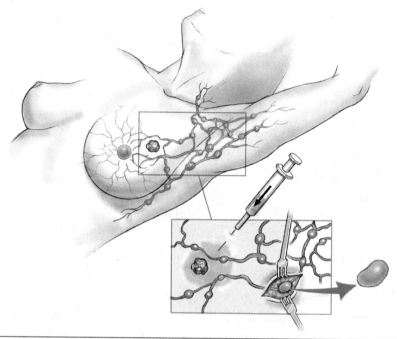

During a sentinel node biopsy, the surgeon injects a radioactive substance or blue dye to help locate the sentinel nodes (the lymph nodes closest to the tumor). The nodes can then be removed through a ½-inch-wide incision and sent to the pathology lab for analysis.

injected to help the surgeon locate the sentinel nodes during surgery. These nodes are removed through a small incision (about ½ inch) and analyzed in a lab. If they're cancer-free, then additional lymph nodes do not need to be removed.

Side effects of this biopsy can include lymphedema, or swelling of the arm; a buildup of tissue fluid at the site of the surgery; numbness, tingling, and pain at the site of the surgery; and difficulty moving the affected body part.[16]

After conducting the procedure, if the lymph nodes are negative, it's a good sign the cancer has remained confined within the breast. If they test positive, your surgeon may remove them as part of your lumpectomy or mastectomy, or in a separate procedure.[17]

In the past, if one or two lymph nodes tested positive in women with breast cancer, as many as possible were removed in what's called an

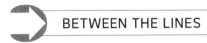

BETWEEN THE LINES

is breast cancer being overtreated?

You have breast cancer, so it needs to be treated. Right? That's the general thinking when it comes to breast cancer—or any form of cancer, for that matter. But a 2012 Harvard Medical School study published in the *Annals of Internal Medicine* estimated that 15 to 25 percent of all breast cancers are overdiagnosed. That is, they're identified and treated even though they would not have caused harm in a woman's lifetime (because they were so small and so slow-growing that they may never have turned into full-blown cancer). The study did not include ductal carcinoma in situ (DCIS), a noninvasive form of cancer regularly treated even though it's unlikely to grow inside the body. If it had, the rates of overdiagnosis would likely be even higher.[18] Meanwhile, an earlier study suggested as many as one in three breast cancers are overdiagnosed.[19]

Elements of breast cancer treatment such as chemotherapy and radiation carry a number of risks, including developing other forms of cancer and even death, not to mention the psychological cost of a diagnosis. If a cancer is unlikely to cause harm, some experts say, there's no reason to undergo such treatment. It may be that "watchful waiting," which involves careful monitoring in conjunction with your doctor, is the best approach for certain breast cancers.

Experts agree that it's important to discuss with your doctor whether watchful waiting makes sense in your case. It may not, so you have to trust your doctor. Refusing treatment because you've read about studies like this may allow your cancer to spread and reduce your chances of a good outcome and cure.

---

axillary lymph node dissection. This changed, however, after a 2011 study that showed no benefit from the removal of numerous nodes when women with only one or two positive nodes underwent lumpectomy with radiation. It's a change that has improved outcomes after surgery,[20] since the procedure can have significant side effects: The removal of more than 10 axillary lymph nodes results in a painful swelling in the arms called lymphedema in as many as 30 percent of women.[21]

Surgery: Before and After

In preparation for your surgery, whether a lumpectomy or mastectomy, you may have several consultations with your surgeon and his medical team. Some women also undergo what's called neoadjuvant therapy, which is hormone-blocking therapy or chemotherapy, prior to surgery. These treatments can shrink a tumor, permitting you to undergo a lumpectomy instead of mastectomy.

Before your procedure, you will be asked to sign a consent form, and you'll be asked about any medications or supplements you take. Nonsteroidal anti-inflammatories such as ibuprofen, blood thinners such as aspirin and warfarin, and some supplements like vitamin E can interfere with blood clotting, so you'll be asked to take a break from these for at least 5 days prior to surgery. You'll receive local or general anesthesia. Lumpectomy may take 1 to 2 hours in the operating suite, while mastectomy can last 1 to 4 hours. If breast reconstruction is performed on the same day, it will add more time to the procedure.

After surgery, you'll be monitored as you emerge from anesthesia. Then you'll be shown how to care for your incision and your drain (if one was placed) and given exercises to do to help with circulation. If lymph nodes were removed, you may be asked to begin moving your arm to reduce stiffness, numbness, and tingling. These symptoms usually fade, but it's very important to incorporate exercise into your recovery to avoid permanent stiffness or other issues near the underarm.[22]

RADIATION

Radiation therapy (or radiotherapy) helps eradicate any remaining cancer cells from your body after a lumpectomy or mastectomy. Cancer cells grow much more quickly than most cells in the body, and radiation can effectively target and kill these cells, reducing recurrence following surgery by as much as 70 percent.[23]

There are two common types of radiation therapy: external beam radiation and brachytherapy (pronounced brak-e-THER-uh-pee), or internal radiation, in which radioactive pellets are placed in the breast tissue near the location of the excised tumor. *External beam radiation*, which is most common, requires daily doses over 3 to 6 weeks. Though the treatment itself takes just a few minutes, the appointment as a whole may take about $\frac{1}{2}$ hour.[24] If the time commitment is inconvenient or difficult, ask your doctor whether a shorter course of radiation might be better suited for you. *Brachytherapy* allows your doctor to deliver higher doses of radiation to more specific areas of the body. It usually causes fewer side effects, and the overall treatment time is shorter than with external beam radiation. How long the radioactive pellets are left in the breast is determined by your doctor. (Some may never be taken out; over the course of several weeks, they stop giving off radiation.)

While radiation usually accompanies lumpectomy, it is recommended following mastectomy only when there is a high risk of recurrence (see "Mastectomy" on page 100). Radiation is not recommended when you're pregnant, if you've already had a course of radiation to the area, or if you have a condition such as lupus or scleroderma that makes you very sensitive to the effects of radiation.[25]

Also, while radiation following lumpectomy may not be recommended for women older than 70 (because some studies have suggested it does not significantly improve outcomes), experts are debating this. A study of more than 7,000 women ages 70 to 79 published in the August 2012 issue of the journal *Cancer* reported that women in this group who received radiation after a lumpectomy were two-thirds less likely to need a mastectomy within 10 years than those who did not receive radiation. The only group in the study, in fact, who didn't benefit from radiation were women ages 75 to 79 with low-grade tumors who also had lymph nodes removed in surgery. After age 80, studies suggest the risk of death from other causes is greater than that from breast cancer recurring, but if you're still in your seventies, in good health, and want to pursue this option, be sure to ask your doctor about it.[26]

Side effects and risks: Radiation treatment itself is painless, but it does have side effects, such as burning in the skin similar to a sunburn, skin sores, fatigue, lowered white blood cell counts (making you more susceptible to infection and illness), and sore throat.[27] Heart and lung problems may also develop. One 2013 study of nearly 2,000 women in Denmark and Sweden who underwent radiation between 1958 and 2001 showed a correlation between radiation dose and later coronary events, such as heart attack.[28] Other studies have suggested a relationship between radiation and lung cancer.[29] Experts point out that such risks have dropped dramatically as radiation technology has improved, and research is ongoing about ways to further reduce them.[30]

If you're having brachytherapy, your body may give off a small amount of radiation for a short period of time. You may be asked to stay at the hospital or limit visitors, particularly pregnant women and children.

Making the Right Decision—For You

The choices you'll face as you deal with a breast cancer diagnosis aren't always easy, and they may involve balancing risks and benefits. Deciding upon a surgery–whether lumpectomy or mastectomy–and whether to pursue radiation involves a number of complex considerations. The information presented in this chapter will help you make the best, most informed decisions you can, which will ultimately contribute to your peace of mind. You'll also find it helpful to consult with your doctors and talk with other women as you make decisions. Support groups are likely to be available in your area or online, and many women find they provide significant assistance and relief in the journey from diagnosis to treatment.

Each woman approaches medical decisions differently. You may feel best fully researching your options, and if so, know that the information presented here is the most up-to-date data on breast cancer treatments available and represents the consensus of experts worldwide. On the other hand, you may simply be looking for help understanding your medical team's terminology and advice and prefer to let them make major decisions. Either way, take heart in knowing that by being informed and taking an active part in your own health decisions, you're doing the best you can to maximize your recovery and outcome.

In the next chapter, we'll look at adjuvant therapies, such as chemotherapy, immunotherapy, and hormone therapy, which can further improve your chances of a healthy recovery. These medical advances represent some of the most exciting recent developments in breast cancer treatment, though they have risks and side effects of their own.

Recovering Direction

At age 35, Crystal Brown-Tatum was many things: a mother to a 13-year-old daughter, a successful owner of a bustling Houston-based public relations firm, and a bride-to-be. She was not, however, worried about the small lump she'd felt in her armpit one evening while taking a shower. "Even though my grandmother had been diagnosed with breast cancer just 5 years earlier, I didn't think to be worried, let alone to have it checked out," she said.

That was August 2006. Within 8 months, that small lump had not only grown but was beginning to hurt. Crystal's new husband encouraged her to clue in her doctors. The day she received her results–stage IIIA breast cancer–Crystal had just wrapped up a busy few days of lobbying in Washington, DC.

Crystal's initial shock turned to anger at getting cancer, for sure, but also at herself for ignoring the lump for so long. "Women of color are less likely to get breast cancer, but they're more likely to die from it," she says matter-of-factly. "I had no idea at the time; you didn't see young black women in many breast cancer brochures or articles. Still, I thought, *How could I not know this?*" Her treatment consisted of a lumpectomy, chemotherapy, and radiation.

Crystal now puts her PR skills to use as a volunteer with Sisters Network, Inc., the only national African American breast cancer survivorship organization in the United States. She also wrote and self-published a book about her experiences, appropriately titled *Saltwater Taffy and Red High Heels*. Her intended audience was black women, but she says it's been well-received by all women.

She'd like women who've been diagnosed to know . . . *this doesn't mean you're going to die tomorrow. Listen to your doctor, connect with people, and be careful of Internet searches—really save your questions for your doctor.*

Breast cancer is . . . *a way to really define who you are.*

Tomorrow will . . . *be better than today. The mistakes of today don't have to be made tomorrow—you're stronger.*

"If you think you can win, you can win.
Faith is necessary to victory."

—WILLIAM HAZLITT

CHAPTER 7

SYSTEMIC TREATMENT: CHEMOTHERAPY AND TARGETED THERAPIES

If local therapy—surgery and radiation—targets the tumor itself, systemic therapy works to rid the body of any remaining cancer. Cancer cells can travel via the lymphatic system and blood vessels to other parts of the body, and it's these cells that systemic therapy targets. Systemic therapy, also known as adjuvant therapy, reduces the chance cancer will recur in the same spot or in other places. As a result, many women undergo one of the treatments described in this chapter.

Systemic therapies include a growing range of options: chemotherapy (drugs that target and kill cancer cells, also called cytotoxic medications), hormone therapy (such as tamoxifen, raloxifene, and aromatase inhibitors), and immune therapy, such as trastuzumab (Herceptin) and newer drugs. These therapies are highly effective: When surgery and radiation are added to systemic therapies, 80 percent of all breast cancers are cured.[1] On the other hand, with surgery or surgery and radiation alone, 70 to 75 percent of women with negative lymph nodes will survive more than 10 years, while only 30 percent of women with positive lymph nodes will survive within the same period.

In this chapter, we'll explore the range of systemic therapies available to you and provide guidance and advice about therapies you should be discussing with your doctor and health-care team.

IS SYSTEMIC TREATMENT RIGHT FOR YOU?

A number of elements go into determining your course of adjuvant treatment. When deciding which therapies to pursue, you'll work with a medical oncologist, who handles this part of treatment after your surgeon and radiation therapist have taken care of local therapy. These doctors may, or may not, act as a team, but there should be some coordination between them. While all systemic therapy has the goal of eliminating cancer from the body and preventing a recurrence, many specialists have different approaches to cancer treatment, which is not yet an exact science.[2] If you're not comfortable with the suggestions of your oncologist or radiologist as you're evaluating options, seek a second opinion.

Below you'll find the primary factors doctors use to determine which systemic therapy will be most helpful for your particular cancer type and stage. These are divided between prognostic and predictive factors. Prognostic factors affect the overall current outlook for your cancer while predictive factors consider how it will respond to treatment.[3]

Age and menopausal status. If you're under 35, breast cancer can be more aggressive. Whether or not you've entered menopause will also affect treatment, determining the type of drugs available to you and their side effects. For example, aromatase inhibitors can be used only in postmenopausal women, while premenopausal women may be asked to consider removal of their ovaries, called oophorectomy, or medical treatment to suppress ovarian function, called ovarian ablation.

Lymph node status. If your axillary nodes test positive for cancer, it's a sign systemic therapy is definitely warranted, since it indicates a likelihood cancer cells may have traveled to other places in the body.

Tumor size and grade. Tumors larger than 5 centimeters will need more aggressive treatment since they are more likely to recur. The grade of a tumor depends on the cancer's degree of advancement and can range from 1 to 3. Low-grade cancer cells, at grade 1, look fairly similar to normal breast cells and are slow-growing; grade 2 cancer cells are moderately differentiated (somewhat abnormal); grade 3 cancer cells are poorly differentiated (very abnormal), fast-growing, and least resemble normal breast cells. High-grade cancers have a worse prognosis and are more likely to recur after treatment, but they're also more responsive to chemotherapy. Plus, if high-grade cancers don't recur within 5 years, they're unlikely to recur down the road.

Cell proliferation. The rate at which tumor cells divide is a measure of the cancer's aggressiveness; a higher rate means you'll want to consider additional therapy.

HER2 status. One recent breakthrough in breast cancer research is the discovery of human epidermal growth factor receptor 2, or HER2, which is a cell-growth-regulating gene that has mutated to become an oncogene, a protein that transforms ordinary cells into cancer cells. Cancers that are positive for HER2 are more aggressive and have a worse prognosis than HER2-negative cancers, but an effective immunotherapy drug, trastuzumab, is available to treat HER2-positive cancer.

Hormone receptor status. Some cancers respond to the hormones estrogen and progesterone. The presence of these hormones in the body makes cancer grow more aggressively. Hormone-blocking drugs deprive cancer cells of these hormones, helping to shrink tumors and prevent recurrence.

WHAT COMES FIRST: RADIATION OR SYSTEMIC THERAPY?

The timing of various therapies depends on your individual condition and diagnosis, but generally, chemotherapy comes before radiation. If you and your doctors have elected not to use chemotherapy, you'll start radiation within a few weeks—generally 4 to 6—of your surgery. (Partial-breast radiation, in which only the section of the breast with the tumor receives radiation, starts just after surgery; while intraoperative radiation is given just after the tumor has been removed, while you're still under anesthesia.) If you've elected to undergo chemotherapy, it begins 4 to 8 weeks after surgery and then, after a break of 2 to 4 weeks depending on the chemotherapy medication you used, is usually followed by radiation. Targeted and hormonal therapies then follow radiation.[4]

While this order is common, it's also possible to have some combination of chemotherapy, radiation, and hormonal or targeted therapies *before* surgery. In this case, it's called neoadjuvant therapy (adjuvant therapy involves much of the same drugs and treatment, but *follows* surgery). Chemotherapy and radiation are most common before surgery, but hormonal and targeted therapies are increasingly being tested, particularly in clinical trials.[5] A number of studies have shown there is no difference in outcomes if radiation and chemotherapy are performed before or after surgery, whether in overall mortality, recurrence, or progression of the cancer.[6]

Where neoadjuvant therapy can help, however, is in shrinking a tumor before surgery, which allows some women to have a lumpectomy rather than a mastectomy. One 2007 meta-analysis (a study that combines and examines the results of multiple trials) looked at the outcomes of 5,500 women with stage I, II, or III cancer: Twenty-six percent were able to have a less-invasive surgery than they'd anticipated after undergoing neoadjuvant therapy.[7]

Neoadjuvant therapy has other benefits, too. A significant benefit is that since it's easy to see whether the tumor has shrunk in response to a specific treatment, doctors can know quickly whether a particular treatment is effective for your cancer. In fact, this method is so effective in comparison to traditional methods (which require removing the tumor and then waiting to see if the cancer returns over a period of years) that the FDA is considering allowing some cancer drugs to be tested via neoadjuvant therapy in small trials.[8] If they're effective, they could be fast-tracked to the market and then followed in a larger trial over a longer period of time. Here, the benefit is again immediacy, since researchers can see whether a drug is effective in a small group of a few hundred women before they undergo surgery, whereas standard trials of new drugs require 10 to 15 years of follow-up in several thousand women. It's a promising method for testing cancer drugs, since it could considerably reduce the time and expense required to find out whether a drug is effective while, researchers hope, providing a benefit to women who have access to newer treatment methods.

At the end of the day, a combination of therapies may work best. Recent small studies suggest combining radiation and chemo—whether before surgery, as neoadjuvant therapy, or after, as simultaneous treatments, switching back and forth between the two—may in fact be more effective than spreading out the therapies sequentially.[9] An advantage of combining these therapies is that it will take 4 to 6 weeks less time than standard therapy, which generally takes about 4 to 7 months for both treatments performed sequentially. Check with your doctor to determine whether such modified treatments might be options for you.

SYSTEMIC THERAPIES

Whether or not you're a candidate for systemic therapies depends on a number of factors—from your prognosis to the type of tumor you have. Some women may undergo radiation therapy and then move straight to hormone therapy without chemotherapy. Others do better with a combination of chemotherapy and radiation, or both of these combined with hormone or other targeted therapy. Some combinations of therapies have been shown to be more effective with certain types of cancers, so your medical team will tailor your treatment to your specific tumor's molecular analysis and other characteristics.

Weighing Treatments: Questions to Ask

When you're making a decision about which treatment avenue to pursue, consider the advice of your doctors along with these questions.

What's the goal of the therapy? Is it to eliminate the cancer, for example, or simply to extend life? Ask your medical team what the chances are that the therapy will accomplish this goal for women with your specific cancer (grade, stage, and molecular subtype).

What evidence is available that shows the therapy causes the cancer to shrink or stop growing? How long does this effect—often called response duration—last?

Has the therapy been shown to prolong life? If the goal of treatment is to do so, what do studies show is the average gained survival time?

What are your chances of a cure with, or without, the adjuvant therapies being recommended to you?

What are the benefits of the adjuvant therapies you're choosing between? What are the risks, such as side effects or long-term complications? Weighing risks and benefits will help you decide whether a treatment is worth it to you.

How will the therapy affect your overall quality of life? Will it improve it? The answers to these questions will depend on side effects and other psychological, physical, and social factors. They're worth asking when weighing any proposed therapy.[10]

CHEMOTHERAPY

Chemotherapy (a shortening of the words *chemical therapy*) simply refers to a collection of drugs that are toxic to cancer cells. It's recommended for women with advanced stage (III or IV) cancer or for women whose tumors are not hormone-responsive and thus not treatable with hormone therapy. It's also often recommended for women whose lymph nodes test positive for cancer cells or whose tumor was large,[11] and may be used prior to surgery to shrink a tumor.

Chemotherapy drugs work by killing off or interfering with the replication of rapidly dividing cancer cells. These drugs often increase survival or reduce chances of recurrence, though by how much is up for debate.

A prominent American expert on breast cancer, Susan Love, MD, estimates that chemotherapy reduces the risk of breast cancer recurring by one-third,[12] while other experts put that figure higher[13] or lower.[14] To calculate whether chemotherapy will be beneficial to you according to Love's estimate, take your chances of recurrence and divide by three, then subtract the result from your total chance. For example, if your chance of recurrence is 60 percent, after chemo, your chances of recurrence will drop to 40 percent. If you're at all unsure about the benefits of chemo, ask your oncologist or another doctor to go to adjuvantonline.com.[15] This Web site—meant for use by health professionals—asks for a battery of complex health information and is useful for thinking through general risk issues. Because the side effects of chemotherapy can be significant (see page 120), it's worth putting time into understanding just how much it will benefit you—and whether or not it will be worth it. There's also a test, Oncotype DX, that may be able to predict your expected benefit from chemotherapy. (See "Genetic Profiling: The Promise of Individualized Medicine" on page 122.)

At the end of the day, chemotherapy's benefits may well be preferable

should you join a clinical trial?

Interested in contributing to science, as well as seeking new treatments for breast cancer? You might consider participating in a clinical trial.

Clinical trials can provide access to experimental cancer drugs not yet on the market. The costs of any medical care are often covered by the study, so this may mean carefully planned, standardized care at a larger health center than you're able to access in your community (though you must be able to travel to the research center).

Medical research uses two primary types of studies to find new therapies: observation and intervention. In an observational trial, participants are followed over a period of time as they go about their daily lives. Researchers might track diet, exercise, medications, or other habits to find out more about a particular condition. In an interventional trial, which tests a new drug or treatment, about half of participants will be given the new treatment being tested–called the intervention arm–while the other half receive a placebo or some form of standardized care, called the control arm. A placebo is an inactive (inert) substance used as a control in an experiment, study, or test to determine the effectiveness of the intervention.

Clinical trials of new drugs only take place after multiple previous trials have been done, both in vitro (in test cells) and in vivo (in animals such as mice)–so they're safe, to a degree. But there are certain risks with any experimental drug, since researchers are

to you, but taking the time to think about the trade-offs will help you make an empowered, informed decision.

Chemotherapy Side Effects

Chemotherapy's storied history is in part a result of its side effects. Because it targets all rapidly dividing cells in the body, it can affect the hair, mucous membranes (mouth, throat, and digestive system), and conducting a trial because they still don't know enough about how it affects people or if it is better than standard treatments. Still, strong ethical and institutional safeguards govern how trials are conducted. If a drug is discovered to cause harm or not have any effect, a trial is stopped. With an interventional trial, you might be in the control rather than intervention arm, so you'd receive a placebo or standard treatment if the trial is for a medication. For women who've unsuccessfully tried many treatments, or for those interested in novel therapies, however, a clinical trial might be appealing.

HOW TO FIND A CLINICAL TRIAL

The National Institutes of Health lists all current medical studies at clinicaltrials.gov. You can search the trials by location and condition; each trial listing includes contact information, recruitment status, and eligibility criteria. The Web site BreastCancerTrials.org offers a matching service for breast cancer trials that are currently recruiting. Fill out a short profile with your condition and what you're looking for, and the site will report on which of the hundreds of trials might fit your specific needs. You can also set up an alert to be notified about new trials. The Dr. Susan Love Research Foundation runs an organization called Army of Women that connects women interested in participating in trials to new options. Its goal is to recruit a million women for breast cancer research, and women with and without breast cancer can participate. Find out more at armyofwomen.org.

blood-producing cells. These can cause hair loss, nausea, vomiting, diarrhea, anemia, mouth sores and infections, and low blood cell counts. Different chemotherapies can have different side effect profiles. Not everyone experiences these side effects, and many of them can be relieved, for example, with immune system–stimulating drugs or antinausea remedies.[16] All these symptoms subside, however, once therapy is complete.

Chemotherapy can also cause fatigue and an irritation of the hands and feet called hand-foot syndrome, as well as induce premature menopause or infertility in women who have not yet stopped menstruating. Though changes in fertility are sometimes reversible, the older you are, the more likely they are to be permanent. Paradoxically, it is still possible to become pregnant while on a chemotherapy regimen, and some drugs could cause birth defects in the fetus. To be safe, make sure you're on a very reliable method of birth control for the duration of treatment (although sex may be the last thing on your mind right now). If you'd like to try to preserve fertility, let your medical team

genetic profiling: the promise of individualized medicine

Doctors have long hoped for ways to know before administering a treatment whether it would work on a particular individual. For breast cancer and chemotherapy, that day may have arrived. Oncotype DX (oncotypedx.com), MammaPrint (mammaprint.co.uk), and Mammostrat (tinyurl.com/cwwn7ma) are three new tests that analyze the genetic profile of a tumor and use the information there to predict whether cancer will recur or metastasize (spread to other areas of the body). Tumors with a higher risk for recurrence or metastasizing are more likely to respond to chemotherapy, so these tests can help women decide whether to undergo or avoid chemotherapy, along with its side effects, without concerns that this decision will significantly affect their health.

Oncotype DX, the first of these tests, was introduced in 2004[17] and has been rapidly adopted by doctors and patients. It's available for women with ductal carcinoma in situ (DCIS) or stage I or II estrogen receptor positive (ER+) tumors who plan to get hormone therapy. It's currently recommended for women whose lymph nodes test negative for cancer cells. It may also be helpful for women with lymph node positive cancer (if you fit into this group, ask your doctor about the test), and it's being studied in other types of breast cancers.[18]

know very early on in your therapy. There are treatment regimens that may make it more likely, such as avoiding chemotherapy in favor of estrogen-blocking drugs.[19]

Longer-term or more serious risks of chemotherapy include neuropathy (nerve and, rarely, spinal cord damage), damage to the heart (called cardiomyopathy), increased risk of damage to the bone marrow or leukemia within 10 years of treatment, and problems with concentration and memory called chemo brain, which typically last for a few years (these problems may also occur with radiation).[20] Risks for these conditions vary considerably.[21]

The test assigns a low, intermediate, or high recurrence score to your cancer and has consistently strong results predicting who will be helped by chemotherapy. Its recurrence score has been shown to be more accurate in predicting recurrence than even pathologic staging,[22] which refers to an analysis of your tumor by size, grade, and lymph node status (see "How to Read Your Pathology Report" in Chapter 5).

MammaPrint[23] also shows significant predictive power. It can be used for cancers that are estrogen positive or negative, unlike Oncotype DX. In a recent small study of 427 breast cancer patients, 219 were classified as low risk by the test, and of these, 97 percent were cancer-free 5 years later. For the 208 participants classified as high risk, 91.7 percent were cancer-free after 5 years.[24] Mammostrat, another test that uses a slightly different method to calculate risk, can be used for women with ER+ tumors only and was introduced in 2010.[25]

Meanwhile, studies show a genetic test newly available in Europe,[26] known as PAM50, is highly accurate in predicting the return of breast cancer in the body within 5 to 10 years.[27] If it moves into general use, look for more news about PAM50 in the United States in the next few years.

Drugs and Scheduling

Chemotherapy drugs are administered intravenously or with a pill that you take once a day. You may be treated with a single drug or with a combination. Most experts agree that combination regimens are more effective but carry higher risks of side effects. Ask your doctor to carefully explain the side effects of each drug so that you're aware of the risks and benefits of each. For example, doxorubicin (once the brand name Adriamycin[28]) is associated with heart damage,[29] while cyclophosphamide (Cytoxan[30]) is more likely to lead to infertility. Since some of these side effects can be long term, it's important to get clear answers from your medical team regarding the drugs you're using.

Standard combinations of chemotherapy drugs include cyclophosphamide, methotrexate (Trexall), and 5-fluorouracil (also called fluorouracil, or 5-FU)–together commonly referred to as CMF; doxorubicin and cyclophosphamide–or AC; and doxorubicin and paclitaxel (Taxol) or

PERSONAL PRACTICE

sorting out the science

It's easy to become confused by all the science surrounding breast cancer, particularly when it comes to systemic therapies. Knowing what type of breast cancer you have (for example, whether you have ER+ or ER- or PR+ or PR-; see Chapter 5) will help you to figure out which treatments may be best for you.

But this is also why you have chosen the health-care team you did. While you're reading this chapter, highlight sections of interest to you. Jot down, in your journal, notes about treatments that seem intriguing to you so you can discuss them with your doctor. Remember that the science regarding breast cancer treatments is constantly changing as new medical advances are made. By discussing what's important to you with your doctor, you may be able to help steer your course of therapy, which will give you a greater sense of control over your life at this challenging time.

docetaxel (Taxotere)–or AT.[31] (The *A* in the last two abbreviations stands for Adriamycin, the former brand name for the now-generic doxorubicin.) Drugs with different functions or mechanisms of action are combined to increase the efficacy of treatment.

Chemotherapy is generally administered in cycles of several weeks, depending on the drug or drug combinations. You'll start on the first day of each cycle, then continue treatment–by IV or pill, both of which are painless aside from inserting the IV–daily or weekly, generally for 2 to 3 weeks. Each cycle is followed by a rest period to allow the immune system to recover, then begins again. Cycles continue for a total of 4 to 6 months. You may be given a "dose-dense" schedule, which simply speeds up the cycles by shortening the intervals between treatments. Studies suggest this method increases survival rates and reduces the chance of recurrence.[32]

TARGETED THERAPY

Advances over the past several decades in breast cancer treatment now mean that sophisticated drugs are available to target cancer cells at their core. Such targeted therapies interact with–and incapacitate–cancer cells at the level of proteins, enzymes, molecules, and hormone receptors. Research is ongoing into this effective form of treatment, but for the moment, there are two primary types in common use for breast cancer: hormone therapy and immune therapy.

Hormone Therapy

Endocrine therapy, or hormonal treatment, for breast cancer focuses on depriving cancer cells of estrogen and progesterone, which stimulate growth. There are two ways to do this. The first is to suppress the production of hormones in the ovaries, and the second is to block receptors for these hormones on the surface of cancer cells.

Breast cancer provided the first breakthrough in targeted therapies for cancer in 1958,[33] when receptors for estrogen were discovered on the surface of cells. When tumor cells contain these receptors–which about 70 percent do[34]–they're called estrogen-sensitive, or estrogen receptor positive (ER+); if they don't, they're called estrogen receptor negative (ER-). Tumor cells that have receptors for progesterone are called progesterone-sensitive, or progesterone receptor positive (PR+); if they don't have progesterone receptors, they're called progesterone receptor negative (PR-). Most estrogen-sensitive cancers are also progesterone-sensitive.[35] (For more information, see "How 'Molecular Analysis' Is Changing Breast Cancer Treatment–For the Better" in Chapter 5.)

Specific drugs have been developed to prevent estrogen from reaching tumors at the cellular level. Selective estrogen-receptor modulators (SERMs) interfere with receptors, which act like gates to the cell, blocking estrogen's entrance. Aromatase inhibitors act via a different mechanism, preventing the enzyme aromatase from converting hormones into estrogen. Another medication, fulvestrant (Faslodex), works by a different mechanism, destroying the estrogen receptor on tumor cells altogether.

Hormone-blocking drugs are generally taken for a total of 5 years and can be exchanged for one another if tolerance is a problem.

Here's a look at the various kinds of hormone-therapy treatments.

SERMS

SERMs block the effects of estrogen in the breast tissue by literally "sitting" in the estrogen receptors in breast cells. If a SERM is in the estrogen receptor, there's no room for estrogen, and it can't attach to the cell. If estrogen isn't attached to a breast cell, the cell doesn't receive estrogen's signals to grow and multiply, thereby cutting off a cancer's ability to grow and thrive. There are three SERMs: tamoxifen (Nolvadex), raloxifene (Evista), and toremifene (Fareston).

Tamoxifen can be used to shrink tumors or following surgery. Studies of tamoxifen have demonstrated that it lowers the risk of any recurring invasive breast cancer by one-third and of estrogen-responsive cancers, in particular, by 45 percent.[36] Disadvantages associated with tamoxifen include an increased chance of uterine cancer (it triples the risk), blood clots, and impaired vision and cataracts (in less than 1 percent of women).[37] It's approved for use in women 35 and older and can also help prevent postmenopausal osteoporosis. Toremifene is a drug similar to tamoxifen approved only for treating metastatic breast cancers.[38] While tamoxifen is generally recommended for 5 years, two large studies published in 2012 and 2013 suggested 10 years of therapy can reduce breast cancer recurrence and death by an additional 25 percent over its benefits at 5 years.[39]

Raloxifene is used mostly in prevention, not treatment, and has fewer

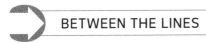

breast cancer and fertility

If you are planning to become pregnant, you may find yourself asking, "Is breast cancer going to end my chances?"

The simple answer? It's complicated. That's why it's very important to be proactive by talking to your health-care team before you begin treatments about the impact of your diagnosis and treatment plan on your fertility. You may also want to discuss whether or not you might pass on a genetic predisposition to breast cancer to future offspring.

Your age and diagnosis—the type and stage of your breast cancer—will influence your doctors' advice and recommendations concerning your fertility. Your treatment plan is especially important. While surgery and radiation don't affect fertility, chemotherapy can. Some drugs—such as cyclophosphamide (Cytoxan)—have been shown to cause premature ovarian failure, very early menopause, or other side effects.

If you learn you're unlikely to become pregnant after recovery from breast cancer, explore options for fertility preservation. Talk to your health-care team, especially your oncologist and patient navigator. Get as many opinions as possible. Speak to your gynecologist and possibly a specialist in reproductive endocrinology. Many centers coordinate these referrals. And check these resources.

Fertile Hope (fertilehope.org) is a national Livestrong Foundation initiative offering reproductive information and support to cancer patients and survivors concerned about infertility.

The Oncofertility Consortium (oncofertility.northwestern.edu) is a national, interdisciplinary initiative exploring the reproductive future of cancer survivors. It addresses the complex health-care and quality-of-life issues concerning young cancer patients whose fertility may be threatened.

Young Survival Coalition (youngsurvival.org) is a global organization dedicated to the critical issues faced by young breast cancer patients. It offers resources, connections, and outreach.

serious side effects than tamoxifen. In trials, it lowered the risk of breast cancer by about 40 percent without raising risk for uterine cancer or blood clots, though some studies have shown stronger reductions, in the range of 60 to 70 percent, for the risk of developing estrogen-sensitive breast cancer.[40] It's approved for use in postmenopausal women. Like tamoxifen, it can prevent postmenopausal osteoporosis. Side effects include fatigue, hot flashes, night sweats, vaginal discharge, and mood swings. SERMs are pills you take usually once a day.[41]

Aromatase Inhibitors

This class of drugs is newer than SERMs and seems to be slightly better at preventing recurrent breast cancer after surgery, but unlike SERMs, they may increase osteoporosis because they stop the production of estrogen altogether.[42] There are three types of aromatase inhibitors: anastrozole (Arimidex), letrozole (Femara), and exemestane (Aromasin). These are also used to treat late-stage breast cancer, but whether they can reduce breast cancer risk overall is still being tested. It's important to note that aromatase inhibitors can only be used by postmenopausal women since they cannot stop the ovaries from making estrogen.[43]

After initial treatment (for example, surgery and possibly chemotherapy and radiation therapy), many studies—and experts—typically make the following recommendations:

- **An aromatase inhibitor is the best hormonal therapy to start with.** When treating early-stage, hormone receptor positive breast cancer, aromatase inhibitors seem to have more benefits and fewer side effects than tamoxifen.

- **Switching to an aromatase inhibitor after taking tamoxifen for 2 to 3 years** (for a total of 5 years of hormonal therapy) offers more benefits than 5 years of tamoxifen alone.

- **Taking an aromatase inhibitor for 5 years after taking tamoxifen for 5 years** continues to reduce the risk of the cancer coming back, compared to no treatment after tamoxifen.[44]

Aromatase inhibitors are pills you have to take typically once a day. They tend to cause fewer of the serious side effects (like blood clots, stroke, and endometrial cancer) than tamoxifen, but they can cause more heart problems, more bone loss (osteoporosis), and more broken bones

a vaccine for breast cancer?

Breast cancer research is evolving every day. Unproven but brimming with potential, vaccines are one technique on the cutting edge of cancer research. They work by harnessing the power of the immune system to fight cancer cells. Critics say immunotherapy is just too complex for a disorder like cancer; there's a lot that's possible to get wrong. For example, in early 2013, a report from the MD Anderson Cancer Center at the University of Texas in *Nature Medicine* suggested that mineral oil, a common ingredient used as a chemical base for many experimental cancer vaccines, actually interferes with the vaccination process, leading immune cells to attack the vaccination site rather than the tumor.[45] And that's just one tiny piece of a treatment with countless elements to perfect.

But advocates say the science may be just around the corner, and judging by the 10 different breast cancer vaccines currently in development at different research centers, they may be right.[46]

Some results have generated excitement. While most experimental drugs have yet to make it through initial trials, which test a drug in a small group of people, one vaccine, E75 (also called NeuVax), is currently recruiting for a Phase III trial that will test the vaccine in 700 people.[47] A Cleveland Clinic team has developed a vaccine that needs only one administration to effectively prevent breast cancer in mice and is now hoping to test it in humans.[48] And in early 2013, researchers at the University of Cincinnati announced they'd developed an oral breast cancer vaccine in mice, the first-ever report of an oral delivery method for a cancer vaccine.[49]

Meanwhile, the MD Anderson researchers who discovered that mineral oil didn't work report that replacing it with saline causes cancer vaccines to suddenly begin shrinking tumors in mice. They plan to begin a clinical trial of the modified vaccine in people in late 2013.[50] While breast cancer vaccines aren't yet ready for their debut, they may not be far away.

than tamoxifen–at least for the first few years of treatment. One of the most common side effects is joint pain or stiffness.[51]

Ovarian Suppression

Another way to prevent hormones from reaching cancer cells is to prevent the ovaries from producing them altogether. This is accomplished via what are called gonadotropin-releasing hormone (GnRH) agonists. GnRH is a hormone that plays a role in preventing hormone production. In the case of breast cancer, this means shutting down the ovaries so there's less estrogen to fuel the growth of hormone receptor positive breast cancer. (GnRH isn't just used for breast cancer, though. For example, GnRH agonists are used to treat prostate cancer in men by decreasing the amount of testosterone in the blood.)[52] There is some concern, however, that these drugs can interfere with the effects of chemotherapy.[53]

GnRH agonists include goserelin (Zoladex), leuprorelin (Lupron), and triptorelin (Trelstar). They're given in injection form, typically once a month. It's important to note that once you stop GnRH therapy, the ovaries begin functioning again, although the time it takes to recover can vary from woman to woman.[54] Side effects include those that typically accompany menopause: hot flashes, mood swings, loss of libido, osteoporosis, vaginal dryness, weight gain, and headaches.[55] Women taking Lupron may also experience bone pain.

Immune Therapy

Trastuzumab (Herceptin) revolutionized cancer research when it gained FDA approval in 1998.[56] It's a targeted therapy that attaches itself to the HER2 receptors on the surface of breast cancer cells to block them from receiving growth signals and, in the process, disabling the protein HER2. About 20 to 25 percent of cancers have this protein, which promotes abnormal cell growth and results in fast-growing cancers that are more likely to spread.[57] (Trastuzumab–pronounced *trass-two-zoo-maab*–is in the drug class known as monoclonal antibodies; the protein is also referred to as HER2/neu.) Trastuzumab also works by alerting the immune system to destroy cancer cells onto which it's attached, hence the moniker *immune therapy.*

It has been shown to reduce the recurrence of HER2-positive breast cancers by about 40 percent and is considered highly effective.[58] But as many as half of HER2-positive cancers don't respond to treatment with trastuzumab, and cumulative drug resistance is a problem among those who do respond.[59] Pertuzumab (Perjeta), another kind of targeted therapy, combined with trastuzumab may be more effective.

Trastuzumab is approved by the FDA for women with metastatic HER2-positive disease and for women with earlier stages of HER2-positive disease as adjuvant therapy (treatment after initial treatment, such as surgery) either alone or as part of a regimen with chemotherapy.

Trastuzumab is administered intravenously, which means it's dripped into your body via a needle inserted into a vein. The first dose takes about 90 minutes to administer. After that, it takes only about 30 minutes to administer the other doses, which are usually given every 3 weeks in a doctor's office. Side effects include flulike symptoms in 40 percent of those who take it: fever, chills, muscle aches, and nausea.[60]

Are All Treatments Covered by Insurance?

After reading about all the treatments–both local and systemic–available to breast cancer patients, you're probably wondering who's paying for the cost of these treatments. The answer is that most costs are covered by insurance (after deductible and co-pays), but they're also often denied. For example, in the case of Herceptin (a brand-name version of trastuzumab), insurance may deny it, but there's always an avenue for appeal. The company that makes Herceptin, Genentech, set up a hotline (866-449-4372) to help you get insurance coverage for it or, if you don't have insurance, to figure out a way to get the therapy you need.

But many if not all of the drug companies offer financial help like this, which is something many survivors don't realize. You'll find out more about which companies do this in the next chapter. You'll also get practical advice on how to navigate the complex financial issues that come up once your diagnosis is confirmed.

Riding On

In 2009, when Elizabeth MacGregor was being treated for invasive ductal carcinoma, she'd hear other cancer patients talk about fighting a battle or surviving a war. "That imagery just didn't work for me–I felt like I was the *battlefield,* not a soldier," says the 50-year-old attorney.

So she reached into her athletic past and opted to think of her cancer experience as a relay race, where she and other cancer patients were a team helping science advance. "I thought, *If I'm lucky and I'm cured, I win. But if I don't survive, the contributions I've made through my cancer journey are meaningful, too,*" says Elizabeth.

That belief helped power her through the roughest moments of her treatment, which included a mastectomy, six rounds of chemotherapy, a course of the drug Herceptin, and a 5-year regimen of tamoxifen.

Having cancer meant she had a condition she couldn't control. Desperate for something to wrestle some mastery over her health, the self-described information gatherer asked her oncologist about every tip and study she found. Her answer was simple: exercise.

That's when Elizabeth had her "aha moment." Two months before her diagnosis, she'd bought a commuter bike to ride to work, a 28-mile round trip. "I grabbed on to the idea that here was one thing I could take charge of," she says. "I decided to ride as if my life depended on it."

Her first rides after chemo were short and slow, but soon she was commuting halfway to work (hopping on the Metro to reach her office) and then all the way. She lost 35 pounds in the process. Today, she rides about 600 miles a month and is a certified cycling instructor.

"Riding helped me be an active participant in my cancer treatment," she says. "I consider every day a gift and try to live in the moment."

She'd like women who've been diagnosed to know . . . *it's important to ask for help from loved ones.*

Breast cancer is . . . *something I hope is cured and prevented in the future.*

Tomorrow will . . . *be a day that I try to appreciate and live to the fullest.*

*"The importance of money
flows from it being a link between
the present and the future."*

—JOHN MAYNARD KEYNES

CHAPTER 8

DEALING WITH FINANCIAL CONCERNS

Some of the worst discomfort accompanying a breast cancer diagnosis isn't emotional or physical. It's the pain that patients feel from the sting of their out-of-pocket costs for medical care. If you're like the thousands of cancer patients with limited or no resources to cover your medical treatments, you're no doubt feeling anxious about surviving the high cost of breast cancer. Even if you have a good insurance plan and other means to cover out-of-pocket costs and expenses right now, you may still be worried about paying for the other inevitable expenses that will eventually come up.

Since everyone's financial situation is unique, we can't make your choices during your breast cancer journey. But we can help you map out options for dealing with your costs.

- **Make healthy financial choices,** especially when mounting an unmanageable debt makes you feel like you're stuck in a maze.

- **Avoid financial stumbling blocks to treatments and other services.**

- **Move in the direction of more cost-effective care,** and even track down some health-care and daily-living resources that are free.

- **Become your own advocate,** and point yourself to organizations and services that advocate for patients and their rights.

Our goal is also to help you find answers to questions about the financial side of breast cancer such as: *What are all the costs—not just the medical ones—that I have to consider? How can I make sure my treatment plan is affordable? Where do I go and what can I do if I don't have insurance or I can't pay my premiums? Does having breast cancer mean that I'm going to lose my savings, my job, or my house? Does it mean that I may go bankrupt?*

Before you read anything else in this chapter, we want you to know one thing: There are plenty of resources available to you, and some of these include financial assistance. You just need to reach out to the organizations that are there to help. As you move through this chapter, think about people you can recruit to help you make phone calls, wade through the paperwork, and even negotiate cheaper medical costs. We cannot stress enough that you can't do it all on your own. Also, if at any point while reading through this chapter, you need to stop and take a break, do so. But be sure to pick up where you left off; understanding how to navigate your new financial landscape is critical to reducing anxiety, which is essential for your healing.

THE HIGH COST OF BREAST CANCER

Cancer is one of the five most costly medical conditions in the United States, and even patients with insurance personally feel the financial squeeze of treating their disease.[1] That's why it's important to understand what kinds of rising costs may impact your breast cancer journey and what you can do about them.

For example, according to the National Cancer Institute (NCI), a division of the National Institutes of Health, breast cancer costs for women and men, their families, and society reached $16.5 billion in 2010. Since then, the costs of all types of cancers have risen, and they're projected to keep increasing. In fact, one NCI projection is that the costs for cancer will be at least $158 billion to $207 billion in 2020—and that doesn't include other expenses, such as pay lost from not being able to work.[2]

Invariably, studies like this can make you feel extremely anxious about your out-of-pocket costs. One review determined that breast cancer survivors—even after treatment—found that their direct medical costs (for example, physician fees) ranged from $300 to $1,180 per month during active treatment and were about $500 per month 1 year after diagnosis. Nonmedical out-of-pocket costs (such as those for transportation to/from doctors' appointments and parking) ranged from $137 to $174 per month in the year after diagnosis and $200 to $509 per month 1 year or more after that.[3]

Your financial situation is unique. But it is important to understand medical and other out-of-pocket costs directly related to your breast cancer journey and to know where to go for services and professional advice that can have a positive effect on your bottom line.

Dealing with finances can be overwhelming, to say the least. You may find it helpful to skip around this chapter to find the information most relevant to your personal financial situation and the answers to your most urgent questions. Below is a quick-start guide to the contents of this chapter:

- **Your Health-Care Rights in a Nutshell** (below) explains how the Affordable Care Act will impact your wallet in general and specifically as a woman or a senior.

- **Understanding Your Financial Future** on page 139 discusses the various treatment costs you may need to take into consideration, from doctors' appointments to home health care.

- **Your Financial To-Do List** on page 140 offers a step-by-step approach to getting all the information you need from the right people so that you can reduce the cost of your care.

- **No Insurance? Here's What to Do** on page 143 points you to the resources in "Finding Financial Help" (page 148), which lists more than 20 organizations that can help lighten your financial burden with grants, personal services, and guidance on how to navigate the medical billing system.

YOUR HEALTH-CARE RIGHTS IN A NUTSHELL

The Affordable Care Act (ACA), signed in 2010, offers well-defined choices for consumers and new ways that insurance companies can be held accountable. The 10 key features of the law that you need to know are as follows:

It provides coverage to Americans with preexisting conditions like cancer (after 2014). Until then, the ACA helped states develop interim insurance plans for people with preexisting conditions like breast cancer.

It keeps young adults covered. If you're under 26, you're eligible to be covered under your parent's health plan even if you have breast cancer.

It ends lifetime limits on coverage. Lifetime limits on most benefits are banned for all new health-insurance plans, ensuring that people with breast cancer have access to needed care throughout their lifetimes.

It ends preexisting condition exclusions for children. Health plans can no longer limit or deny benefits to children under 19 due to a preexisting condition, such as cancer.

It ends arbitrary withdrawals of insurance coverage. Insurers can no longer cancel your coverage just because you got diagnosed with breast cancer or because you made an honest mistake on your insurance application form.

It reviews premium increases. Insurance companies cannot charge you more during your plan year for a breast cancer diagnosis. They can, however, raise the rates for your next plan year, but not by more than 10 percent without having the reasons for the rate increase reviewed either by your state's rate review program or the federal rate review program.

It restricts annual dollar limits on coverage. Annual limits on your health benefits have been phased out, so breast cancer patients like you won't have to put off treatments until the new plan year because you've reached a so-called annual limit.

It removes insurance company barriers to emergency services. You can seek emergency care at a hospital outside your health plan's network.

It covers preventive care at no cost to you. You may be eligible for recommended preventive health services like screenings for breast cancer recurrence, with no co-payment necessary.

It guarantees your right to appeal. You now have the right to ask that your plan reconsider a denial of payment.[4] If payment is still denied after you make your appeal, the law permits you to have an independent review organization decide whether to uphold or overturn the decision. Additionally, your state may have a health-care consumer assistance program that can help you file an appeal or request a review.

(To locate a program in your state, go to familiesusa.org/resources/program-locator/.)

New Rights for Women Under the Affordable Care Act

For the first time, as a woman with breast cancer, you have unique benefits under the new law.[5]

Insurance companies can no longer deny coverage to women. Before the new law went into effect, most insurance companies selling individual policies to women could deny coverage or charge them more because their breast cancer was a preexisting condition. From 2014, it becomes illegal for insurance companies to discriminate against anyone with a preexisting condition.[6]

Women can choose their doctor(s). Now all Americans joining new insurance plans can choose from any primary care provider or OB-GYN in their health plan's network or emergency care outside of the plan's network without having a referral.[7]

Women can receive preventive care without co-pays. Since August 1, 2012, about one in three women, or 47 million, under the age of 65 may no longer incur out-of-pocket costs for preventive services like mammograms. For example, if the health-care law were not in place, the average out-of-pocket cost for a mammogram would be $39. Because of the ACA, millions of women no longer have to share the cost through co-payments, coinsurance, and deductibles.[8]

Women pay lower health-care costs. Before the law, women could be charged more for an individual insurance policy because of their gender. As of 2014, insurers can no longer charge women higher premiums than men.[9]

5 Things You—And Your Family—Need to Know

You may be able to get health insurance if you don't have it already. If you've been uninsured for at least 6 months and have been diagnosed with a health condition like breast cancer, you may be able to get health insurance through the federal Pre-Existing Condition Insurance Plan (for more information, go to pcip.gov).

You can appeal insurance decisions. If a new insurance plan doesn't pay for services you believe are covered, you now have clear options to appeal the decision.

Insurance companies can't drop you because they don't want to

insure you. If you made an honest mistake on your coverage application, insurance companies can no longer drop you when you get sick.

You can't be discriminated against because you have breast cancer. Starting in 2014, new group and individual plans won't be able to exclude you from coverage or charge you a higher premium for a preexisting condition, like breast cancer.

You may be eligible for tax credits. Starting in 2014, if your income is less than the equivalent of about $88,000 for a family of four today, and your job doesn't offer affordable coverage, you may get tax credits to help pay for insurance.[10]

3 Things Seniors with Breast Cancer Should Know

Your Medicare benefits can't be taken away. Your existing guaranteed Medicare-covered benefits won't be reduced or taken away. The same applies to your ability to choose your own doctor.

The "donut hole" is changing. If you have high prescription drug costs that put you in Medicare Part D (known as the donut hole), you're entitled to a 50 percent discount on covered brand-name drugs until your out-of-pocket costs reach $4,750. After that, you pay $2.65 per month for generic drugs and $6.60 per month for brand-name prescription drugs–or 5 percent of the medicine's retail cost (whichever is higher). The donut hole will be closed completely by 2020 (at which point, you'll pay a flat 25 percent for covered brand-name and generic drugs). However, between now and 2020, you're guaranteed to get continuous Medicare coverage for your prescription drugs at a cost.[11]

Mammograms are free. Some preventive services–like mammograms once every 12 months and diagnostic mammograms when medically necessary–are now covered by Medicare and will cost you nothing (not even a co-pay). And you won't need to meet your deductible first. You'll also be able to have a free annual wellness exam, essentially a basic physical performed by your primary care physician.[12]

To learn more about the health reform bill, go to healthcare.gov/how-does-the-health-care-law-protect-me. If you need help sorting through health insurance and the health reform bill, the American Cancer Society has a staff of trained experts available to answer questions 24 hours a day, 7 days a week, free of charge. Their toll-free number is 800-227-2345 (ask them, too, to send you their free guide to the ACA).

UNDERSTANDING YOUR FINANCIAL FUTURE

To begin managing your finances now and know what may or may not be available for use in the future, we strongly recommend that you become familiar with the medical and nonmedical costs of breast cancer. By doing so, you'll be better able to see a bigger and more personalized overall picture of potential financial burdens. The best place to begin is to go over this list of the typical medical services for which you may be charged.

Doctors' appointments. This includes payments for the care you receive each time you visit a doctor at her private office or a clinic. If you have insurance, you'll probably be responsible for the co-pay (if your doctor is part of your health-care plan) established by your insurance provider, not by your doctor.

Lab tests. These tests—for blood, urine, and more—are paid for separately. If you use a lab in your health-care plan, you'll typically have a co-pay established by your insurance provider and the lab. If you have your blood work sent to a different lab, however, you may be responsible for the total cost (so make sure your health-care providers know which lab to use).

Treatment costs. This category covers a wide range of procedures (see the list that follows) and additional medical care that you may receive. Some may last for a few days or weeks; others can go on for months and even years. You may also have costs related to clinical trials and expensive medications that may not be covered by health insurance or assistance programs. This list covers most (but not all) of the line items that can show up on your bills:

- **Clinic visits** for treatments.

- **Imaging tests,** including mammograms and other x-rays; CT scans and MRIs that result in separate bills for the radiologist, equipment, and any medicines/dyes used.

- **Radiation treatments,** which may include implants, external radiation, or both.

- **Chemotherapy,** which may include the costs of the drugs and charges billed by the infusion center (a place where chemotherapy is administered).

- **Drug costs,** which vary, depending on where and when they were ordered. The costs associated with inpatient, outpatient, prescription, nonprescription, and procedure-related drugs cover a wide range of expenses. Some are onetime; others will be ongoing for a short period of time or much longer.

- **Hospital stays,** which include a long list of related charges. These may be for drugs, tests, and procedures, as well as nursing care, doctor visits, physical therapy, and consultations with other specialists.

- **Surgical procedures,** which will include costs besides those for the surgeon, anesthesiologist, and pathologist. There will be separate charges for the operating room, equipment, medicines, and any other costs incurred during surgery.

- **Home health care,** which can include equipment, drugs, visits from nurses and therapists, and other costs associated with caring for you at home.[13]

YOUR FINANCIAL TO-DO LIST

Reading through a list of cancer treatment costs is enough to unnerve anyone. The key, though, as we've said before, is not to panic. Instead, make a pact with yourself to slowly and methodically check off everything on the to-do list that follows as soon as you can. Again, ask for help to do this; you can't and don't need to do it on your own. Have someone else take notes at your appointments, ask questions, request additional information, and help clarify confusing or conflicting details. Here's how to get started.

Step 1: Make appointments to see your patient financial services representative at your treatment center. During this meeting you may sense or even fear that your treatment plan is unaffordable. Remember, there is no sense in worrying until you have the full picture. Your treatment center's rep can fill in information based on data about your financial situation and resources and can respond to all your questions about insurance coverage, billing, and more. If no rep is available, consider contacting a local rep from Medicaid or a social worker.

Ask your rep about ways you can lower your medical expenses to prepare for future discussions with insurance, billing, and other

organizing your paper trail

Organizing your medical records and other important papers related to your breast cancer—and especially your finances—saves time and money. This can reduce stress and promote healing throughout recovery.

So make a commitment to getting your bills and financial documents in order. If the whole task or any parts of it are too difficult for you, don't hesitate to shout "Help!" and ask a friend to pitch in. You don't need to share financial details unless you want to.

Get a file box or accordion-style file folder to hold paper statements, and set up a virtual file on your computer that will contain statements sent to you by e-mail or ones you've scanned. Back up your virtual file weekly on a flash, external hard drive, or "cloud" such as Dropbox (dropbox.com) so files can be restored and also available on other electronic devices.

- Set up a file folder for each month. Store statements from insurance companies and doctors describing ongoing or completed services and the dates they occurred.

- Make a file for paid bills and invoices. Write "paid," the date, and check number or credit card used on the top before you file it.

- Create a "Waiting to Be Filed" folder. You'll be amazed how much paperwork you'll have, and you won't have time to file it immediately. This gives you a place to put it to stay organized.

Check that copies of your health and disability insurance policies are current. If not, call your insurance provider to get a new copy or go to their Web site and download a copy. Next, make copies of these policies and highlight your account numbers for quick reference. Put them in a separate folder.

- Tell someone you trust where to find this information if you're not available.

representatives. If you feel awkward asking questions, bring along a copy of this list and give it to the person(s) you're talking to:

- Are payment plans available?
- Are there other hospitals or treatment centers nearby that charge less for the same treatments?
- Does this hospital or treatment center have a special fund to help patients who cannot afford to pay?
- Do any local government or private agencies provide financial assistance?
- Can you give me free samples of prescription medications and some nonprescription ointments, supplements, or other items that I will need? (See "Pharmaceutical Companies That Can Help" on page 151.)
- Can you prescribe less expensive generic (or similar) equivalents of the drugs I must take?
- What have I forgotten to ask?

Why do this? This is your chance to discuss the projected costs of upcoming treatments, procedures, imaging, therapies, drugs, everything. Be sure to bring a list of questions (or a copy of this page) and take notes (or bring along someone who can take notes for you).

Step 2: Deal with your insurance coverage once you've spoken to your financial services rep and health-care team. Do the following to keep on top of your insurance as you undergo treatment and recovery:

Have copies of your policies handy. If you can't find the original policies, call the customer service numbers on the back of your insurance cards and order new ones from each provider. In each case, ask if they can e-mail you a copy as well. Plan to keep your policies in the financial file box we describe on page 141.

Keep a photocopy of your insurance card(s) in the folder with your policy. That way, if you lose or misplace it, you'll have one you can use until a new one arrives.

Scan your insurance card(s) and even your policy, if possible, and file the copies on your computer, smartphone, and other portable devices. If you store your medical and backup information on a cloud, make sure copies are saved in a medical file there, too. That way, the information

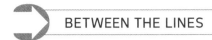
no insurance? here's what to do

If you do not have private or government (Medicare or Medicaid) medical insurance, do not make assumptions about whether or not you can afford your medical care. Even without insurance, it's important to talk to your medical team about those questions. In the pages ahead, we'll also discuss ideas, recommendations, and programs that can help you to:

- Locate services, medications, referrals, and professional advice at reduced costs or free of charge

- Avoid making uninformed, careless, or risky decisions that may result in unnecessary financial burdens (and even compromise your care and recovery)

So if it helps to skip to that section right now (on page 148), do that, and come back to this section later.

---

will sync to your computer, smartphone, or tablet so you can access it anytime, anywhere.

If you're covered by a group plan at work, make an appointment with the person in charge of employee benefits to review your health-insurance benefits. Plan to also review your other employee benefits at this time. If a spouse or partner's policy covers you, ask that person to make the appointment and then accompany you.

If there's a possibility you may lose your benefits through unemployment, call your current insurance company to learn about COBRA (Consolidated Omnibus Budget Reconciliation Act of 1986), which is a way to continue your existing coverage by paying for monthly costs on your own.

Call each insurance company you deal with and ask to have a case manager assigned to you, whether you pay for private insurance or receive medical insurance as an employee benefit. Case managers provide a wide range of services for patients, such as coordinating your health-insurance approvals and locating support services. Once you have that person's name, phone number, and e-mail address, call her to introduce yourself and set up an appointment in person or by phone.

Let that person know that you need a copy of the Summary of Benefits and Coverage–essentially what you're covered for–and the Uniform Glossary, which contains terms commonly used in health-insurance coverage like *deductible* and *co-payment*. They're part of the patient rights and protection sections of the ACA. (Keep the Summary of Benefits and Coverage handy in your medical file box.) Then explain that the reason for your meeting will be to review your plan(s) and discuss:

- Where you can and cannot go for treatment (in network and out of network)
- Your co-payments, deductibles, waiting periods, and the effect of the ACA on all your benefits (see page 135)
- What you should and should not do when you file claims to get reimbursed for out-of-pocket expenses
- Who you should contact if a treatment is not preapproved or paid for
- Your options for services not covered by your treatment plan (for example, MRI, genetic testing, acupuncture, holistic or naturopathic care, and chiropractic care)
- What to do if you cannot pay your bills or continue paying your premiums

Why do this? When you don't understand something, you're more likely to become worried and overwhelmed. Understanding up front *every* aspect of your insurance coverage puts you in control and helps prevent the unnecessary anxiety that can interfere with your healing. When you know the ins and outs of what's covered, when it's covered, and why, you're also better able to speak to your doctors, hospital billing departments, your insurance case manager, and your insurance company about your bills.

Step 3: Prepare now for the bills you'll be receiving by meeting with patient representatives (also called financial counselors) in the billing departments at your medical practices, hospitals, treatment centers, and imaging centers. Do this after you've discussed your treatment plan with your doctor(s), health-care team, and insurance provider in order to get another perspective on the bigger financial picture. When you meet, be sure to:

Bring copies of your insurance policies and treatment plan so the representative can review them.

Ask to see examples of the kinds of statements you'll receive from that office. If you've already been treated at this office or facility, the representative can print out your statements and go through them in detail.

For example, there are codes (numbers) by each expense on your bill. Each code is an explanation of services or treatments you've received from your doctor, treatment center, or hospital. When the wrong code is inadvertently checked or the right one is left unchecked, it can make the

billing mix-ups do happen

Billing mistakes and mix-ups happen all the time for different reasons. But until you know for sure what's going on with your bill, the notices for payment can make you very anxious.

Let's assume you have insurance, and the last time you saw the doctor you made your regular co-payment at the office. Unexpectedly, you get a large bill for your doctor's examination and some tests. After looking over the statement, you're pretty sure you're being billed for something that's covered. But you don't know for sure, and that makes you anxious and maybe angry.

Don't stay anxious and don't ignore the bill. Instead, call the number on the bill and discuss the charges with a customer service representative or your case manager.

The reason: Sometimes a bill comes mistakenly only because the medical office hasn't received a payment from the insurance company yet. Or perhaps all or a portion of the bill is unpaid because of an unresolved question about the coverage between the insurer and the office that treated you. In either of those cases, the computer at the doctor's office or billing center doesn't know the details. It only knows to follow instructions to automatically send statements and notices for payment.

Only by being proactive can you stop that cycle. You may even discover that the problem has already been resolved and a corrected statement is in the mail.

difference between a treatment being approved or denied. The more you become aware of the codes used, the easier it will be for you to understand these bills (and potentially spot billing mistakes before they cause extra anxiety).

Why do this? Billing mistakes happen all the time (see "Billing Mix-Ups Do Happen" on page 145). The more you understand about your bills, the better able you are to catch mistakes that could cost you and your family.

STAYING ACTIVE AND INVOLVED

One important reason to pay attention to your financial health is that some of your expenses don't have dollar signs in front of them. Instead, they can be physical, emotional, and even spiritual tolls that result from anxiety about medical bills and can seriously compromise your treatments and your health.

For example, when patients become swamped by anxiety and feel hopeless about unpaid bills, they may try to save money and start missing doctors' appointments, declining therapies, skipping lab tests, or withdrawing from family, friends, and supportive communities.

Researchers at Duke University and Dana-Farber Cancer Institute in Boston surveyed 216 patients who sought help paying for their cancer care through the HealthWell Foundation, a national nonprofit that helps qualifying underinsured patients afford high-cost medications. Most participants were women (88 percent), and 76 percent had breast cancer. Two-thirds of the patients had Medicare, and 83 percent also had prescription drug coverage. One person had no coverage. The investigators discovered that even with health insurance to cover certain expenses, patients' out-of-pocket expenses averaged $712 a month. Included were costs for co-pays, prescription medicines, lost wages, travel to/from appointments, and other expenses, representing a significant financial burden for 30 percent of the patients and a catastrophic burden for 11 percent.[14]

According to Amy P. Abernethy, MD, an oncologist and senior investigator of the study, "This study provides a patient-centered view of a reality of modern-day cancer care–something that we call 'financial toxicity.' We used to think about chemotherapy toxicity in terms of bad side effects. . . . Now we are starting to think in terms of how treatment

creating a budget

After getting a picture of your medical expenses, let's focus on managing your nonmedical costs. Try using this worksheet to mark down specific items that have both short- and long-term effects on your finances.

Here's a list of nonmedical expenses that may affect your wallet. As you ponder your circumstances, be sure to write down additional categories that come to mind.

- Buying or making payments on insurance premiums: medical, disability, life, . . .
- Daily living: mortgage, utilities, groceries, child care, auto, . . .
- Lost or reduced income: number of hours, full-time/part-time, sick leave, personal/vacation days, unemployment, . . .
- Legal issues: medical, estate planning, employment related, . . .
- Wellness costs: yoga, meditation, acupuncture, massage therapy, vitamins and supplements, . . .

choices impact real aspects of daily living such as the ability to buy groceries or not."[15]

We hope you never feel such despair over your finances that you take any cost-cutting route that can seriously compromise your treatments and health. You may qualify for streams of relief if you know where to look for them. So let's begin moving in that direction.

HOW TO BECOME FINANCIALLY PROACTIVE

Whether you have private health insurance (group or individual) or government insurance (Medicare or Medicaid), it's probable that you've already received and/or paid some co-pays and bills. And if you don't have insurance, you may be already receiving invoices or warning notices requesting full or partial payment for services that led to your diagnosis and treatments received so far.

In either case, if you've done the preliminary "legwork" we've suggested, you now have people and places to turn to with questions and concerns. Sometimes problems that look enormous cause lots of anxiety. Then, it's only after a phone call or e-mail that you may find out it's a problem that can be easily resolved.

Reach out to people you can talk to. As soon as anything happens that can affect your financial situation (and credit rating) negatively, make arrangements to talk to a social worker or counselor on your health-care team or at your hospital. Or refer to the section below.

When you go to appointments, bring copies of the bills and other statements causing concern. Make sure to have the contact information for the case managers and financial counselors with whom you've spoken already. If the person you'll be talking to is out of state or online, ask for a case number and where and to whom to send the information.

FINDING FINANCIAL HELP

If financial setbacks become a reality for you, contact the following organizations that address your particular concerns. In addition to sound advice, many provide financial, travel, prescription, lodging, and other forms of assistance.

AARP, 888-687-2277, aarp.org/health, is for people 50 and over seeking information about Medicare and other health-insurance programs.

American Cancer Society, 800-227-2345, cancer.org/treatment, provides links and information about numerous sources of financial assistance and information about health-care services, legislation, and programs. The searchable database offers resources for financial assistance and free support based upon ZIP codes and/or cities and states. Use this link to access the database: tinyurl.com/qy3cn2t.

For example, the American Cancer Society has 31 Hope Lodges nationwide that offer cancer patients and their caregivers free lodging when their best hope for effective treatment is in another city. Their Road to Recovery program provides transportation to and from treatment for people who have cancer who do not have a ride or are unable to drive themselves. Volunteer drivers donate their time and the use of their cars so that patients can receive the lifesaving treatments they need.

Cancer Financial Assistance Coalition (CFAC), cancerfac.org, is a coalition of financial assistance organizations joining forces to help cancer patients experience better health and well-being by limiting financial challenges. Their mission includes advocating on behalf of cancer patients who continue to bear financial burdens associated with the costs of cancer treatment and care. Because the CFAC is a coalition, it cannot respond to individual requests for financial assistance.

To find out if you qualify for financial assistance, go to the Web site, search the database, or contact the organizations that deal with breast cancer for guidance and information. The CFAC database provides information about organizations and services available in your ZIP code and state.

Cleaning for a Reason, 877-337-3348, cleaningforareason.org, is a nonprofit serving the United States and Canada that partners with professional maid services to offer house cleanings to help women undergoing treatment for cancer. The insured and bonded companies offer each patient 4 free cleanings, one a month for 4 consecutive months, as a way to give back to their community. Patients can apply online for the service where and when it's available.

Faith-based organizations may have local or regional offices and can provide direct assistance or refer you to other local or state agencies that do. Some of these organizations include Catholic Charities, Lutheran Services in America, and Jewish Family Services. Check your phone book or online for listings in your area.

Linking A.R.M.S., 877-465-6636, is a partnership between Susan G. Komen for the Cure and Cancer*Care*. For those who are eligible, Linking A.R.M.S. provides financial assistance grants. They can be used for oral chemotherapy and hormone-therapy medications, pain and antinausea medication, medical equipment, and lymphedema support and supplies. Call the breast cancer helpline, above, for more information.

Medicaid, medicaid.gov, offers benefits provided by your state. You can find the toll-free number for your state on the Web site.

National Cancer Legal Services Network, nclsn.org, provides a directory of 40 organizations in states nationwide that provide free legal help for people and families affected by cancer. For the directory, go to is.gd/HTaOaD.

For example, in North Carolina, the Cancer Pro Bono Legal Project is a collaboration between the University of North Carolina and Duke University law schools, the cancer centers at the two universities, as well as the North Carolina Bar Association and North Carolina Society of Healthcare Attorneys. Law students assist pro bono attorneys who work with patients on documents related to advance directives, financial power of attorney, and health-care power of attorney. Additionally, the students and attorneys offer cancer patients monthly seminars on legal topics that include insurance rights, employment rights, Social Security disability insurance, and financial planning.

Partnership for Prescription Assistance (PPA), 888-477-2669, pparx.org, provides free information to help qualifying patients without prescription drug coverage get free or reduced-cost prescription medicine. Others offering a similar service may charge fees. At the PPA Web site, you can access information about 475 public and private programs, including nearly 200 offered by biopharmaceutical companies.

For example, Rx Outreach (rxoutreach.com) is a patient-assistance program that helps patients with all kinds of illnesses access more than 400 prescription medications. Patients must qualify based on income.

PPA will also point you to additional resources and services such as:

- Medicare prescription drug coverage
- Medicaid programs, including the Children's Health Insurance Program
- Co-payment programs
- Participating patient-assistance programs
- Free/low-cost health clinic finder
- Savings cards (when your prescriptions aren't covered by insurance)

Patient Access Network Foundation, 866-316-7263, panfoundation.org, provides up to $7,500 annually to women and men with metastatic breast cancer when costs are prohibitive, limiting access to breakthrough medical treatments. In order to be eligible:

pharmaceutical companies that can help

Many pharmaceutical companies help breast cancer patients cover the costs of their prescriptions and chemotherapy. For those who qualify, these patient drug assistance programs are available at either a reduced cost or for free. Criteria include your financial circumstances and other factors, such as age. Talk to your health-care team and contact the manufacturer.

Note that not all programs are ongoing. Medications may or may not be available at the time you contact the pharmaceutical company.

- AstraZeneca, 800-292-6363, tinyurl.com/c2932d6, Arimidex (anastrozole), Faslodex (fulvestrant), Zoladex (goserelin), and the AZ&Me program

- Bristol-Myers Squibb, 800-332-2056, tinyurl.com/qv2cr6, Ixempra (ixabepilone) and several programs

- Celgene, tinyurl.com/nvurhvy, Abraxane (protein-bound paclitaxel) and Celgene Patient Support Program

- Eli Lilly, 855-559-8783, tinyurl.com/7vyn6ms, Evista (raloxifene), Gemzar (gemcitabine), and Lilly TruAssist program

- Genentech, 866-422-2377, tinyurl.com/pja83m9, Avastin (bevacizumab), Herceptin (trastuzumab), Xeloda (capecitabine), and four programs, as well as Xeloda Access Solutions (888-249-4918)

- GlaxoSmithKline, 888-663-4752, tinyurl.com/lqypexp, GSK Cares program; additionally, the Commitment to Access program for cancer and specialty medicines (866-265-6491).

- Novartis, 800-277-2254, tinyurl.com/p8djtbn, several patient assistance programs

- Pfizer, 866-706-2400, tinyurl.com/ya8eckz, several patient assistance programs

- Patient's income must fall below 500 percent of the federal poverty level (poverty levels change every year; go to the US Department of Health and Human Services Web site to check if you qualify: aspe .hhs.gov/poverty/13poverty.cfm)
- Patient must have Medicare insurance coverage
- Medication must treat the disease directly
- Patient must reside in and receive treatment in the United States

Patient Advocate Foundation, 800-532-5274, patientadvocate.org, offers legal and advocacy help for disputing insurance claim denials and provides financial assistance information. It also offers an online tool that can help you find resources if you are underinsured and/or looking for insurance and other types of assistance.

Patient Services Incorporated, 800-366-7741, patientservicesinc.org, provides assistance with the cost of MRI screenings for breast cancer. To find out if you qualify, use the online eligibility tool.

The Pink Fund, 877-234-7465, thepinkfund.org, provides short-term financial aid to breast cancer patients in active treatment. The organization will make a direct bill payment for the maintenance of health-insurance premiums and nonmedical bills, such as a mortgage or rent payment, a car payment, utility payments, and car insurance payments. The Pink Fund does not, however, make payments for any medical treatments, prescription drugs (including hormone therapy), medical co-pays, insurance deductibles, breast prostheses (artificial breasts after breast removal surgery), wigs, food, gas, or car repairs. You can find out whether or not you qualify for assistance and fill out an application to prequalify online.

Social Security Administration, ssa.gov, offers disability benefits. To find out if you qualify, contact your local office.

Transportation can be arranged by most city, county, and state agencies at a low cost or even for free. Contact your city, county, or state transportation department to find out about services in your area. Long-distance transportation, when necessary for treatments at distant medical centers, is available for patients who meet the provider's qualifications. In some cases, the cost of a caregiver is covered, too. For more information, contact the following providers:

- **Air Charity Network,** 877-621-7177, aircharitynetwork.org, is a volunteer network connecting those in need with free flights to specialized health-care facilities.

- **Angel Bus,** 800-768-0238, angel-bus.org, is a nonprofit providing nonemergency, long-distance ground transportation to patients with financial need. They'll also provide free gas cards to offset fuel costs for those who drive to/from treatments.

- **Corporate Angel Network,** 866-328-1313, corpangelnetwork.org, is a nonprofit organization that flies patients free of charge in empty seats on corporate jets. Patients can fly as often as necessary, and financial need is not required.

- **Lifeline Pilots,** 800-822-7972, lifelinepilots.org, coordinates free flights through volunteer pilots for financially distressed passengers with medical needs.

- **Mercy Medical Airlift,** 800-296-1217, mercymedical.org, provides free air transportation (they can also coordinate ground transportation) to distant medical treatment facilities.

- **National Patient Travel Center,** 800-296-1217, patienttravel.org, provides information about all forms of free long-distance medical transportation and provides referrals to all sources of help.

- **Raquel's Wings for Life,** 940-627-1050, raquelswingsforlife.com, is a nonprofit organization that transports cancer patients (and their families, if necessary) to the medical center they need. [16]

Remember that when it comes to managing your financial health for the best outcome possible, you need to make informed and realistic decisions. When you do, you won't become stuck in a financial maze and cut off from resources. Instead, you'll find helpful and healing places to turn to that you might have never known about otherwise.

Following Her Intuition

Jewell Biddle had to dampen her anxiety. Years of serving as a prosecuting attorney and judge, plus a divorce, left her "extremely stressed." And she paid the price for it–she developed cysts, which she and her doctor monitored very closely. When she traded the gavel for a job as an insurance agent, her stress decreased, but the cysts were still a problem.

Then in July 2002, while her regular doctor was unavailable, a different physician reviewed her recent ultrasound and told her everything looked fine. Jewell had no reason *not* to believe him, but she insisted that her regular doctor take a look anyway. "Only she knew my history with all of these cysts; only she had my trust," says Jewell.

Good thing the former judge followed her instinct. Jewell's doctor spotted three different tumors in three quadrants of the right breast. She had stage III breast cancer. "The minute I heard the diagnosis, I thought, *I'm going to beat this*," says Jewell, now 66.

She chose an aggressive course of treatment that included a bilateral mastectomy (even though cancer was present in just one breast, both breasts were removed as a precautionary measure), removal of lymph nodes, and four rounds of chemotherapy. An infection with a high fever between her second and third rounds of chemo sent her to the hospital. "That was the closest I felt to death," she recalls. Four months after her last treatment, her index finger swelled, signaling lymphedema.

During that treatment, Jewell defied orders to not exercise. "I understood why they didn't want me to exercise, but it seemed like down the road, not exercising would do me more harm," she says. She started hiking the trails near her home and remains an avid hiker. Like others who've had cancer treatment, Jewell experienced post-traumatic stress disorder (PTSD) symptoms and says hiking helped relieve them.

She'd like women who've been diagnosed to know . . . *you can beat this. Find doctors and surgeons you really trust, and don't be afraid to be assertive in your medical care.*

Breast cancer is . . . *a terrible diagnosis but beatable.*

Tomorrow will . . . *be terrific.*

PART FOUR

LIVING *with* BREAST CANCER

I n the chapters that follow, you'll find a handy guide to life with breast cancer. The months ahead won't be easy, but with our advice, you'll be prepared to cope with the challenges. Learn what to eat to boost your energy when treatments leave you feeling fatigued, or when it's tough to eat at all. Our simple exercise plan will help you keep strong and limber, even if you're dealing with lymphedema. Find out about complementary treatments like acupuncture, healing touch, and reiki, and talk to your doctor about whether they're right for you. And find ways to lower the stress you're probably feeling these days—and connect with a support group that can lighten your load and enrich your life.

*"Let your food be your medicine and
your medicine be your food."*

—HIPPOCRATES

CHAPTER 9

DIET AND
NUTRITION

If your diagnosis jump-started your desire to overhaul your diet to better
your odds of becoming a long-term survivor, you're not alone. One
study of women with breast cancer found that only 9 percent initially
believed that an unhealthy diet contributes to disease. Yet, after getting
their diagnosis, 32 percent (nearly one-third) of the women chose to significantly modify their dietary habits[1]–for good reason.

A healthy diet provides the fuel your body needs to work properly day
in and day out. But, now, this fuel becomes even more important in helping your body to recover and heal posttreatment. Studies also show that
eating a combination of the right foods can help prevent your breast cancer from recurring. In fact, some studies indicate that the right diet (along
with lifestyle modification) may be able to prevent breast cancer, altogether, in up to 35 percent of cases.[2]

The most comprehensive review of research looking at the relationship of nutrition and diet (as well as exercise) to all kinds of cancer was
published in 2007. The associations between diet and breast cancer,
specifically, revealed that plants are the building blocks of an anticancer diet. More specifically, this study found that fruits, vegetables,
whole grains, and other food from plants provide an array of cancer-
protective compounds, such as vitamins, minerals, and other key nutrients like antioxidants. (See "Antioxidants to the Rescue!" on page 186.)
They're also essential to managing your weight–and avoiding weight

gain—which is one of the most important things you can do to reduce your risk of cancer.[3]

But we know that making changes to your diet right now can be extremely challenging, especially when you feel like everything you're doing is a challenge and a change. This may be especially true if you're getting radiation or chemotherapy and/or are just feeling fatigued, depressed, or anxious. In fact, this is the time you're probably craving your favorite comfort or soul foods—not kale, red peppers, and bok choy! But baby steps are what's most important when it comes to lifestyle changes. Make small changes that will last in your diet rather than overhauling everything you eat all at once, feeling completely miserable about it, and then giving up on your new eating plan after just a week or two.

The first step is to read this chapter. In it, we'll give you sound information about why a healthy diet—with the right nutrients—is a healing recipe for success on your breast cancer journey. We'll provide evidence that when you add anticancer foods to your diet and subtract unhealthy ones, you lower your risk of a recurrence and/or dying from breast cancer. We'll also offer suggestions for getting the fortifying nutrients you need throughout your treatments—especially during troubling times when side effects can make even the most delicious food look unappetizing and difficult to eat.

WHY DIET MAKES A DIFFERENCE

Here are just a handful of the studies and what they concluded about the benefits of a healthy diet and its association with lower risk for breast cancer.

Cruciferous Vegetables Are Key

One study looked at Chinese breast cancer survivors diagnosed with stage I to stage IV breast cancer over the course of 4 years.[4] The researchers concluded that eating green leafy (cruciferous) vegetables, such as kale, broccoli, Brussels sprouts, and cabbage, during the first 36 months after their diagnosis was associated with:

- 62 percent reduced risk of total mortality
- 62 percent reduced risk of breast cancer mortality
- 35 percent reduced risk of breast cancer recurrence

For Dairy, Go Low-Fat

Opt for low-fat milk, yogurt, and cheese. One 15-year study of almost 1,900 breast cancer survivors, conducted at Kaiser Permanente Division of Research in Oakland, California, found that those who ate one or more servings of high-fat dairy daily (as opposed to low-fat dairy foods) had a 49 percent higher risk of breast cancer death compared to survivors who ate up to half a serving a day. And of all the women in the higher-intake group, those who ate greater amounts of high-fat dairy had a 64 percent higher risk of dying from any cause compared to those who consumed little or none.[5]

Cut Down on Overall Fat

In an effort to determine how fat affects a woman's breast cancer risk, researchers at the National Cancer Institute questioned 188,000 post-menopausal women about how often they ate high-fat foods. Of those surveyed, 3,500 developed invasive breast cancer. The researchers found that dietary fat intake was directly associated with the risk of postmeno-pausal invasive breast cancer.[6] Moreover, this risk of developing breast cancer rose 15 percent if fat intake doubled.[7]

Eat Brightly Colored Foods

Carotenoids are micronutrients that give an orange-yellow and red pigment to fruits and vegetables like carrots, apricots, mangoes, squash, papaya, and sweet potatoes, and are also found in many dark green vegetables like kale, spinach, and collard greens. Lycopene is a carotenoid that's found in tomatoes, watermelon, and pink grapefruit. Studies have found that these micronutrients have anticancer properties that inhibit tumor development and help keep certain breast cancers from spreading.

In one study, a research team at Harvard Medical School examined eight published studies involving 7,000 people. Their investigation concluded that women whose carotenoid levels were in the top 20 percent reduced their risk of breast cancer by 15 to 20 percent compared to those whose carotenoid levels were in the lowest category. This indicated that while there's some benefit from having a moderate level of carotenoids, there's even *more* benefit at a higher level.[8]

Go Easy on Alcohol

The National Institutes of Health and AARP teamed up to study the effects of alcohol consumption on breast cancer risk in postmenopausal women. The researchers found that as few as one or two drinks per day increased the risk of women developing estrogen positive (ER+) and progesterone positive (PR+) breast cancer. (See "How 'Molecular Analysis' Is Changing Breast Cancer Treatment–For the Better" on page 92.) Moreover, when compared to women who didn't drink at all, those who had three or more glasses of alcohol daily increased their risk by as much as 51 percent.[9]

Consider Working with a Nutrition Expert

These studies probably help reinforce any desire you have to change your diet. We want to reassure you that you're in the right place to get started. This chapter will take you through exactly what to eat and what not to eat. But if you still have questions at the end of this chapter about what's right for you (and you know you'll need someone to help motivate you throughout your entire journey, particularly when eating well becomes a challenge), you may want to seek out the advice of a nutrition expert. We'll tell you how in "When to Consult a Nutrition Expert."

A nutrition expert can help tailor your diet to your breast cancer and to your treatment protocol because, when it comes to breast cancer, one diet definitely does not fit all. As you move through your healing journey, it becomes even more important to factor in the many ways diet can benefit and, at times, even compromise your diagnosis–and overall health. A quick example is grapefruit. It's loaded with vitamin C and other nutrients that make it a healthy choice. However, studies show it can weaken the effect of certain drugs and interact with others. So until you talk to a nutrition expert or doctor to see if you fall into this category, it may be wise to choose a vitamin C–rich kiwifruit instead.

But at the end of the day, common sense should always prevail. If a news report begins touting the health benefits of coconut milk, don't rush out to buy it just yet. Or if you hear about a miracle "detoxing diet," skip it. Stick to what's tried and true, and don't pay attention to the latest fads.

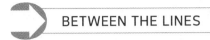

when to consult a nutrition expert

As you begin making dietary changes, a nutrition expert can point you to health-promoting foods that provide enough calories and nutrients to help you feel better—and heal from the physical and emotional impact of breast cancer. (A medical nutrition expert is often covered by insurance, including Medicare and Medicaid.)[10]

If one of these specialists is not already a member of your health-care team, ask your doctor or oncology nurse to enlist one for you or to give you a referral. Or go online. The Academy of Nutrition and Dietetics provides a directory of registered dietitians (eatright.org/programs/rdfinder) that allows you to search for nutrition experts by location and specialty.

If you can't consult with a local specialist, talk with one at no charge by calling the American Cancer Society (ACS) at 800-227-2345. The ACS also offers a two-part online nutrition course for cancer patients at tinyurl.com/adgf56a. And download the free booklet *Nutrition for the Person with Cancer during Treatment: A Guide for Patients and Families* at is.gd/zLQgmg.[8]

Why It Makes Sense: A well-balanced diet can be one of the most effective, safe, and natural ways to offset deficiencies that trigger disease and affect healing. An expert who reviews your diagnosis, treatment plan, medications, and medical history can work with you to create a safe dietary plan to fortify and sustain your body—and maintain your energy level throughout your healing journey.

Say you love spicy food and your diet regularly includes lots of curries. A nutrition expert with knowledge of breast cancer will be able to tell you that if chemotherapy is part of your treatment, you may experience side effects, such as painful mouth or throat sores, that don't interact well with these kinds of foods. He may advise that for now, cool, creamy foods (like milkshakes or smoothies) are better for you. Moreover, you may also feel nauseated or find you can't keep your favorite foods down. An expert can guide you when you can't anticipate these reactions on your own.

GETTING THE BIG PICTURE: HEALTHY FOOD 101

If the old saying is true that "a picture is worth a thousand words," begin looking closely at the "still life" in front of you when you sit down to eat. Hopefully, more than half the picture is a combination of fruits, vegetables, and whole grains. If not, it's probably time to paint a new one that will give you the healthiest mix of protein, fats, carbohydrates, fiber, and other nutrients that your body needs to recover.

If that doesn't sound appealing because you're a meat and potatoes person or prefer lots of white pasta and bread, look at it this way: The best news about the healthy foods we'll be talking about in this chapter is that they go to work for you starting from the time you eat them. They can help you to heal by:

- Boosting your immune system
- Fueling your body to go the extra mile–especially during treatment
- Helping you to better deal with depression, anxiety, and the side effects of your treatment
- Helping you to maintain, or lose, weight
- Reducing your chance of a recurrence during treatment–or years after

YOUR GUIDE TO HEALTHY EATING

Here's a crash course in the amazing ways food works to keep you cancer free. It's a lot of information, so feel free to tab pages, write in the margins, or keep notes in your journal. And be sure to keep a running list of questions for your health-care team so you don't forget to ask them on your next visit.

Protein

Protein supplies amino acids, which help to keep your immune system healthy; repair cells; and create cells, hormones, and enzymes. Of the 20 amino acids that your body needs to function properly, only 12 are produced internally. The remaining eight have to come from your daily diet.

During your treatments, your body needs enough protein to recover, heal, and keep other illnesses at bay. Depending upon your diagnosis, treatment plan, and overall health, you may even need additional protein. Healthy sources include lean meat, fish, poultry, low-fat dairy products, beans and legumes, and nuts and seeds.

When deciding which types of protein you should include in your diet, it's always best to check with your doctor first about whether you should eliminate all red meat or keep meat lean and to a minimum. The same applies to fish and soy products.

Red meat consumption may be linked to breast cancer.[11] Research focusing on countries that have low red meat consumption–like Japan, Korea, and China–suggests that limiting your intake helps prevent breast cancer.[12] As Western fast food and diets have become increasingly popular in these countries, breast cancer numbers have risen, especially among those women who have increased their consumption of red meat.

In another study, researchers looked at whether red meat and poultry might cause breast cancer. They found preliminary evidence that both seemed to boost the risk of breast cancer in white women but not in black women.[13] Researchers also found that an increase in weekly consumption of red meat (to about 18 ounces or more) and poultry (to about 7 ounces or more) appeared to raise breast cancer risk in white women.[14] Keep in mind when you read these findings that these studies are limited by the study population that it addresses. You can likely find different studies reaching different conclusions. Use common sense and discuss your diet with your doctor or a nutritionist before drastically changing your diet. A nutritionist can be particularly useful in helping you convert your dietary habits to a more well-balanced approach.

Soy, which comes from the soybean plant, can be a versatile, protein-rich substitute for meat, eggs, and other animal sources of food in your diet. (At the supermarket you can buy an array of soy products ranging from tofu and soy milk to tempeh, veggie burgers, and miso soup.) While soybeans have more protein and fat than other beans, they're low in carbohydrates. They also contain nutrients, such as valuable amino acids, essential fatty acids, soluble fiber, vitamins, and minerals, including calcium and iron. Soy is also the richest known source of isoflavones–plant estrogens with properties that resemble your natural estrogen.

And herein lies the root of the debate that's ongoing about whether or not soy is good for you. One study, conducted at the State University of New York at Buffalo and at Roswell Park Cancer Institute in Buffalo, found that soy and other plant-based compounds called isoflavones may be associated with a reduced risk of developing certain types of breast tumors. In fact, women with newly diagnosed breast cancer who consumed the highest amounts of isoflavones had a 30 percent decreased risk of having an invasive tumor and a 60 percent decreased risk of having a grade 1 tumor. Additionally, the premenopausal women who consumed certain types of isoflavones lowered their odds by 70 percent of having a large (greater than 2 centimeters) tumor.[15]

But on the flip side, there are studies that demonstrate that higher concentrations of estrogen in your body can increase your risk for breast cancer. For example, some studies demonstrate that soy isoflavones mimic the action of estrogen and cause an increase in cell proliferation in breast tissue, acting as a precursor for breast cancer.[16]

And then, as if the debate over soy wasn't confusing enough, there are researchers who say that whether or not you should eat soy really depends on the type of breast cancer you have. This particular study, which looked at the effects of dietary soy isoflavones on Korean women diagnosed with HER2+ or HER2- breast cancer, found that soy—mostly from black soybeans—was not associated with the risk of breast cancer recurrence in HER2- breast cancer patients.[17] But it was associated with the risk of cancer recurrence in HER2+ breast cancer patients. Also, while there was some concern that the natural phytoestrogens in soy might interfere with the effectiveness of breast cancer hormone-therapy treatments (like tamoxifen and/or anastrozole, which work by depriving cancer cells of the estrogen they need to grow and thrive), one study found that it did not affect this type of systemic therapy.[18]

The bottom line when it comes to soy is this: More research still needs to be done. But if you're going to eat it, do so in moderation (no more than one to two servings a day), and stick with whole-food sources of soy, like edamame (or soybeans), instead of processed sources of soy (like soy milk or veggie burgers) because, in general, whole foods are healthier than processed ones.[19]

Seafood is a healthy source of high-quality protein and other essential nutrients that can help prevent cancer. One study looked at the diets of menopausal breast cancer patients with a combined hormone receptor status. The researchers found that a diet rich in seafood (as well as vegetables) is associated with a decreased breast cancer risk in Korean women. Those whose diets were based on meat and starch did not have that benefit.[20] Also, strong evidence from some animal studies indicate that fish oils slow the development—and decrease the growth of—breast tumors.[21]

In a 2013 review of 21 studies conducted on 883,585 women, Chinese researchers found that those women with the highest intake of omega-3 fatty acids from seafood had a 14 percent lower risk of breast cancer. In fact, just a miniscule increase in omega-3-rich seafood every day (0.1 gram or 0.004 ounce) was associated with a 5 percent lower breast cancer risk. The researchers say that this study offers "robust" evidence that marine omega-3 fatty acids are associated with a decreased risk of breast cancer.[22]

The one caveat with seafood: Avoid fish with high levels of mercury (a known neurotoxin). Because it's hard to know which ones are safe, here are some general guidelines.

- Limit your intake of shark, swordfish, king mackerel, or tilefish; these are all high in mercury. Fish that are low in mercury include shrimp, canned light tuna (which has less mercury than albacore or "white" tuna), salmon, pollock, and catfish.

- Eat no more than four servings of fish per week, even if it's low in mercury. One serving of fish is about 3 ounces (or the size of your palm). But if you're eating fish with mercury or that's been caught in local waters (where chemical contamination is a concern), limit your total fish intake for that week to 6 ounces.[23]

- Download apps such as Safe Seafood (seafoodapp.com) or Seafood Watch (tinyurl.com/87qo52) from the Monterey Bay Aquarium if you have a smartphone. Both list fish to avoid or eat in moderation and include those that are always safe to eat. The Monterey Bay Aquarium also has regional and sushi pocket guides that you can download from their Web site (montereybayaquarium.org) onto your computer.

If you don't eat fish or can't stand the smell because you're nauseated from chemotherapy, omega-3 fish oil supplements are a good substitute (look for ones that don't have a fishy smell or aftertaste). One study of 35,000 postmenopausal women found that those who regularly took omega-3 fish oil supplements were one-third less likely to develop breast cancer than those who don't take fish oil. They also found a lower risk of breast cancer in women who took these supplements, even among those who are traditionally believed to be at higher risk, including women who are obese, heavy drinkers, and physically inactive.[24]

Fats

Fats supply your body with energy and transport fat-soluble vitamins (like A, D, and E) and other nutrients. They also supply you with fatty acids that help to manufacture new cells and hormones. There are four basic kinds of fats: saturated fats, trans fats, and monounsaturated and polyunsaturated fats.

Saturated fats come from animals and are found in beef, pork, veal, poultry, dairy products, and eggs. Foods from plants that contain saturated fat include coconut, coconut oil, palm oil, and palm kernel oil (often called tropical oils), and cocoa butter. For decades, saturated fats have been a known factor in high cholesterol and heart disease.

Trans fats, also known as trans fatty acids, are formed during a process called hydrogenation, where liquid vegetable oils are transformed into solid fat. Foods in your pantry or refrigerator that contain trans fats are usually processed foods that contain "partially hydrogenated" oils or fats such as margarine and shortening. But it's also found in fried foods and in commercial baked goods like cookies, crackers, pastries, doughnuts, muffins, pies, and cakes (just another reason to limit your intake of these foods). The trans fat content of foods is printed on the package on the nutrition facts label. Look for "0 gram trans fat."

Trans fats raise cholesterol levels, and they may also increase breast cancer risk. In one study of 25,000 women, those women who had the highest levels of trans fats in their blood were about twice as likely as women with the lowest trans-fat levels to develop breast cancer.[25]

Monounsaturated and polyunsaturated fats, also called unsaturated fats, are the healthy ones found in fish, nuts, seeds, and plant oils like olive oil and canola oil. These fats can help lower your blood cholesterol. In the case of olive oil, it may significantly reduce your risk of breast cancer, according to some studies.[26]

Omega-6 fatty acids are found in seeds, nuts, and oils like soybean oil, safflower oil, corn oil, and sunflower oil. Like omega-3 fatty acids, omega-6 fatty acids are important for brain function and normal growth and development.[27]

Experts agree that a healthy diet contains a balance of both these fatty acids. But research shows that an imbalance of them—where you have more omega-6s than omega-3s—may actually cause inflammation and disease. There is even some research that suggests a diet rich in omega-6 fatty acids may also promote breast cancer development.[28]

One study looked at data from the Malmö Diet and Cancer Study, a screening survey of almost 12,000 middle-aged people in Malmö, Sweden. Baseline information about the participants' dietary habits was collected, and then they were followed for more than 10 years. During that time, 430 women who were over 50 at the start of the study were diagnosed with invasive breast cancer. The researchers concluded that "a significant increased risk was observed among those with high intakes of omega-6 polyunsaturated fatty acids."[29]

Carbohydrates

Carbs are your main source of energy and, because they enter your bloodstream as glucose, carbohydrates provide quick energy. There are two types of carbohydrates: *simple carbohydrates*, such as sugar, molasses, and honey; and *complex carbohydrates*, such as grains, vegetables, fruits, and beans.

When choosing which carbs you want in your diet, complex carbohydrates should always be at the top of your list. Vegetables, fruits, whole grains, and beans and legumes are among the healthiest sources of complex carbohydrates (and they provide you with filling fiber, too).

All forms of sugar (white and brown, natural and organic) as well as molasses and honey are high-calorie "simple" carbohydrates that are often called empty calories. That's because they don't provide your body with the essential vitamins or minerals that it needs right now. But they do contribute to weight gain and obesity, which is a risk factor for breast cancer. And they may actually contribute to the growth of cancer, too. In 2008, researchers at the Duke University School of Medicine found that cancer cells avoid cell death–allowing them to grow unhindered–by metabolizing glucose.[30]

Fiber

Fiber comes from the parts of veggies, fruits, and grains that you can't digest. For that reason, it's often referred to as roughage. Adequate amounts of fiber can help maintain bowel health, lower blood cholesterol levels, control blood sugar levels, and aid in weight loss. It may also lower your risk for breast cancer. In a review of studies assessing dietary fiber and breast cancer risk, researchers in China and the United States found that diets rich in fiber were associated with the lowest risk for breast cancer. The analysis, which looked at 712,195 participants, showed that for every 10 grams (0.35 ounce) of fiber intake, women reduce their breast cancer risks by 7 percent.[31]

Another study, conducted by the Fred Hutchinson Cancer Research Center in Seattle, found that, among the 688 breast cancer survivors involved in the study, those who consumed more than 15.5 grams (0.55 ounce) of insoluble dietary fiber (one of two types of fiber; see

tips for eating when it's hard to do

The side effects of breast cancer vary, but some of the most common ones are mouth sores, a loss of appetite, nausea, and/or vomiting. (We discuss this in detail in Chapter 7.)

First, if you're having any of these side effects, don't assume you "should" be. Call your health-care team. If what you're experiencing is normal, follow these tips.

For Appetite Loss

Graze. Instead of eating three large meals, snack on nutritious foods or eat smaller meals. It's not how much is on your plate that counts, but *what's* on your plate.

Go instant. Sometimes an instant meal–like an energy bar with well-balanced ingredients or a store-bought nutritional shake– works fine. Try a few of these store-bought items now so you'll you'll know which ones to get when you need them.

Drink water with your meals and drink any other beverages at least half an hour *after* meals so they don't diminish your appetite.

Exercise. Moving, even a slow walk around the block, will help stimulate your appetite. But always exercise moderately unless your doctor suggests otherwise. (Too much exercise can rob your body of the nutrients and stored energy you need.)

For Nausea and Vomiting

The best way to deal with this may be taking antinausea medication (also called antiemetics) your doctor recommends, either prescription or over the counter. Here are other things that can help.

page 170) daily were 49 percent less likely to experience a recurrence compared to survivors who ate less than 5.4 grams (0.19 ounce) daily.[32]

You need both types of fiber–soluble and insoluble–to keep things moving smoothly through your digestive tract.

Avoid fatty, greasy foods. These can be particularly hard to digest now.

Eat foods at room temperature. Hot or cold foods can make your stomach queasy when it feels off-kilter.

Avoid strong odors by asking family members not to cook spicy dishes with garlic, onions, fish, bacon, or other pungent foods.

Eat like a baby. Go bland with crackers, toast, applesauce, gelatin desserts, rice, or a baked potato sans butter. Clear broths, skinned chicken, and soft fruits and vegetables may be easily digested, too. Ginger ale at room temperature and herbal teas can also help settle your stomach.

For Mouth Sores

Eat cold food and drink cool drinks. They won't hurt or cause further irritation, like hot food or drinks can. Room temperature food may also help.

Eat food that's soft and soothing. Use your blender to make your own "baby food," or buy some jars at the supermarket. Other options: yogurt, oatmeal, cooked grains, mashed potatoes, ice cream, milkshakes, puddings, custards, gelatin, and frozen fruit bars. Don't worry about whether these foods (like ice cream) are healthy–just worry about eating enough to give your body energy.

Skip acidic food, citrus juices, spicy food, and salty food. All can be irritating.

Keep ice pops in your freezer. They'll help if your mouth is dry. Ice chips work well, too.

Soluble fiber behaves like a sponge. It attracts water, then dissolves to form a gel. That, in turn, slows the movement of food through your gut, which keeps you fuller longer, helping to control your weight. It may also help control diabetes and cholesterol.

Foods that contain soluble fiber include oats (oatmeal, oat cereal, and oat bran); fruit (like apples, berries, oranges, and pears); vegetables (like cucumbers, carrots, and celery); beans and legumes (like peas and lentils); nuts; and seeds. Psyllium–a plant–is also a source of soluble fiber and is found in over-the-counter supplements like Metamucil.

Insoluble fiber doesn't dissolve in water. It adds bulk to your diet (needed to prevent constipation) because it passes through your digestive system intact. Unlike soluble fiber, insoluble fiber speeds up the passage of your food through the digestive system.

Healthy sources of insoluble fiber include vegetables (like broccoli, cabbage, carrots, and zucchini); whole grains (like wheat bran, whole wheat, barley, bulgur, and brown rice); the skins of fruit (like apples and pears); and nuts and seeds.

Essential Nutrients

Essential nutrients are vitamins, minerals, fatty acids, and amino acids that keep us healthy. Because your body doesn't manufacture them, they have to come from outside sources such as fruits, veggies, grains, nuts, and other natural foods. You can also get them from fortified foods such as milk, orange juice, and bread, as well as from supplements.

Here's a list of the essential nutrients, what they do, and the healthful foods that are rich in them. Unless your doctor tells you to take a multivitamin or specific nutrients in supplement or liquid form, we recommend that you get your nutrients from whole-food sources.

Vitamins

Vitamins A, B, C, D, E, and K are all needed for metabolism, and several (vitamins A, C, and E) contain antioxidants, substances that protect cells from damage caused by free radicals (see "Antioxidants to the Rescue!" on page 186).

- **Vitamin A** is important for good vision, a strong immune system, and healthy skin. In clinical studies, fenretinide (a type of vitamin A called a retinoid) is being studied specifically for its anticancer

should you take dietary supplements?

After all you've heard about the importance of nutrients, you're probably wondering whether or not it's wise to take supplements during your breast cancer journey. Supplements may help, but they may not, so it's important to talk your doctor or nutrition expert about supplements you're currently taking and the ones you're thinking about taking.

- High-dose antioxidant supplements may be linked to health risks and may interfere with your breast cancer treatments. For example, supplementing with high doses of beta-carotene may increase the risk of lung cancer in smokers. Supplementing with high doses of vitamin E may increase risks of prostate cancer and stroke.[33]

- Information about supplements may not be complete or reliable. And they can interact with medications and other supplements.

- The word *natural* on a label does not always mean *safe*. For example, the herbs comfrey and kava may cause liver damage.

- The term *standardized* (or *verified* or *certified*) does not guarantee product quality or consistency.

- Herbal supplements may contain dozens of compounds, the active ingredients of which may not be known.

- What's on the label may not be what's in the bottle—and you may be taking less, or more, than you realize. For example, herbal supplements may not contain the correct plant species, and amounts of the active ingredient may be lower or higher than the label states.

- Some dietary supplements may be contaminated with other herbs, pesticides, or metals, or adulterated with unlabeled ingredients.[34]

properties. Scientists believe that fenretinide may help to inhibit breast cancer by allowing ceramide (a waxlike substance) to build up in tumor cells, thereby killing them. In a Phase III breast cancer prevention trial that included 15 years of follow-up, fenretinide was found to reduce the incidence of second breast malignancies in pre-menopausal women.[35]

Sources of vitamin A include cod liver oil, eggs, and plants rich in beta-carotene (which gives many fruits and vegetables their yellow or orange color) like carrots, sweet potatoes, cantaloupe, pumpkin, mangoes, kale, spinach, collard greens, and goji berries. Two points to keep in mind: Eating some fat with vitamin A–rich foods helps enhance absorption, and too much vitamin A can be toxic. Never supplement vitamin A without your doctor's advice.

- **Vitamin B** is actually a group of vitamins that play important roles in cell metabolism and division, as well as immune and nervous system function. Vitamins B_6 and B_{12} from food (not supplements) have also been shown to reduce the risk of pancreatic cancer,[36] and some clinical studies show an increased intake of vitamin B_{12} together with folate and vitamin B_6 may lower the risk of breast cancer.[37]

  There are eight distinct B vitamins (B_1, B_2, B_3, B_5, B_6, B_7, B_9, and B_{12}) that are often found in the same foods. Together, these eight are referred to as the vitamin B complex. The B vitamins are found in whole, unprocessed food like whole grains, brewer's yeast, bananas, lentils, potatoes, and beans. You can also get concentrated sources of the B vitamins in turkey, tuna, red meat, and liver. It's important to note, however, that unlike the other B vitamins, B_{12} is not available from plant sources. Therefore, vegans should consult with their doctors to determine if they need to take a supplement and, if so, in what doses.

- **Vitamin C**, also known as L-ascorbic acid or L-ascorbate, is an anti-oxidant that helps neutralize unstable oxygen molecules that might damage DNA (see "Antioxidants to the Rescue!" on page 186). It's also an essential building block of collagen, which is found in blood vessels, skin, and tissue (as well as bone). You need collagen for healthy teeth and gums and to help wounds heal, making this a crucial nutrient as you move through your recovery process.

Almost all the studies done on vitamin C and breast cancer look at its role as an antioxidant. A few studies in animals and test tubes indicate that very high blood levels of vitamin C might shrink tumors.[38] Most conclude, however, that there's not enough evidence that vitamin C can reduce a recurrence or mortality. One study did focus on high, intravenous doses of vitamin C and found that, in this case, vitamin C helped to reduce inflammation, but its effect on survival in breast cancer patients is unclear, and more studies need to be done.[39]

Because our bodies can't produce our own vitamin C, it must come from outside sources, such as citrus fruits (oranges, lemons, limes, and grapefruits), strawberries, cantaloupe, tomatoes, potatoes, cabbages, and green peppers. It's also found in fortified foods like breakfast cereals, fruit drinks, and dairy products.

- **Vitamin D** is found in cells throughout the body. Muscles need it to move, nerves need it to carry messages between the brain and every body part, and the immune system needs vitamin D to fight off invading bacteria and viruses. Your body also needs it to absorb calcium and build strong bones.

  You can get vitamin D from exposure to the sun (which is why it's called the sunshine vitamin). You can also get it from natural food sources like fatty fish (e.g., sardines, salmon, and mackerel), beef liver, and egg yolks; and from fortified foods (like milk, yogurt, orange juice, cereals, and milk substitutes such as soy milk, almond milk, and coconut milk). But it's hard to get enough vitamin D from diet alone, so discuss with your doctor whether or not you should take a vitamin D supplement.

  A growing body of research supports the theory that a vitamin D deficiency is a risk factor for breast cancer, and the vitamin may even be able to play a role in its prevention.[40] For example, one study conducted in 87 counties across the United States concluded that breast cancer patients who lived in the Northeast (where there's less sunshine year-round) had poorer breast cancer outcomes than those who lived in the Southwest.[41] The theory is that because there's less sunshine, these women had less exposure to vitamin D.

  Another study in Russia had similar results.[42] Moreover, some studies have found that breast cancer patients who got their diagnosis or began treatment in the summer or fall also had better outcomes. In this case, the researchers theorized that the benefit came from being exposed to more sunlight at the time of diagnosis.[43]

Several studies done in labs prior to actual clinical testing on women have suggested that vitamin D may prevent breast cancer development, reduce the risk of recurrence, and reduce mortality in women with early-stage breast cancer.[44] One of these studies, conducted on mice at Georgetown University Medical Center, reported that vitamin D significantly reduced development of estrogen receptor positive (ER+) breast cancer in lean and obese mice. But the vitamin didn't provide the same result in receptor negative (ER-) cancer. Additionally, when the obese mice with ER- breast cancer were given vitamin D in their diet, they fared worse than the lean ones. Lead investigator Leena Hilakivi-Clarke, PhD, cautioned that vitamin D supplementation can be tricky. That's because studies on the effect of vitamin D in different types of cancer demonstrate there's no simple connection between use and benefit.[45]

- **Vitamin E** is actually eight different compounds (alpha-, beta-, gamma-, and delta-tocopherol and alpha-, beta-, gamma-, and delta-tocotrienol), not that you need to remember all of them. What's important to know is that nuts, seeds, and vegetable oils (like wheat-germ oil) are among the best sources of vitamin E. You can also get vitamin E from green, leafy vegetables (such as spinach) and fortified cereals. It's loaded with antioxidants and, in laboratory studies, two types of vitamin E (alpha- and gamma-tocopherols) exhibited anti-inflammatory effects. It can also help wounds to heal, lower cholesterol, have a positive effect on platelets and your cardiovascular system, and act as an anti-inflammatory.

In preliminary studies, done in test tubes or culture dishes (in vitro studies), vitamin E has been shown to be involved in immune function—as well as cell signaling, regulation of gene expression, and other metabolic processes.[46] Vitamin E also seems to inhibit the activity of something called protein kinase C, an enzyme involved in cell proliferation and differentiation into smooth muscle cells, platelets, and monocytes (a type of white blood cell).[47] All are important studies that point to a potential link between vitamin E and healthy cell functioning. But to date, there isn't solid evidence that any form of vitamin E can reduce the risk of breast cancer or increase survivorship. More research definitely needs to be done.

Because high levels of vitamin E can be toxic, we strongly advise that you do not take supplements without checking first with your health-care team. Long-term use of doses higher than 400 to 800 milligrams daily can increase your risk of a stroke and cause side effects such as fatigue, dizziness, weakness, headache, blurred vision, and rashes.

- **Vitamin K** is sometimes called the clotting vitamin because it helps you form blood clots when you're wounded. Your body produces vitamin K in the large intestine and also gets it from food sources such as green tea, cruciferous vegetables, liver, soybean oil, wheat bran, yogurt, cheese, and fermented soy products like miso, *natto* (a traditional Japanese dish made from fermented soy), and tempeh.

  Studies indicate that besides clot formation, vitamin K may also reduce bone loss, decrease your risk of bone fractures, and help prevent arteries and other soft tissue from calcifying.[48] Vitamin K can help prevent osteoporosis and may be beneficial if the treatment you are on is associated with bone loss.

feeling overwhelmed?

Is your head spinning from all the nutrition information in this chapter? Go ahead, tab the page, give your eyes (and your mind) a break, and come back to the information here when you get a chance. The goal in this chapter is not to have you overhaul your diet in one day but to give you the tools to make small changes throughout your entire healing journey.

Also, feel free to jot notes in your journal or highlight interesting studies, tips, and foods throughout this chapter (this is *your* guide, after all!).

Dietary Minerals

Dietary minerals are potential allies in the fight against breast cancer. Like vitamins A, C, and E, minerals act as antioxidants that fight free radicals (unstable molecules in the body that attack cells and can trigger disease). Since our bodies don't manufacture dietary minerals, we need to get them from the plants in our diet or from supplements. Some of the key minerals include sodium, calcium, magnesium, iron, zinc, and selenium. It's important to note that excess amounts of some minerals can have a negative effect (for example, too much magnesium over time can cause kidney problems), which is just another reason to check in with your doctor or nutrition expert before adding any to your diet.

Although most studies say that more research is needed to support the use of supplemental minerals in the anticancer brigade, several have pointed to their efficacy. One study, for instance, conducted at the National Institute for Environmental Medicine in Stockholm, Sweden, looked at whether dietary selenium was associated with survival among 3,146 women diagnosed with invasive breast cancer. Researchers found that dietary selenium taken before the women's diagnosis could improve breast cancer–specific mortality as well as overall mortality.[49]

While all minerals are important to your body, we'll mention the key ones here.

- **Calcium** is the most well-known mineral, and for good reason. You need it (along with vitamin D) for strong bones and to prevent osteoporosis. Calcium is also critical for the health of your muscles, heart, and digestive system, and it supports the function of blood cells, too. Moreover, while dairy products are one of the best sources of calcium, you can also get this essential mineral from almonds and leafy greens like kale.

- **Iodine** is a key mineral used by the body to make thyroid hormones, which control the body's metabolism. It's found naturally in some foods like fish (cod and shrimp), dairy products (milk, yogurt, and cheese), and grains (breads and cereals), and it's also found in iodized salt. But iodine also plays a key role in breast tissue. For example, women with fibrocystic breast disease–characterized by lumpy, tender breasts–seem to have improved symptoms after supplementing with iodine for 6 months. High levels of iodine can cause thyroid gland inflammation and even thyroid cancer, so never supplement without talking to your doctor or nutrition expert first.

Some researchers also believe iodine plays some role in breast cancer, pointing to the fact that iodine consumption has dropped in the United States since the 1970s, and breast cancer rates have increased.[50] (Iodine was used in the processing of flour before that time; now it's not. Plus, most of the salt used in food processing today isn't iodized.) Other researchers point out that Japanese women consume 25 times more dietary iodine (thanks to eating seaweed) than North American women, and have lower breast cancer rates.[51] In one study done on rats, researchers found that adding iodine-rich seaweed to their diets delayed the onset and number of mammary tumors.[52] None of the iodine research is conclusive, however; all scientists agree that more research needs to be done.

- **Iron** is critical to pretty much everything your cells do in your body. For example, it carries oxygen from your lungs throughout your body, and it helps your muscles store and use oxygen. If you don't get enough iron, every part of your body is affected, and you can develop iron deficiency anemia, which can cause even more fatigue than you already may be feeling right now. But don't rush to supplement just yet (and definitely not before you discuss it with your health-care team).

  Several studies point to the risks associated with too much iron in the body. Research published in the journal *Lancet Oncology* suggests that high iron levels in the body after menopause actually correspond to an increased rate of breast cancer.[53] Another study found that high quantities of iron in breast tissue in women who already had fibrocystic changes may cause tissue changes that lead to malignant breast tumors.[54]

- **Selenium** is a key antioxidant that's vital to immune system function. It works in conjunction with other vitamins and minerals to prevent free-radical damage to the body. It's found in Brazil nuts, sunflower seeds, fish (like sardines and salmon), meat (like beef, liver, pork, chicken, and turkey), eggs, mushrooms, brown rice, and onions.

There have been numerous studies conducted on selenium and cancer.[55] In one study published in the *Journal of the American Medical Association*, men and women taking selenium supplements for 10 years had 41 percent less total cancer than those who didn't take the supplement.[56] And with regards to breast cancer specifically, one study found that women who carry a mutation of the BRCA1 gene had more chromosome breaks (in the most simple terms, these are fragile areas in a cell's DNA that physically break and don't heal back together correctly[57]) than women who did not carry the mutation. When women with the BRCA1 mutation were given selenium for 3 months, the number of their chromosome breaks was reduced to normal.[58]

Another study of breast cancer patients who had had a mastectomy found that their blood levels of selenium were lower than in healthy patients. But researchers also found that there was a higher concentration of selenium in the cancerous tissue. The researchers theorized that this may be a result of selenium's attempt to defend the body against the carcinogenic process.[59]

Despite the evidence in favor of selenium, still be sure to sit down with your doctor or medical nutritionist to figure out if you should be supplementing beyond what you're already getting in your diet.

• **Magnesium,** like other minerals, is essential to good health. According to the National Institutes of Health Office of Dietary Supplements, it's needed for more than 300 biochemical reactions in the body. It helps maintain normal muscle and nerve function, keeps heart rhythm steady, supports a healthy immune system, and keeps bones strong. Magnesium also helps regulate blood sugar levels and promotes normal blood pressure. About 50 percent of the body's magnesium is found in bone; the other half is found inside the cells of body tissues and organs.

You can get magnesium through whole grains, legumes like black beans, vegetables (particularly dark green, leafy vegetables like spinach, collard greens, and Swiss chard), and nuts and seeds (such as pumpkin seeds, sunflower seeds, cashews, and almonds). Researchers have found that even a slight, ongoing magnesium deficiency can lead to bone loss and may possibly even play a role in high blood pressure, cardiovascular disease, diabetes, and yes, even cancer.

A study conducted at the School of Public Health at the University of Minnesota found that diets rich in magnesium reduced the occurrence of colon cancer among women.[60] An earlier study published in the *Journal of the American Medical Association* found that women with the highest magnesium intake had a 40 percent lower risk of developing colon cancer.[61]

Magnesium was also found to help reduce hot flashes by 41 percent in breast cancer patients (a common side effect of chemotherapy and treatments that block estrogen like tamoxifen, raloxifene, and aromatase inhibitors), according to one small pilot study. The breast cancer patients increased their magnesium dosage to 800 milligrams per day, and researchers found that other symptoms of estrogen reduction like fatigue, sweating, and distress improved as a result.[62]

- **Zinc** is involved in cellular metabolism, and it plays a role in immune function (why you often find it in over-the-counter cold remedies), wound healing, cell division, and normal growth and development. Oysters are chock-full of zinc, as are meat and dark meat chicken. Certain types of seafood–like crab and lobster–are good sources. Other sources include beans such as chickpeas and kidney beans, nuts like cashews, whole grains, fortified breakfast cereals, milk, yogurt, and cheese. A deficiency in zinc can impair immune function and, in some cases, may trigger breast cancer.[63]

  In a study published in the journal *Science Signaling*, researchers found that when something goes wrong with the body's zinc delivery system (how zinc moves in and out of cells to ensure correct levels are maintained), highly aggressive forms of breast cancer can result.[64] Researchers at Pennsylvania State University reported that glands in the breast have unique zinc requirements because they have to be able to transfer high levels of zinc through breast milk during breastfeeding. When zinc is deficient, researchers concluded, cellular functioning of the breast is compromised and can result in breast cancer (and the spread of it as well).[65]

Essential Fatty Acids

These are the sources of omega-3s and omega-6s that we discussed on page 166. These essential fatty acids are critical, and studies show they may help prevent the spread of malignant cells.[66] In a study conducted by Fox Chase Cancer Center and the University of Pennsylvania, women with triple negative breast cancer seemed to particularly benefit from omega-3s. The research team found that omega-3 fatty acids and its metabolites (smaller molecules) weakened the critical mechanisms of all types of cancer cells. But that wasn't all. In the triple negative ones, it reduced the spread of the cells by a whopping 90 percent.[67]

Essential Amino Acids

These are critical to every function in the body, but they cannot be made by the body. They must be supplied through food, every day. There are nine amino acids that are considered essential: histidine, isoleucine, leucine, lysine, methionine, phenylalanine, threonine, tryptophan, and valine. Although you probably haven't heard of most of these (and you probably don't need to remember them, either), what's most important to remember is that amino acids are the building blocks of protein and are responsible for the strength, repair, and rebuilding of your body. Good sources of essential amino acids are animal sources: lean meat, eggs, and dairy. If you're a vegan, however, know that soybean protein is a complete source of essential amino acids.

Harvard University researchers analyzed data from the Nurses' Health Study, a study involving more than 121,000 women, and found that women who ate plenty of eggs while they were teenagers (between the ages of 12 and 18) were less likely to get breast cancer when they got older. Researchers theorized that eggs may reduce the risk of breast cancer because they're rich in essential amino acids, and some experts believe that diet during the teen years is critical because that's when the breasts are developing.[68]

Additional research with amino acids and breast cancer has focused on starving cancer cells of the essential amino acids they need to survive and spread. A study conducted at Georgia Regents University (formerly Georgia Health Sciences University) in Augusta found that this method worked to reduce the growth of ER+ breast cancer cells.[69]

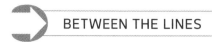

food and your mood

Eating the right food is good medicine for your body—it helps prevent heart disease, diabetes, and other chronic and life-threatening conditions like cancer. But did you know that eating walnuts as part of a healthy diet might help ease stress—and boost your mood, too?

In one study, participants followed three different diets for 6 weeks each. They were also subjected to stress either by giving a speech or immersing a foot in cold water. The results showed that when they followed a diet that included walnuts and walnut oil, their blood pressure and stress responses were lower.[70]

Mounting evidence also supports the idea that replenishing nutritional deficiencies with healthy, whole foods may help ease depression, too. For example, researchers in France and London found that 60 percent of the people with the most "northern European" eating habits (which included higher consumption of sugar, white flour, and animal fats) were more likely to suffer from depression.[71]

One reason is that more sugar, white flour, and fat can intensify inflammation processes in our bodies and brains, which causes molecules to be released that act on our neurons and influence thoughts and mood.[72] The takeaway: The negative effect of a poor diet can cause mood swings that make it difficult to cope with breast cancer.

Besides walnuts, low-fat, high-protein, high-carbohydrate snacks—such as a whole wheat or multigrain English muffin or slice of bread topped with a thin coat of honey or sugar-free jam and peanut butter—may help boost your mood. It's an antiblues recipe that allows tryptophan, an amino acid, to be transformed into serotonin, which lifts mood. More mood-boosting strategies: Eat more fish and add flaxseeds to smoothies—both are rich in omega-3 fatty acids that have been shown to have a positive effect on your mood.[73]

NOW . . . BEGIN YOUR DIET BY FILLING YOUR PLATE WITH PLANTS

Remember when your mother said, "Eat your vegetables. They're good for you," and you rolled your eyes? Turns out that she was right. All those vegetables we've been talking about, along with fruits, grains, and beans, are now considered an essential driving force behind every healthy diet. That's especially true of the green, leafy members of the cruciferous family–broccoli, cabbage, kale, collard greens, Brussels sprouts, and bok choy. In fact, because they're so full of healthful and healing nutrients, they're called superfoods.

One reason the cruciferous vegetables excel as foundational building blocks is that they're the richest source of *phytochemicals*, antioxidant compounds produced in vegetables, fruits, grains, and beans. The word *phyto* means plants, and there are over a thousand of these compounds. Although they're categorized as nonessential chemicals, meaning they're not needed to sustain life, they are very essential to your breast cancer journey.

Why Plants Are Critical

For many years, scientists have known that plants produce phytochemicals for protection. These compounds help them survive. Now studies of their effect on humans show that phytochemicals have protective or disease-preventive properties that can help us, too.

In one study, investigators examined data from the Black Women's Health Study. They discovered that the incidence of ER- breast cancer was 43 percent lower among women consuming as little as two vegetables per day compared with women who ate fewer than four per week. The conclusion: A high intake of cruciferous vegetables may be associated with a reduced risk of breast cancer in African American women–and even all women.[74]

Other studies have shown that phytochemicals can help to protect us from cancer by stopping potential carcinogens (cancer-forming substances) from forming and/or stopping carcinogens from attacking cells. They also help healthy cells not become malignant.

To add a mix of plant superfoods and phytochemicals to your diet, consult the following chart.

PHYTOCHEMICAL	FOODS IT'S FOUND IN[75]
Sulforaphane	Broccoli sprouts, broccoli, cauliflower, Brussels sprouts, savoy cabbage, red cabbage, kohlrabi, kale, collard greens, and horseradish
Isothiocyanates	Wasabi, mustard, horseradish, capers, watercress, Brussels sprouts, and other cruciferous vegetables
Phenolic compounds	Olive oil, garlic, green tea, dark plums, berries, and artichokes
Flavonoids	Most fruits, vegetables, and herbs; red beans, black beans, speckled beans; red wine; green tea; and the white pulpy inside of an orange
Organosulfides	Garlic, onion, leeks, shallots, and cruciferous vegetables
Isoflavones	Soybeans, legumes, and flaxseeds
Indoles	Cruciferous vegetables

Go Green for Better Health

Cruciferous vegetables are members of the *Brassica* genus. Cabbage, Brussels sprouts, and broccoli are ones that usually come to mind first. But cauliflower, kale, collard greens, mustard greens, arugula, watercress, bok choy, and turnips, as well as radishes, horseradish, and even wasabi (Japanese horseradish) are members of this clan, too.

Although it's important to include a variety of healthy foods in your diet, studies show that these vegetables in particular are hard to beat. That's because they're loaded with essential nutrients, such as carotenoids; vitamins C, E, and K; folate; and minerals. Additionally, they pack a good dose of fiber[76] and are also rich sources of compounds called glucosinolates.

Glucosinolates are the compounds that make several of these vegetables a bit smelly. If cooked Brussels sprouts or cabbage already plays a role in your diet, you know what we mean. More important, there's evidence that glucosinolates may play a role in breast cancer survival, too.[77]

When a team at Vanderbilt University investigated the role of cruciferous vegetables in breast cancer survival, they found that these superfoods were associated with a reduced risk for total mortality, breast cancer–specific mortality, and recurrence. And when women ate more of these vegetables, their risk of death or cancer recurrence decreased.[78]

One more amazing thing about glucosinolates: When you break up the plant cells in cruciferous vegetables by chopping, chewing, or blending them, the glucosinolates come into contact with an enzyme in the plant cells called myrosinase. A chemical reaction follows that produces isothiocyanates, which are now being studied as powerful anticancer compounds that may prevent tumors from growing.[79]

Vegetables

Cruciferous vegetables and veggies with carotenoids, as we've already discussed, may be the superstars of the plant group, but they're definitely not the only shining examples of anticancer veggies on your plate. Here are some other vegetables you can choose from.

Beans and peas (legumes). Generally, legumes are considered unique because all of them—not just soy—are excellent sources of plant protein and also provide nutrients such as iron and zinc. Because their nutrients are similar to ones that come from meats, poultry, and fish, legumes are an excellent source of protein for vegetarians.

To try: Kidney beans, pinto beans, black beans, lima beans, black-eyed peas, white beans, chickpeas, split peas, and lentils.

Resistant starch (RS). These veggies contain carbohydrates, but not the ones you hear about the most that pile on pounds, such as those in bread, pastries, pasta, and processed snacks. Those carbs cause spikes in your blood sugar that trigger chronic inflammation. No, resistant starch vegetables are actually very good for you because they can give you the sustained energy, nutrients, and fiber that you need during your treatments. In fact, even though these healthy carbs have more calories than nonstarchy members of the veggie group, they can help you to lose or maintain weight when they're part of a healthy eating plan.

To try: Corn, black-eyed peas, green bananas, green peas, green lima beans, plantains, potatoes, taro, and water chestnuts.

Others. This category sounds like a hodgepodge because it is. But among these orphaned veggies you'll find some potential anticancer stars such as garlic, which belongs to a class of bulb-shaped plants called allium. This pungent vegetable has antibacterial properties; as for its role in breast cancer, studies show that garlic may block the formation of cancer-causing substances and stop them from being activated, as well as enhance DNA repair.[80]

To try: Artichokes, asparagus, bean sprouts, beets, celery, cucumbers, eggplant, garlic, green beans, green peppers, lettuce, mushrooms, okra, onions, wax beans, and squash.

Fruits

Does an apple a day really keep the doctor away? Maybe. Along with vegetables, fruits should always be part of your anticancer diet for numerous healthful and potentially healing reasons.

In one review of studies, Korean researchers found that eating a lot of citrus fruits may reduce your risk of breast cancer by 10 percent. They noted that the evidence for dietary citrus was consistent across all the studies.[81] At the University of Arizona Cancer Center, a preclinical study of limonene (a chemical in citrus peel oil) demonstrated that it may be able to stop the growth cycle and spread of malignant cells, as well as be used for breast cancer prevention and/or treatment.[82]

But some of the best news about fruits is that they're naturally low in fat, sodium, and calories. They're also the most portable grab-and-go foods you can eat. Now, if you still need more reasons to include more fruit in your diet, check out the most enticing ones, listed below. The only caveat is to remember that even though fructose (the sugar found in fruit) is natural, too much of it (like too much of any food) can upset your stomach and the overall balance in your body.

Fruits contain many essential nutrients, such as potassium, dietary fiber, vitamin C, and folate, which is particularly important because it helps the body form red blood cells.

Fruits are loaded with dietary fiber that can help reduce cholesterol levels and provide a feeling of fullness with fewer calories. (Keep in mind that fruit juices, however, contain little or no fiber, so opt for whole fruit whenever you can.)

Fruits are an excellent source of vitamin C, which is an antioxidant that is key for the growth and repair of all body tissues, which will be important throughout your breast cancer journey.

Grains and Seeds

Although a strong relationship between eating whole grains and seeds and reducing your risk of breast cancer has not yet been established, one scientific review of studies suggests that grains and seeds may be protective because they're:

BETWEEN THE LINES

antioxidants to the rescue!

Antioxidants in food play a role in preventing breast cancer, defending the body against something called free radicals.

Here's a quick lesson in how they work: Let's start with oxygen. After we breathe it in, it travels from our lungs to every single cell, helping turn food into energy.

But oxygen can also have negative effects, whether you're healthy or not. Body cells are stable when their molecules have a full set of electrons. When oxygen enters the picture, though, these cells can lose an electron, becoming unstable or oxidized—the same chemical reaction that causes metal to rust or a cut apple to turn brown. Losing an electron to a passing oxygen molecule converts that cell's molecule to an unstable, damaging atom called a free radical.

The body's main defense against free radicals? Antioxidants—produced in the body or obtained from food sources. Their job is to donate missing electrons to free radicals and return them to normal.

Free radicals attack cells, changing their structure and function. This cellular damage is part of the aging process—and may even contribute to the development of cancer.

Free radicals can be created in the body as a result of exposure to the sun's ultraviolet light or through environmental exposure to cigarette smoke (even secondhand smoke), car exhaust, factory pollution, pesticides, and insecticides. Poor diet (not enough fruits and vegetables and/or too much fat) can lead to the production of free radicals; so can lack of sleep and stress.

But in the case of cancer, free radicals can actually help

- Concentrated sources of dietary fiber, resistant starch, and oligosaccharides—carbohydrates thought to protect against cancer
- Rich in antioxidants
- Significant sources of phytoestrogens, which are thought to be particularly important in the prevention of hormone-dependent cancers[83]

destroy cancer cells. This is how chemotherapy and radiation work, to a certain degree, which is why scientists from Memorial Sloan-Kettering Cancer Center urged that using supplemental antioxidants during chemotherapy and radiation be avoided, since they might reduce the effects of therapy, allowing cancer cells to grow instead of being destroyed.[84]

Carotenoids. Chock-full of antioxidants, carotenoids are responsible for the red, orange, and yellow coloring of tomatoes, oranges, and bananas.

Polyphenols. These are the largest antioxidant family in vegetables and fruits. They include compounds called anthocyanins, flavonols, catechins, flavones, isoflavones, and proanthocyanidins.

Anthocyanins. Responsible for the deep red, purple, black, and blue hues in raspberries, blueberries, strawberries, cherries, cranberries, and grapes, anthocyanins have shown potential in fighting breast cancer. A study at the University of Porto in Portugal found anthocyanins significantly reduced cell production within 24 hours, acting as a breast cancer inhibitor.[85]

Catechins. These antioxidants are found in green and black tea. A University of Mississippi study examined the affect of EGCG (a major green tea catechin) on breast cancer in mice and found it helps inhibit cancer cell growth.[86]

Other sources. Herbs (like cloves, cinnamon, oregano, and turmeric) are full of antioxidants, as are nuts (rich in the antioxidant vitamin E), coffee beans, and dark chocolate.

One Swedish study set out to determine the relationship between dietary fiber and postmenopausal breast cancer. The research team found that, in women who had the highest intake of dietary fiber, there was a 13 percent lower risk of breast cancer. But, according to researchers, the type of breast cancer women had made a difference. Those women who had lobular tumors seemed to get this benefit from fiber more so than those who had ductal tumors. And women who had ER- and PR- tumors seemed to see this benefit from fiber more so than those with ER+ and PR+ tumors.[87]

In 2010, a researcher in Finland who reviewed Nordic studies of rye reported evidence that rye bread and other products made from whole grain rye flour, which is rich in fiber and phytoestrogens called lignans, are likely to contribute to a reduced risk of breast cancer.[88]

And in 2013, a Canadian research team reported the results of the first study to look at flaxseed alone and breast cancer. The investigators used a questionnaire to determine how much flaxseed and flax bread 2,999 women with breast cancer and 3,370 healthy control women ate as part of the Ontario Women's Diet and Health Study. After a series of variables were factored into the data, the team found that flaxseed was associated with a significant reduction in breast cancer risk.[89]

Best Sources of Grains and Seeds

Try switching out the grains you typically eat–particularly if they're "white" unhealthier grains–for healthier varieties. For example, you can easily use brown rice as a substitute for the white kind in some of your recipes. Quinoa, which is considered a complete food, is one of the oldest sources of grains (or seeds) on the planet. It can be eaten hot or cold–and for breakfast as well as dinner. The same is true of chia seeds, which are often labeled "ancient grains." Throw them in your blender when you're making a smoothie and you'll never know these crunchy tidbits are there.

Grains and products to try include the following:

Amaranth	Bulgur (cracked wheat)
Brown rice	Chia
Buckwheat	Millet

Oatmeal	Whole wheat bread
Popcorn	Multigrain crackers
Rolled oats	Whole wheat crackers
Quinoa	Whole wheat pasta
Sorghum	Whole wheat sandwich buns and rolls
Whole grain barley	
Whole grain cornmeal	Corn tortillas
Whole rye	Whole wheat tortillas
Multigrain bread	Wild rice

What about Dairy?

If you ask several different oncologists whether dairy products are healthy additions to your diet right now, you won't get a consensus. That's because there's evidence both for and against dairy. For example, in research from the Susan G. Komen for the Cure breast cancer organization, an analysis of data from more than 20 studies found no link between dairy products and breast cancer risk.[90]

However, data from the Nurses' Health Study II says the opposite. It found that women who ate two or more servings of high-fat dairy products (like whole milk or butter) every day had a higher risk of premenopausal breast cancer.[91] Additionally, there are a growing number of other reasons to consider limiting or excluding dairy products from your diet. Some products—whole milk and many types of cheese—have a relatively high saturated fat content, which may increase your risk of breast cancer. And nonorganic dairy products may contain carcinogenic contaminants, such as pesticides, growth factors, hormones, steroids, and other additives fed to cattle. Organic dairy products may well be an option to reduce exposure to the above additives. However, there is no research proving an organic diet can keep you cancer-free. In the end, whether or not to use organic dairy products is up to your personal preference.

Due to the conflicting findings on how dairy foods affect your breast cancer risk, be sure to consult your oncologist or nutrition expert when making a decision about including dairy products in your diet.

NUTRITION CHECKLIST FOR
YOUR BREAST CANCER JOURNEY

While reading through all the nutrition advice in this chapter can be overwhelming at first, here's a simplified list of healthy-eating advice that you can follow now to help food become an agent of healing for your body.

Keep an eye on portion size. The last thing you want to do right now is gain weight. Obesity is associated with an increase in estrogen levels in the body and a greater risk for breast cancer. Always remember to check package labels to see what the serving size is. One healthy energy bar may actually be two servings at 250 calories each instead of one.

Try to eat at least five (or, if you can, nine) servings of fruits and vegetables a day. One serving is a medium fruit or half a cup. Focus on eating brightly colored vegetables and fruit (especially deep green, orange, red, and yellow ones). And try to eat berries, too, which are loaded with antioxidants. Note that frozen fruits and vegetables are healthy, too (they're flash frozen at the peak of their freshness), and are often a more economical choice than fresh.

Eat whole grains like amaranth, millet, quinoa, steel-cut oats, and brown rice. If you're eating cereal or bread, look for the words *multigrain* or *whole wheat* over *wheat flour* or *white flour.*

Always opt for fat-free or low-fat dairy products, such as milk, yogurt, cheese, or nondairy almond beverages that are fortified with calcium and vitamin D.

Be aware of sodium. Compare the sodium content in different brands of soups, breads, and processed foods you're eating. Choose products with the lowest numbers. Too much sodium in your body causes you to retain water. Since you're already at risk of lymphedema, this is one good reason to keep your daily intake to a minimum. Remember: Your body only needs 200 milligrams of sodium a day, yet 1 teaspoon of salt contains about 2,300 milligrams.

Avoid processed foods with lots of additives and/or artificial ingredients when other choices are available. A good rule of thumb: If you can't pronounce the ingredient or don't know what it is, don't eat it.

Drink water, and avoid drinks with added sugar (including soda). Sugar has been shown in studies to cause inflammation and inhibit immune functioning–which is something you don't need right now on your healing journey. Plus, too much sugar can cause weight gain, which we've already mentioned is a risk factor for breast cancer and breast cancer recurrence. Don't like the taste of plain water? Add frozen berries, cold cucumbers, or even a splash of fruit juice to it.

Eat lean protein. Skip steaks (and limit your intake of red meat), and include sources of lean protein, such as seafood, poultry, eggs, beans, peas, and unsalted nuts and seeds.

Eat seafood at least two to three times a week. Opt for fish that's high in healthy omega-3 fatty acids–like salmon, sardines, halibut, and mackerel–and low in mercury, a known neurotoxin.

Use olive oil and other oils with healthy omega-3 fatty acids (like canola oil) to replace unhealthy solid fats such as butter and lard. Omega-3s are important for breast cancer prevention (and breast cancer recurrence prevention) because they've been shown to balance estrogen levels, decrease breast cancer cell growth, and decrease spreading of breast cancer cells. They also help decrease inflammation that may be present in the body for a variety of reasons, including chemotherapy and radiation.[92]

Replace food containing saturated fat with choices that have monounsaturated and polyunsaturated fat (found in olives, olive oil, avocados, flaxseeds, walnuts, and fish oil). Some research suggests that the oleic acid found in olive oil may help reduce breast cancer risk.[93] Other studies show polyunsaturated fats can improve cholesterol levels and may help lower blood pressure.[94]

Lower your intake of dietary cholesterol. Read package labels so you can keep it to less than 300 milligrams a day. High cholesterol foods include cheeseburgers, macaroni and cheese, ice cream, steak, and liver.

Eliminate trans fats by avoiding fast food like french fries and processed foods like cookies and pastries. It's also found in solid shortening and stick margarine. (As of 2006, food manufacturers have been required by the FDA to list trans fats on food labels.[95]) One study of 25,000 women found that women who had the highest levels of trans fats in their blood were about twice as likely as women with the lowest trans fat levels to develop breast cancer.[96]

 Scan here or visit prevention.com/ugbcrecipes for fresh, fast, and delicious recipes that meet these guidelines.

CHAPTER 10

THE EXERCISE PRESCRIPTION

Are you tempted to skip exercise on your journey to recovery? Is it one of the last things that you want to do right now? If so, that's understandable, especially if you're out of sorts from bouts of fatigue and other side effects–or feeling stressed or depressed. But exercise may be one of the best things you can do for your health and future.

Research conducted as part of the large Nurses' Health Study and published in the *Journal of the American Medical Association* shows the importance of exercise, even at low levels, for survivors. The researchers followed 2,987 female registered nurses until 2002; all had been diagnosed with stage I, II, or III breast cancer between 1984 and 1998. They found that the women who exercised 3 to 5 hours a week had better survival rates than their sedentary counterparts. To their surprise, the women who worked out the longest or hardest came up short. Instead, it was the nurses who did lower-intensity activities (the equivalent of walking at a 2 to 2.9 mph pace for an hour) who saw the best survival numbers.[1]

Exercise isn't the only risk-reducing factor you have control over. Investigators at the University of California San Diego Moores Cancer Center found that eating a healthy diet and exercising moderately helped survivors cut their risk of dying in half, regardless of their weight. The study looked at 1,490 women who were 70 or younger, had been diagnosed with early-stage breast cancer, and had completed their primary treatment. Researchers tracked their diet and physical activity for between 5 and 11 years. The results showed that even over-weight survivors who ate at least five servings of vegetables and fruit a day and walked briskly for 30 minutes, 6 days a week, reaped the full benefit. (Unfortunately, it was only the women who took up both healthy habits who saw the significant reduction in mortality risk.)[2]

We could list study after study showing similar results (just keep reading), which is why our goal in this chapter is to encourage and inspire you to start–or continue–exercising, whether you're in the middle of treatment or moving on with your life. We'll explain what to keep in mind, whom to talk to, and how to go about being active again.

To make it easier for you, we've included workout plans that can be done during treatment or recovery (with your doctor's okay, of course). We've even added options for people who are less mobile and/or just starting out. Now let's get going so you can start feeling better today.

EXERCISE GETS A GREEN LIGHT

Reducing your risk of dying or suffering a recurrence of cancer is a big deal, but exercise impacts patients' lives in many other positive ways, day in and day out. Recent research has shown that working out also helps breast cancer patients and survivors deal with fatigue and nausea; improves their strength, flexibility, balance, stamina, and emotional well-being; and helps them manage their weight. Here's some more good news.

Better Quality of Life

A review of 40 controlled clinical trials with 3,694 cancer patients (including women with breast cancer) analyzed the impact of activities like resistance training, walking, biking, yoga, qigong, and tai chi on patients' lives. In every study, the participants were randomly assigned to either exercise or nonexercise (control) groups. The people who worked out consistently reported improved quality of life and said they were bet-ter able to deal with issues related to:

- Body image
- Self-esteem
- Social interactions
- Sleeplessness

- Sexuality
- Anxiety
- Fatigue
- Pain[3]

Improved Self-Esteem

In a study at Southern Connecticut State University in New Haven, 45 women with breast cancer who had been diagnosed within the previous 2 years participated in an individualized exercise program that included both strength and cardiovascular activities. Investigators conducted in-depth interviews to determine how the women perceived exercise at various stages of the program. All the participants–whether they were in the middle of treatment or had entered recovery–credited the program with helping them feel better, regain control, and move forward.[4]

Reduced Anxiety

A review of 56 studies involving 4,800 patients before, during, or after treatment for a variety of cancers again compared active and inactive groups. (Activities included walking, resistance training, cycling, yoga, and qigong.) The exercise group fared better than the sedentary group. In some cases, moderate to vigorous exercise prompted more impressive results than lower-intensity activities. Researchers concluded that exercise may have beneficial effects on a cancer patient's quality of life, physical and social functioning, and fatigue. (Breast cancer survivors in particular experienced a greater reduction in anxiety with exercise than other cancer patients did.)[5]

IS EXERCISE SAFE RIGHT NOW?

No doubt there have been many times since your diagnosis when you've been in pain both physically and emotionally. Maybe just thinking about exercise makes you wince. But more important, you may be wondering whether working out is safe. In the past, physicians cautioned cancer patients to avoid exercise; they worried it would be too taxing and cause more harm than good. Today, the medical community's recommendation is a resounding "Go for it!" Be sure to talk to your doctor about whether this is the right time for you to get started.

"Because so much has happened since you got your diagnosis, you may already feel like you're running a marathon, just to get through treatment and recovery," says Mary Gemignani, MD, MPH, a breast surgeon and our lead physician for this guide. "Your main goal now is just to be more active. Exercise shouldn't make you feel run down, so whatever your level of fitness is or was, start slowly."

Because everyone's situation is different, it's very important to speak with your oncologist before you start a fitness program. He will consider the following factors before clearing you to exercise or establishing activity restrictions.

- The type of surgery you had—lumpectomy, mastectomy, removal of lymph nodes, or reconstructive surgery
- Treatments, such as radiation and chemotherapy
- Medications
- Side effects and other problems, such as tender areas, fatigue, or lymphedema (see page 197)

KNOW THE GUIDELINES

While experts now routinely recommend exercising during and after cancer treatment, it's still not clear if there's an optimal type or amount patients should do, so the common advice is: Do what you can tolerate. Most workout prescriptions for breast cancer patients have followed guidelines established for the general population by the American College of Sports Medicine (ACSM), an organization that promotes exercise and certifies and educates fitness professionals. Based on an extensive review of the relevant research, the ACSM, in conjunction with other health organizations, says the following exercise guidelines are "generally appropriate" for both patients and survivors.[6] However, your program should be tailored to your individual situation in cooperation with your health-care team. Naturally, you should gradually build up to these numbers—they're a goal to aim for, not a starting point. The overarching message is to avoid inactivity, and do what you can.

Do 30 minutes of exercise, 5 days a week. You want to accumulate 150 minutes per week of moderate-intensity aerobic exercise (a level where you can maintain a conversation as you work out).

Alternatively, accumulate 75 minutes of vigorous exercise per week, or do a combination of moderate and vigorous exercise. That's a level where you can only say a few words with each breath.

Perform resistance training twice a week. Strength (or resistance) training builds strength and bone density. Chemotherapy can cause women to lose bone density, which is why this type of exercise is particularly important for survivors. It may also help with lymphedema (see "Good News for Lymphedema Patients").

Stretch after your workouts or at least two or three times a week.

Because everyone responds differently to cancer treatments, you may need to modify your exercise plans on "down" days, such as after radiation or chemotherapy, when you're extremely fatigued or experiencing vomiting or diarrhea. Although current research suggests you can exercise safely during chemotherapy or radiation, it's wise to wait until after you've gone through at least one round, so you have an idea of how you respond.

The ACSM has also established some cautionary exercise recommendations specifically for cancer patients.

Exercise with a partner, caregiver, or exercise professional for safety reasons when possible.

Avoid public fitness facilities, where there may be an increased risk of exposure to viruses and bacteria. This is particularly important if you're going through chemotherapy or radiation or have had lymph nodes removed. All increase your risk of infection.

Avoid swimming and hot tubs if you have an active in-dwelling catheter (a tube that goes into the body), such as a central venous catheter or a peripherally inserted central catheter.

Stop exercising and contact your doctor if you have any of the following symptoms during exercise or after a workout.

- Disorientation, dizziness, blurred vision, or fainting
- Sudden onset of nausea or vomiting
- Unusual or sudden shortness of breath
- Irregular heart rate, palpitations, or chest pain
- Leg or calf, bone, or unusual joint pain or pain not caused by a previous injury
- Muscle cramps or sudden onset of muscular weakness or fatigue

good news for lymphedema patients

Lymphedema (blockage of, or damage to, the lymph vessels that causes swelling) is a potentially debilitating side effect of treatment; built-up fluid in the affected arm can be painful and make it difficult and frustrating to perform everyday tasks. It's reasonable to wonder whether exercise, especially resistance training moves, can worsen it.

But recent research shows that lymphedema patients *should* exercise. The Physical Activity and Lymphedema (PAL) study published in the *New England Journal of Medicine* concluded that slowly progressive weight lifting did not aggravate limb swelling among breast cancer survivors with lymphedema. In fact, after a year of supervised weight training, participants had increased strength and fewer flare-ups and symptoms than people who didn't exercise.[7]

Kathryn Schmitz, PhD, MPH, the PAL lead investigator, believes women with lymphedema should not have to spend the rest of their lives avoiding activities that might overtax their arms. Instead, through weight training and other forms of exercise, they can very slowly increase the amount of stress the affected arm can handle. She cautions to just be smart about how you use your arm and exercise common sense.[8]

If you have lymphedema and would like to start an exercise program, ask someone on your health-care team for a referral to a specialist (a physical medicine doctor, physical therapist, occupational therapist, nurse, or massage therapist) who has been trained in lymphedema management and breast cancer rehabilitation.[9] You want to follow an exercise plan that has been designed with specific guidelines in mind, which might include wearing a compression garment on the affected arm.

READY, SET, MOVE!

After reading about the benefits of exercising during and after cancer treatment–and how to do it safely–we hope you're motivated to get moving. While you may have a goal of someday entering a triathlon or running a marathon, your main plan now should be getting your body used to being active again. Some of you will have an easier time with this than others, but it's not a competition and there's no one right way to do it; baby steps are fine.

If you're an exercise veteran, you're probably missing all the positive side effects of your daily fitness regimen. But don't let your eagerness to get back in the game hurt you: You have to pace yourself and gradually build up to where you left off. The tennis court, golf course, or running path will still be there when you make it back!

easy and inexpensive ways to get moving

You don't have to have a gym membership or invest in pricey exercise equipment to start being more active. You can make your everyday errands, chores, and activities pay bigger health and healing benefits, no equipment required.

Park farther away from the store or mall and walk instead of circling the parking lot to get a spot up front. If you're not up for walking that far yet, pull in just a few spaces back from where you normally would and gradually move away as you feel better.

Take the stairs, at least a flight or two, instead of the elevator.

Rake, pull weeds, and plant in your yard. All are effective forms of exercise that can burn 80-plus calories in just 30 minutes. Squatting and lifting will help strengthen your legs, arms, and back. (If you've had lymph nodes removed, wear gloves to avoid cuts and potential infections.)

For those of you who may be unfamiliar with exercise, here's a quick primer on three must-have aspects of any well-rounded fitness program. You may naturally gravitate to one of them, but ideally you should include activities from all three each week.

Flexibility Exercise

Stretching, yoga, tai chi, qigong, and even Pilates tend to be low intensity, and they help improve your flexibility, balance, and mobility—all important factors for returning to "normal" life again. Yoga and Pilates can be very challenging, but they don't have to be; there are easy options (see page 220 for some basic yoga *asanas*, or moves).

Start mopping, sweeping, scrubbing, or dusting. But first, cue up some music that makes you want to move. Studies have shown music can make you exercise harder and longer—so your home should be spotless!

Add some calf raises (rise up and down on your toes) when you're cooking or brushing your teeth. Or do squats as you're standing there. You can even practice standing on one leg at a time to improve your balance.

Add some exercise to commercial breaks while you're watching TV. Stand up and then squat down until your hips hit the couch (or just go as low as you can); rise up again and repeat. Do up to 10 squats during each break.

Take a walk during breaks at work. And see if you can talk your coworkers into doing informal meetings on walks.

Aerobic Exercise

These invigorating activities are often referred to as "cardio" due to their heart-healthy benefits. They're crucial for helping you maintain your weight or shed extra pounds. (Breast cancer patients often gain weight during treatment.) Because cardio exercise is often done at a moderate intensity or harder, always start slowly and gradually increase your effort

keep track of your progress

Whenever you start something new on your healing journey, it's good to write it in your breast cancer journal. Many women find that keeping a record of their workouts, however brief, helps them reflect on their progress, meet goals, and stay motivated.

There are all kinds of gadgets and apps that record exercise-related data for you if you're not a journal kind of person. A pedometer is inexpensive and easy to use, and it records your steps, distance, and sometimes calories burned—helpful feedback that can motivate you to add a few more steps to your day. Find one at your local pharmacy or sporting goods store.

Of course, there's also an app for all this. Smartphones often have GPS technology and accelerometers built in so you can use a pedometer app to track your steps, mileage, speed, and even your route. Apps like RunKeeper (runkeeper.com) allow you to set goals, do interval training (where you alternate doing more intense work with recovery periods), and see graphs of your progress and other information online.

Finally, there is a growing number of sophisticated (and pricier) gadgets that, besides tracking your steps and general daily activity, also analyze how well you slept and let you log your calorie intake. Some even prompt you to move if you've been sitting too long.

as you get stronger. Some popular aerobic options are:

- Walking (stride right with the beginner-friendly plan on page 219)
- Jogging or running
- Swimming
- Dancing
- Biking
- Hiking
- Circuit training (a combo of aerobic exercise and resistance training)

Resistance Training

Resistance, or strength, training with free weights, resistance bands, or even your own body weight is hugely important because it helps you rebuild muscles that have been weakened through weeks of recuperation and inactivity. Muscle also helps elevate your metabolism, which can give you the upper hand in managing your weight. A comprehensive strength-training program should target muscles in your entire body, including your arms, chest, back, abdominals, glutes (your butt muscles) and hips, and legs (see an example on page 211). Before doing upper-body exercises, though, you should consider any restrictions you have due to surgery or other treatments. In many cases, you might want to wait until the acute phase of your treatment (when you're undergoing surgery, chemotherapy, and/or radiation) is complete before embarking on a strength program. Once you're cleared to do total-body strength exercises, you may want to seek advice from a certified personal trainer who has experience working with breast cancer patients. You can find a certified cancer exercise trainer, who must have a minimum of 10,000 hours of training, through the American College of Sports Medicine at members.acsm.org/source/custom/online_locator/onlinelocator.cfm.

FEEL-BETTER WORKOUTS

To take some of the guesswork out of exercise, we've put together some start-to-finish strength and cardio workouts that you can do at home with minimal equipment. The moves are safe, easy to figure out, and developed by our fitness experts. By the time you finish your journey to recovery, you'll have built (or reestablished) a strong foundation that will make it easier to stick with a healthy exercise habit for life.

The following routines have been designed for you to do as you're going through treatment or recovery, but only if you've been cleared to do resistance-training moves by your oncologist. And always listen to your body–and progress slowly.

How they work: Do these workouts once or twice a week, but not on back-to-back days. Perform one or two sets of 8 to 12 repetitions of each move in order, unless otherwise noted. Rest for as long as necessary between sets. If you're not supposed to do upper-body exercises yet or use any weight, do the starred (*) exercises without weights, follow the modification, or just skip the arms part. Always warm up your body for a few minutes first with some light exercise, such as walking or marching in place, and take some time at the end of the workout to stretch the muscles you've worked. If anything hurts (a muscle "burn" is normal, sharp pain is not), stop doing the exercise. Most of all, try to enjoy yourself! Moving is a gift to treasure.

Tools you'll need: Some of the exercises call for a set of light dumbbells or a broomstick, but they're not mandatory. Start with the lightest weight available, maybe just 1 or 2 pounds; you can also use soup cans or water bottles. (Check with your doctor about the amount of weight you're allowed to lift; she may not want you to go above 10 pounds.) Add a pound every 2 or 3 weeks as you get stronger.

To make it more challenging: If you're ready to work up more of a sweat, do the moves in circuit format, performing one set of each exercise in order and resting for 30 seconds to a minute between sets (rest as long as it takes for your breathing to return to normal). Once you've completed one circuit, do it again.

WORKOUT #1: FATIGUE FIGHTER

The following routine is safe to do during treatment to boost your energy and minimize fatigue. Follow any restrictions established by your doctor and take it slow.

1. PLIÉ SQUAT

WORKS LEGS AND GLUTES

Stand with your feet wide, toes turned out, with hands on your hips. Lower into a squat, bending your knees about 45 degrees and keeping them aligned with your middle toes (don't let them angle in). More advanced exercisers can bend knees up to 90 degrees. Squeeze your glutes as you straighten your legs to return to the starting position, then repeat.

Make it easier: Stand with your feet shoulder-width apart and squat halfway, bending your knees as if you're going to sit in a chair behind you.

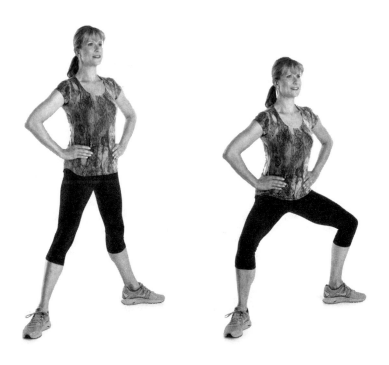

2. BIRD DOG*

Get on the floor on all fours, hands aligned under your shoulders and knees under your hips. Pull your abs in toward your spine. Slowly extend your left arm forward and right leg back, so both are parallel to the floor. Find your balance, then slowly lower them and switch sides, extending your right arm and left leg to complete 1 rep.

Make it easier: Raise either one arm or one leg at a time, not both.

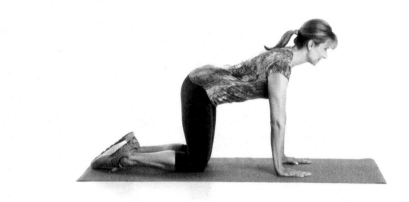

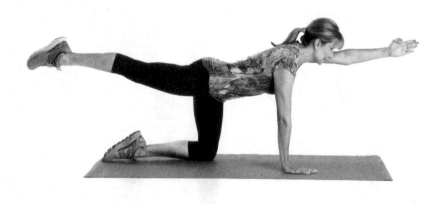

3. SPEED SKATER*

Hold a light dumbbell in each hand at your sides, palms facing forward, and stand with your feet shoulder-width apart, knees bent 45 degrees. Extend your right leg out to the side, then shift your weight over to your right leg as you curl the weights to your shoulders. Bring your left leg in next to the right, knees still bent, and lower your arms. Extend your left leg out to the left and shift your weight over to the left as you curl the weights to your shoulders again on the next rep. Continue shifting from right to left as you lift and lower the weights.

Make it easier: Take out the arm part or don't use any weight.

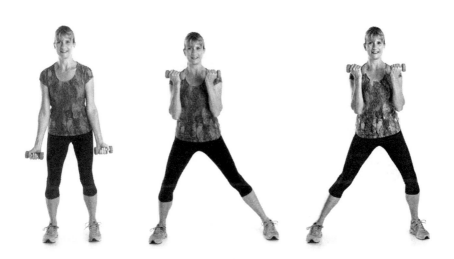

4. ONE-ARM ROW*

Stand with your feet staggered, left in front of right, and hold a very light dumbbell in your right hand. Keeping your back straight, lean forward from your hips and rest your left hand on your left thigh. Extend your right arm straight down, palm facing left. Bend your elbow and draw your right hand toward your rib cage so your elbow rises above your back. Lower the weight and repeat. Switch sides to complete the set.

Make it easier: Don't use any weight.

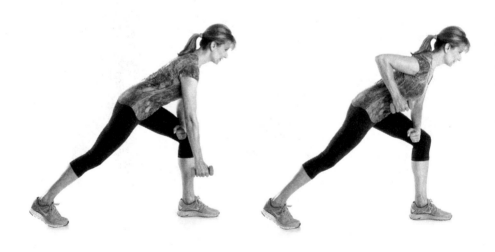

5. TREE FLOW*

WORKS GLUTES AND CORE; BUILDS BALANCE

Balance on your left leg as you place your right foot softly against your lower calf; stand as tall as you can so you don't sink down into your left hip. Extend your arms out to the sides and find your balance (focusing on a spot on the floor or wall will help you stay stable). Bring your left arm down to your left side as you raise your right arm overhead. Switch arms. Do 12 reps, then switch legs and repeat.

Make it easier: Take out the arms, and just balance for 30 seconds to a minute per leg.

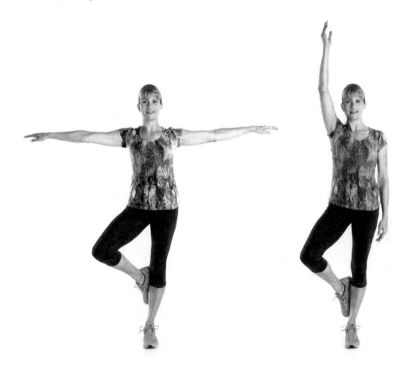

6. WALL PRESS*

Stand a foot or so from a wall and place your palms on the wall so the tips of your fingers are at chest level (the rest of your hands will be slightly below chest level). Bend your elbows and lower your chest toward the wall, keeping your arms tight to your body instead of letting your elbows flare out to the sides. Straighten your arms and repeat.

Make it easier: Only bend elbows about 45 degrees.

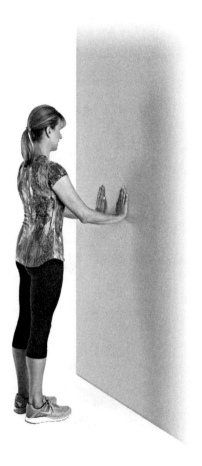
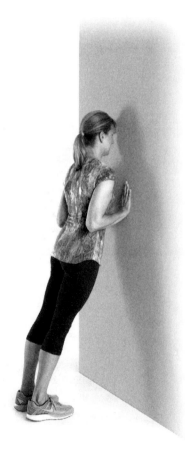

7. BRIDGE*

Hold a light dumbbell in each hand and lie faceup with your knees bent and feet flat. Extend your arms out to the sides at shoulder height, palms turned up. Lift your hips, squeezing your glutes tightly, as you raise your arms and bring the weights together over your chest. Lower your hips and arms to within an inch of the floor and repeat.

Make it easier: Take out the arm part or don't use any weight.

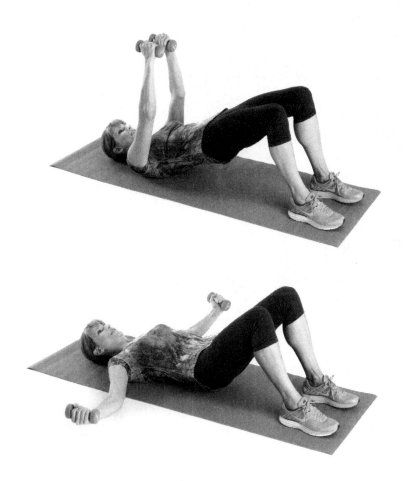

8. SIDE SWEEP*

Sit tall on the floor with your legs wide and straight. Extend your arms out to the sides. Turn to the right and lean over to the side as you contract the right side of your abs tightly. Sit tall again, and repeat to the left side on the next rep.

Make it easier: Clasp your hands in front of your chest and keep your arms tucked close as you turn.

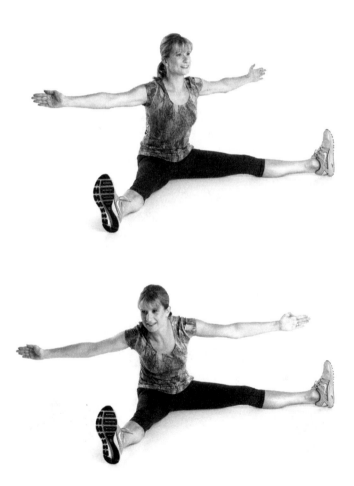

WORKOUT #2:
RECOVER AND REJUVENATE

The following workout is safe to do during recovery to strengthen muscles in your entire body and either get you started on a lifetime habit of exercising or help you return to your previous routine. Follow any restrictions established by your doctor, and take it slow.

1. TWISTING LUNGE*

WORKS LEGS, GLUTES, SHOULDERS, AND CORE

Hold a single light dumbbell with both hands, one on each end of the weight, directly in front of your chest. Lunge back with your left leg and lower until your front thigh is parallel to the floor (or just go as low as you can). As you lunge, rotate your upper body and arms to the right. Return to the starting position, and repeat on the opposite side (lunge back with your right leg and rotate your upper body to the left) on the next rep.

Make it easier: Don't use any weights, or stay in the lunge and rise up and down as you twist to one side then back to the center. Don't bend your knees as far.

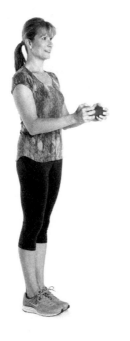
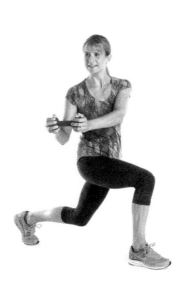

2. PLANK*

Get in a pushup position on the floor with your hands aligned under your shoulders and knees and toes on the floor. Lift your knees so your body is straight from head to heels, and hold for up to 30 seconds. (It's okay if you can only hold it for 5 seconds to start; you can build up!) Rest for a minute and then repeat once. To make it more challenging, raise one leg or arm at a time for a few seconds.

Make it easier: Do this on your knees.

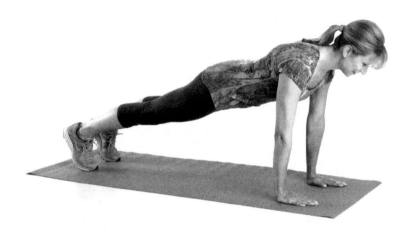

3. SQUAT TO RAISE*

WORKS LEGS, GLUTES, AND SHOULDERS

Stand with your feet shoulder-width apart and hold a single light dumbbell with both hands, one on each end of the weight, in front of your hips. Squat, bending your knees as if you're going to sit in a chair behind you, as you bring the weight to the outside of your right knee. Straighten your legs as you raise your arms up and over to the left. Return to the squat and repeat. Switch sides with the arms halfway through the set (lower weight to the left side as you squat).

Make it easier: Don't squat as low, use less weight, or take out the arm part.

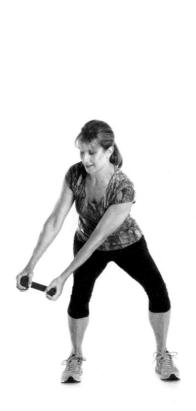
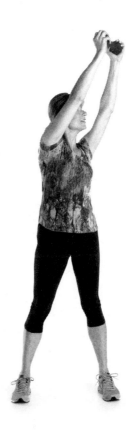

4. DIP*

Sit on the edge of a sturdy chair or bench with your hands gripping the sides and your legs extended halfway so your knees are somewhat bent (the straighter your legs, the more challenging the move). Straighten your arms and shift your hips forward. Keeping your hips close to the bench, bend your elbows behind you and lower your hips a few inches toward the floor. Straighten your arms and repeat.

Make it easier: Do this on the floor with your hands behind you.

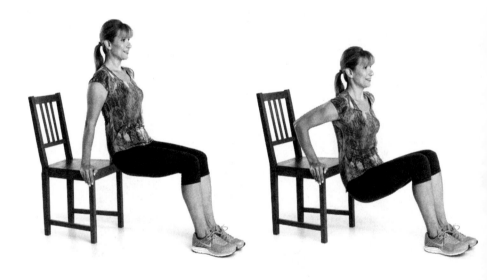

5. BROOMSTICK ROW*

Sit tall on the floor and hold a broomstick or some other stick with your hands shoulder-width apart, palms facing down. (If you don't have a broom or stick, you can fake it and just pretend you do.) Bend your knees, raise your feet a few inches off the floor, sit back about 30 degrees, and hold the stick in front of your chest so it's parallel to the floor. Turn to the right as you bring the right end of the stick toward the floor, as if you were rowing. Return to the center and turn to the left, lowering the left end of the stick toward the floor, to complete 1 rep. Alternate sides.

Make it easier: Keep your feet on the floor.

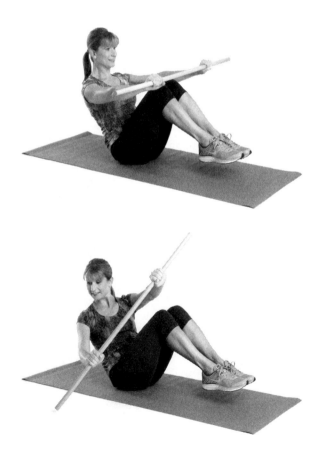

6. BENT-OVER ROW*

Hold a dumbbell in each hand and stand with your feet shoulder-width apart. Bend forward from your hips, keeping your back straight, and extend your arms straight down, palms facing each other. Keeping your torso still, draw your hands toward your rib cage so your elbows rise above your back. Hold for a count, squeezing your shoulder blades together, then lower your arms and repeat.

Make it easier: Do it without the weight or lift one arm at a time.

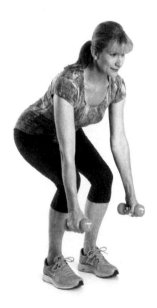 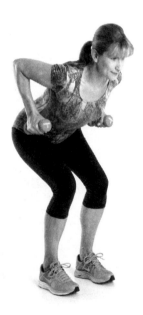

7. STANDING CRUNCH*

Stand with your feet shoulder-width apart, toes slightly turned out and knees bent. Bend your elbows so your hands are in fists next to your chin (boxing position). Shift your weight to your left leg and point your right toes so they're barely touching the floor. Turn your upper body and your arms to the right as you raise your right knee toward your left elbow. Do 12 reps, then switch sides and repeat.

Make it easier: Leave both feet on the floor, and do a standing side crunch with your upper body.

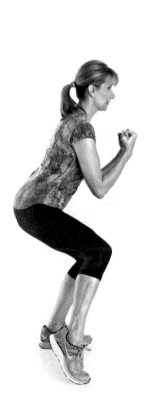
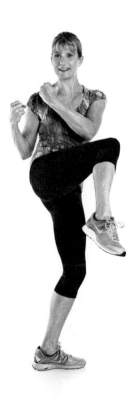

8. PUSHUP

WORKS CHEST, TRICEPS, AND CORE

Get in a pushup position on the floor with your hands aligned under your shoulders and your knees and toes on the floor. Lift your knees so your body is straight from head to heels. Bend your elbows up to 90 degrees and lower your chest toward the floor (angle your elbows in slightly toward your body, not straight out to the sides). Press up and repeat.

Make it easier: Keep your knees on the floor; don't bend your elbows as far.

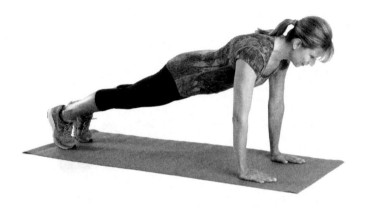

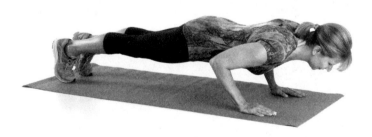

WORKOUT #3:
WALK YOUR WAY HEALTHY

Walking is one of the easiest ways to regain or improve your health. Barring injuries, anyone can do it, and you can alter it to suit almost any fitness level. (Speed walking can be more challenging than running!) When it comes down to it, though, you probably just want a workout that's invigorating and not intimidating, and walking is it!

Follow this 30-minute routine outdoors or on a treadmill, and you'll be amazed how quickly your strength and stamina start to return. If you don't feel up to doing the slightly harder walking bouts here—or walking for 30 minutes—just maintain your pace and back off whenever you need to; you're in the driver's seat. Also, a somewhat hard pace isn't breathless. You should be breathing heavier but still able to maintain your activity. (Don't be surprised if you get winded a lot faster than you used to; that's perfectly normal.) One note: Because you'll be adjusting your intensity using the rate of perceived exertion, or RPE, scale (from 1 to 10, 1 being sitting on the couch and 10 being sprinting for a bus), you can adapt this workout to any cardio activity.

TIME (MINUTES)	WHAT TO DO	INTENSITY	RPE (1–10)
0–5:00	Warm up with easy walking.	Light	3–4
5:00–10:00	Walk at a moderate pace.	Moderate	5 (you can maintain a conversation)
10:00–10:30	Increase your pace slightly or go uphill.	Moderate to somewhat hard	5–6
10:30–12:00	Recover at an easy pace.	Light	4–5
12:00–20:00	Repeat the hard-easy pattern (30 seconds hard, 90 seconds easy) four times.	Hard to somewhat easy	4–6
20:00–27:00	Walk at a moderate pace.	Moderate	5
27:00–30:00	Cool down easy.	Light	3

LIMBER UP WITH YOGA

There are many different styles of yoga–Ashtanga, Bikram, Iyengar, Kundalini, Anusara, and Yin are just a few examples–but the end result is almost always the same: a stronger, more flexible body and improved posture. Besides helping you be more active, yoga is also an excellent way to combat stress, fatigue, sleep problems, and depression. Do any of those sound familiar right now? Try these four basic moves to strengthen and stretch your large leg muscles while calming your brain. Think of it as a big "aaahh" for body and mind. You can do these daily if you want, whenever you need to chill out.

1. WARRIOR

Stand with your feet hip-width apart, arms at your sides. Take a big step back with your right leg, turning toes out slightly, and lower into a lunge; your hips will open to the right. Raise your arms parallel to the floor, left arm forward and right arm back, palms turned down. Look forward over your left arm. Make sure your front knee is aligned over your ankle. Pull your shoulders down and try to reach forward and back through your fingertips as you take five deep breaths from your belly. Switch sides and repeat.

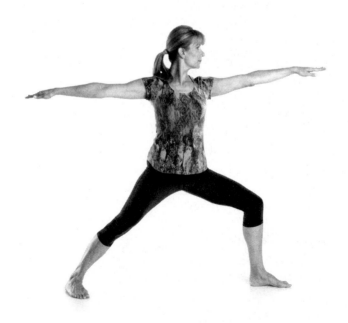

2. TRIANGLE

From Warrior, rise up with your arms still extended and straighten your legs. Step your rear foot a few inches closer to the front foot if necessary and shift your hips back slightly. Bend over from the hips and rest your left hand on your shin or ankle (not the knee) as you extend your right arm straight up; legs remain straight. Look up at your right arm and take five deep breaths from your belly. Switch sides and repeat.

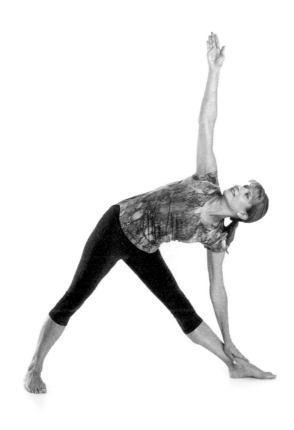

3. CHAIR

Rise up from Triangle and step your feet together so your big toes are touching. Extend your arms overhead, palms facing each other—not touching—then lower into a squat (only go as far as you can). Hold here and take five deep breaths from your belly.

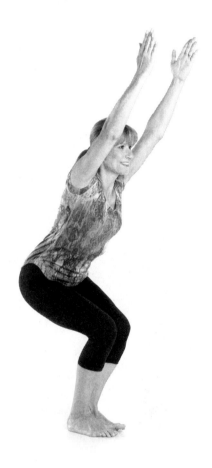

4. SEATED TWIST

Sit tall on the floor with your legs extended. Bend your right knee and place your foot on the floor as close to your hips as you can, toes pointing forward and knee up. Turn to the right, reaching back with your right hand, and rest the back of your left arm against your right thigh, so your arm is bent and fingers point up. Look behind you and take five deep breaths from your belly. Switch sides and repeat.

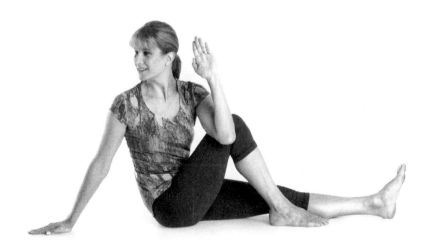

NOT FEELING YOUR BEST?
YOU CAN STILL EXERCISE!

Keep your muscles moving even when you're not ready for a full workout. You can do the Bridge and Side Sweep from Workout #1 in addition to these exercises to keep your muscles moving. One tip: Focus intently on the muscles you're working to increase the strengthening effect.

1. LEG SLIDE

WORKS HAMSTRINGS AND QUADRICEPS

Lie faceup with your arms at your sides and legs straight. Press your heels into the floor and drag them toward your hips (you can lift your hips slightly if you want); press them into the floor again as you extend your legs out straight (wearing socks will make it easier to slide your feet). If you can only go a few inches in each direction, that's a good start. If the floor is too uncomfortable, this move can be done on your mattress. Do 10 reps in and out.

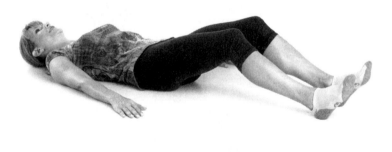

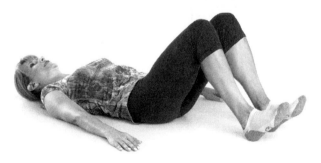

2. SEMICIRCLE CRUNCH

WORKS ABS

Lie faceup with your knees bent and feet flat and place your hands lightly behind your head, elbows wide. You're going to make a 180-degree arc with your upper body: Pull your belly button in as you lift your head and shoulder blades up and over to the right, then straight up, then bring them over to the left. Return to the starting position and repeat, moving left to right this time on the next rep.

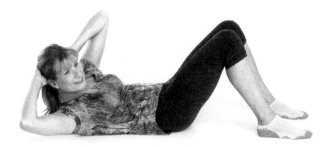

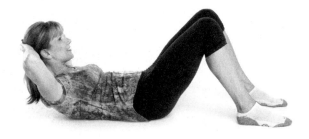

3. BACK AND BELLY COMBO

WORKS CORE AND BACK

Lying flat with your hands palms down at your sides, pull your belly button in toward your spine, as if you were slipping on your tightest pair of jeans. Hold for 5 counts and then release; repeat 5 times. Next, press your arms into the floor (or mattress), keeping your elbows straight. Hold for 5 counts and then release; repeat 5 times.

SEATED WORKOUT

If you're not quite steady enough to stand up and exercise, use these moves to keep your body strong. (Instead of doing the Dips in Workout #2, just straighten your arms and hover your hips above the chair for up to 3 counts; repeat 4 times.) Again, keep your focus on the areas you're working.

1. KNEE TUCK

WORKS ABS

Sit tall (chest high and shoulders down) on the front half of your chair. Grasp the sides lightly with your hands and lean back slightly as you tighten your abs and bring your right knee up to chest height. Lower it as you raise your left knee on the next rep. Alternate sides. If you get really good at this, try lifting both knees at once, even just a few inches. Do up to 5 reps per leg.

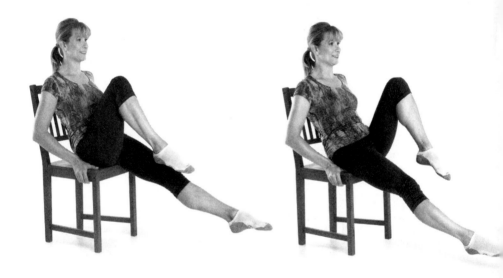

2. LEG EXTENSION

Sit tall with your knees bent 90 degrees and hands on your thighs or overhead. Extend your right leg forward until it's parallel to the floor. Hold for up to 3 counts, squeezing the muscle tightly, then lower and repeat with your left leg on the next rep. Do up to 10 reps per leg.

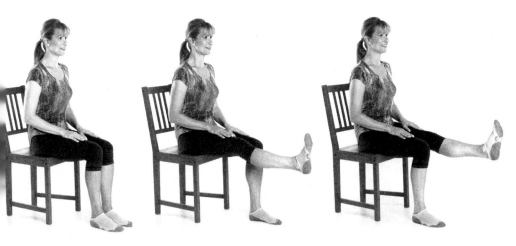

3. TOWEL SLIDE

If you have a chair with wheels, like a desk chair, sit in it and extend both legs forward, toes up and heels on the floor. Keeping the rest of your body still, press your heels into the floor as you bend your knees and try to bring the chair toward your feet. Extend your legs again and repeat. If you're in a regular chair, place your heels on a towel on a slick floor (or wear socks), and draw the towel toward your chair. Straighten your legs and slide the towel out again to return to the starting position. Do up to 10 reps.

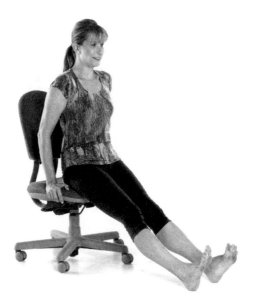 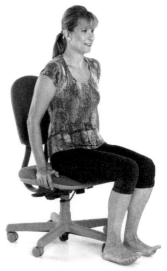

By now, you're probably already exercising or have created a plan to exercise. Remember, keep notes in your journal about how you're feeling overall, how you feel after a workout, and what exercises you enjoy the most (these are the ones you'll come back to again and again). You'll not only get physical benefits from working out during your journey to healing, you'll also experience mental benefits as well—one of which is stress relief. In the next chapter, we'll take you through all aspects of stress, including how it can affect your healing and what you can do, besides exercise, to lower anxiety and improve feelings of self-esteem and body image.

mix it up!

This is an excellent time to cross-train, which essentially means you do a variety of activities. You can strength train one day, walk another, and cycle on yet another day. It keeps your muscles from getting overused and tight and it fends off boredom.

training on a budget

In an ideal world, you'd have a certified personal trainer or physical therapist who's experienced in working with breast cancer patients develop and walk you through your new exercise program. But for many women, that's a budget buster. Even when a doctor recommends physical therapy, the co-pays or other out-of-pocket costs can make it prohibitive. There are some budget-friendly alternatives, though, especially if you're willing to do a little research.

Check out your local hospital or treatment center. If there's an on-site breast cancer center for patients and survivors, you may have free access to yoga, tai chi, dance, and other exercise classes. Many also have a library of instructional exercise videos and books you can borrow.

Ask other survivors or your patient navigator about free or low-cost exercise programs offered elsewhere in your community. Public schools or local colleges, libraries, community recreation centers, and senior centers may offer them.

Use the Internet. Type "videos, exercise, breast cancer" into your browser or YouTube to find free how-to exercise videos that you can watch online. You can also search based on a particular exercise, such as "squat," "plank pose," or "triceps extension."

Buy or rent breast cancer exercise DVDs and books at Amazon, eBay, Netflix, and other online stores. One to try: *Strength and Courage: Exercises for Breast Cancer Survivors* (strengthandcourage.net/dvd/dvd.aspx).

Use your Wii, Xbox 360, PlayStation, or other video game system. These aren't just for kids; they're a good at-home way for adults to have fun burning calories, maintain or reach a healthy weight, build muscle, and improve balance.

The most popular exercise programs are available on all the game systems, and they include step-by-step instructions given by a trainer who lets you know when you've got it right (or wrong). You can adjust the intensity of programmed workouts or customize a routine to match your fitness level. If you don't have a game system, ask around. You're bound to find a family member, neighbor, friend, or coworker who's willing to lend you one or sell it cheap because they've upgraded to a newer model.

That's exactly what Mary Jane Witholter-Zamora did. After being diagnosed with stage IV triple negative breast cancer in 2005, Mary Jane wondered if she would ever be able to lift a bowling ball or swing a golf club again. This was especially true when she got news that the cancer had metastasized to her lung. She was already exhausted from having a mastectomy, chemotherapy, and radiation, and then she heard she would need a lobectomy to remove the lower lobe of her left lung. As she began her recovery, she was too tired to get off the couch or do anything else.

One day, her adult daughters brought over a Wii. Together they began playing the video game version of Mary Jane's favorite sports—bowling, tennis, and golf. "It was a little exhausting," she admits. "But I really got hooked. It was fun and at the same time it helped improve my range of motion and attitude." Finding herself encouraged that someday she would return to those sports again, she began playing on her own. "It was just what I needed to get back in shape—and I've stayed in shape for the last 8 years. It reinforced my positive attitude. Even though I'm back at work and doing my favorite activities, including Zumba and line dancing, for 'real' now, I still play other games to the beat of my Wii."[10]

Bouncing Back

What would you do if you were diagnosed with breast cancer five times in 6 years? When this happened to Lesley Ronson Brown, 62, she told herself to be flexible–and not just because she's a yoga teacher.

Years of hatha yoga training and teaching have kept Lesley resilient. Instead of bouncing back and forth between the extreme highs and lows that go along with cancer, yoga has helped her detach from them.

"My diagnoses included two for cancer in my breast and three for positive lymph nodes in my chest and under my arms," Lesley says. And then she got lymphedema, too. "Each time cancer came back," Lesley explains, "instead of climbing steep mountains or going into deep valleys, yoga took me over rolling hills and to healing places on my mat."

Her first experience with cancer came when she found a golf ball– size lump on the side of her breast. A biopsy confirmed her tumor was malignant and she started chemotherapy. When the pathology report showed that it was Stage IIA invasive ductal carcinoma with one positive lymph node, radiation followed. Lesley thought she was in the clear.

"Yoga has taught me to follow my instincts," she says. "Two years after that first breast cancer, I just didn't feel right. I sensed something was there and an ultrasound confirmed it." Because the recurrence was in the same breast, she had a mastectomy and reconstruction, and the pathology report showed a different type of cancer. In 2009, cancerous lymph nodes in her chest were radiated. A year later, suspicious ones on her left side were removed and eight tested positive for metastatic cancer.

Throughout all this, yoga has remained her driving force to stay positive. You can read her articles on breastcanceryogablog.com.

She'd like women who've been diagnosed to know . . . *it's the end of your world as you knew it, but you have the opportunity to create a new world for yourself.*

Breast cancer is . . . not *the worst disease you could get. Each year there are new treatments and protocols developed.*

Tomorrow will be . . . *a new day, of course!*

*"When we are unable to find tranquility
within ourselves, it is useless to seek it elsewhere."*

—FRANÇOIS DE LA ROCHEFOUCAULD

CHAPTER 11

GETTING STRESS UNDER CONTROL

No doubt, your diagnosis has already caused you enormous amounts of stress and anxiety and probably many sleepless nights. While stress is a fact of life for everyone, you probably feel like you have more than your fair share right now. That's understandable, because the underlying cause of stress in people's lives is change, and you're dealing daily with an illness that is changing and challenging every aspect of life as you know it.

But you can and you *need* to keep your stress under control to prevent it from wreaking havoc on your health, both mental and physical. Even more of a concern for women with breast cancer: The list of evidence linking stress to a weakened immune system and slowed healing grows longer and stronger. In fact, researchers from UCLA's Jonsson Comprehensive Cancer Center discovered a 30-fold increase in cancer spread throughout the bodies of stressed mice compared to those that were not stressed. This led the researchers to conclude that stress can biologically reprogram the immune cells that are trying to fight the cancer. So instead of acting like soldiers protecting the body against disease, they wind up having the opposite effect, helping to spread it.[1] Add to that, the most common stress-related side effects are depression, sleeplessness, chest pain, headaches, and anxiety. You have enough on your plate right now without having to worry about these additional health concerns.

To help ensure that any stress you're experiencing doesn't derail your efforts to become well, this chapter focuses on practical and doable steps you can take to manage it. Included are scientific and practical information, tips, and tools to use on your healing path—and long afterward.

WHAT HAPPENS TO YOUR BODY UNDER STRESS?

To get a handle on stress, it's important to first understand what it's doing to your body and why. When you get stressed, a series of automatic physical and emotional reactions, commonly called the fight-or-flight response, is set into motion. Way back in cavemen days, this bodily response to stress was actually a good thing. Without these reactions, our ancestors would never have had the energy, stamina, or alertness to be able to get away from danger or predators—and stay alive.

Of course, today, we don't live in a world where saber-toothed tigers are hunting us for dinner. Instead, other scary things have replaced them. No doubt, getting the diagnosis that you have breast cancer was one of them. It upset your internal gyroscope and threw your entire world into upheaval. When you got that diagnosis, here's what was most likely going on inside your body.

Your body sensed "danger." When you become fearful and suddenly sense that something life-changing or life-threatening is about to happen, or is actually happening, your body's internal alarm system (that so-called fight-or-flight response) is jump-started by a part of the brain called the amygdala.

Extra cortisol was released. One of the first things that occurs when the body's alarm is sounded is that there's a surge of the primary stress hormone, cortisol, into the bloodstream. It's cortisol that was responsible when you experienced that burst of frenzied, almost panicked, energy after your diagnosis (a result of an increase in blood sugar levels triggered by this hormone). It can also increase your blood pressure. When elevated levels of cortisol remain in the body for prolonged periods of time (what happens if you aren't able to develop stress-busting techniques to cope with your illness), you start to experience lowered immunity and slowed wound healing.

Your body released chemical messengers, called neurotransmitters, into your bloodstream. These include adrenaline, epinephrine, and norepinephrine. It's these neurotransmitters that are the reason that your heart may have started to race, you felt like you couldn't breathe, and you may have even started to hyperventilate when your doctor first told you the news. These neurotransmitters also triggered your reaction if you cried (they regulate your emotional response). They also signal the hippocampus (a nearby area of the brain) to store the entire experience in long-term memory, which is why you'll never really forget when your doctor first spoke these words to you: "You have cancer."

It became harder to fall, and stay, asleep. It's no wonder you haven't been able to get some much-needed rest. Under stress, your body releases a protein called neuropeptide S, which decreases sleep and increases alertness and a sense of anxiety. The body is essentially keeping you awake—and alert—to face the danger it senses. But if you keep your stress levels on high over the course of your treatment and recovery, you won't be getting the rest your body needs to heal.

So what's the answer? The antidote to stress is not to stop any of these automatic reactions from occurring (that would be pretty hard to do) or to get rid of them altogether. Instead, it's learning how to respond to and manage them to help reinforce your body's natural ability to heal itself.

HOW TO GET YOUR STRESS UNDER CONTROL

Today, it's no surprise that some of the most powerful antidotes for stress aren't pills. Instead, they're methods of mind, body, and spiritual awareness that help to calm the body and relax those endless worrying thoughts in your mind. Cancer doctors, top-notch hospitals, and therapists are wholeheartedly embracing these methods—and recommending them to their patients—as important tools for stress relief, recovery, and long-term healing. They include imagery and visualization, meditation and breath work, expressive therapies (music, art, and dance), as well as gentle body movement like yoga, qigong, and tai chi.

What makes these stress-busting methods super practical is that, after learning the basics, you can do them on your own at home, which is great under normal circumstances and even more so while you recuperate from surgery or the side effects of chemotherapy. Some, like meditation, breath work, imagery, and visualization, can even be done while

(continued on page 238)

what's my stress response?

Before you begin learning more about managing stress, take a few moments to focus inwardly and ponder the ways stress affects *you*. Start by writing in your journal about stresses you may have felt from the time you or your doctor suspected breast cancer. Also include your answers to the questions below. If you notice anger, tears, goose bumps, or some other physical response to what you're writing, note that in your journal, too. Questions to consider are:

WHAT ARE THE SIGNS I'M FEELING STRESSED?

- Sleeplessness, fatigue, fogginess, and/or fuzziness?
- High or higher blood pressure?
- Muscle tension?
- Depression?
- Headaches?
- Strange dreams?
- Sore jaw or teeth grinding during sleep?
- Bleeding gums?
- An uncontrollable sweet tooth?
- Mindless eating?
- Belly aches?
- Others?

HOW WOULD YOU BEST DESCRIBE THE STRESS YOU'RE FEELING?

- It's like a pressure cooker in my head ready to blow.
- It feels like a rope around my neck that's slowly tightening.
- It's a stack of worries on a roller coaster ride in my gut.
- It's an ear-piercing alarm causing panic and making my heart race uncontrollably.
- Or write down your own description of how stress is making you feel.

WHEN I FEEL STRESSED, WHAT DO I USUALLY DO TO GET A HANDLE ON IT?

- Try to figure out what's going on
- Have a glass of wine (or two)
- Take a bath
- Go for a massage
- Fill in another way here _____
- Exercise
- Eat
- Take it out on other people
- Write in my journal/diary

WHEN I FEEL STRESSED, WHAT DO I DO TO IGNORE IT?

- Watch TV/movies
- Surf the Web
- Act as though everything's okay (when inside it's not)
- Fill in another way here _____
- Exercise
- Work
- Eat
- Clean the house

Now read the rest of this chapter to learn about stress and explore ways you can manage it. Then once you're done, return to this Personal Practice to consider these questions: If I made a commitment to doing one new thing to help me to manage my stress better, what would it be? Am I ready to make that commitment? If you feel ready to make a commitment, write down what you'll do. Also commit to a day and time when you plan to get started making this healthful and healing change—and try, as best as you can, to stick to this goal.

lying down or sitting in a chair, which helps if you want to practice them a few days before, during, and immediately after your surgery. And yes, we did say *during* your surgery. Listening to guided imagery during an operation can help you heal faster, reduce blood loss and postoperative pain, and boost your immune system.[2]

Of course, one of the most accessible and easiest ways to relieve stress is to get a daily dose of the best medicine of all–laughter. In one small study that looked at the ways nine women with breast cancer used humor, the researchers concluded it was an important coping factor that also played a role in spirituality and the patients' perceptions of the meaning and purpose of life.[3] Other research has shown that humor also has a positive effect on stressful life events and helps to alleviate feelings of depression, insomnia, loneliness, anxiety, and poor self-esteem.[4]

IMAGERY, VISUALIZATION, AND HYPNOSIS

Imagery (also called guided imagery), visualization, and hypnosis share many things in common. Perhaps the most important one is that they effectively use the power of your imagination to accept suggestions and information that reduce stress and strengthen your determination to heal. Although all have been studied for decades, some of the most recent investigations into their efficacy show that, with regular practice, they can:

- Boost short-term immune cell activity
- Lessen headaches and pain
- Reduce stress and anxiety
- Lower blood pressure

The proof they work: What's especially good news for breast cancer patients is that imagery and hypnosis have been shown to lessen the discouraging and debilitating side effects of chemotherapy, such as nausea, depression, and fatigue. The same is true of breast cancer patients undergoing radiation treatments. When investigators from the Continuum Cancer Centers of the New York Beth Israel Medical Center evaluated the impact of guided imagery on patients undergoing radiation therapy for breast cancer, 86 percent of the participants said the guided imagery was helpful, and all said they would recommend the intervention to others. Researchers concluded that incorporating practices such as guided imagery into standard oncology practices improves the overall care for breast cancer patients undergoing radiation therapy.[5]

And here's more support for guided imagery practices. We've all heard about post-traumatic stress disorder (PTSD), but we usually associate this debilitating condition with military personnel returning from the battlefields. But it's not unusual for some cancer survivors to suffer from posttraumatic stress (PTS) or PTSD while they battle breast cancer–and for years afterward.[6] Symptoms include bad dreams; frightening thoughts; feeling emotionally numb; feeling strong guilt, depression, or worry; losing interest in once-enjoyable activities; and feeling tense and/or having angry outbursts. In one study, 23 percent of participants diagnosed with breast cancer in stages I to III had PTSD symptoms when the study began, but plenty more began noticing symptoms within the first 6 months after diagnosis. (For more information about PTS and PTSD, see Chapter 6.)

Encouraging news about the efficacy of guided imagery is emerging from the military sector. In one study, 123 marines with symptoms including nightmares, flashbacks, irritability, and emotional numbness were assigned to receive either their standard PTSD treatment–ranging from individual or group therapy and/or medication–or their standard treatment plus healing touch or guided imagery. After six sessions over the course of 3 weeks, the patients who received standard treatment plus the guided imagery and healing touch therapies had lower levels of depression and cynicism (and greater improvement in quality of life) than those who received standard treatment alone.[7]

When it comes to hypnosis, consider this recent study conducted at New York's Mount Sinai School of Medicine on women about to have a lumpectomy or breast biopsy. One group of women received a brief, one-session hypnosis intervention that included guided relaxation and imagery. The other group did not have the hypnotic procedure. The results? The women who received hypnosis required less sedation and reported less pain intensity, nausea, fatigue, discomfort, and emotional upset. Because of this, they also spent 11 fewer minutes in surgery (with a cost savings of almost $800 per patient).[8] (Keep in mind that hypnosis therapy is sometimes covered by insurance, but it varies by policy and individual case.)

the good side of stress

Our immediate tendency to link the word *stress* to the negative things that happen in our lives, and in the world, is natural. But did you know that the most positive and joyful events in our lives also stress us (and start that cascade of automatic reactions in the body called the fight-or-flight response)? Moving to a new home, getting married, having a baby, starting a new job, or preparing to take the trip of a lifetime are just a few examples of things that can cause the stress response to kick in. Surprisingly, even getting a thumbs-up that you've successfully completed chemotherapy or radiation can be one of them, too. We'll talk more about why that particular one can be stressful in Chapter 15.

How to do them: Most people would say that the practices of imagery, visualization, and hypnosis are similar to meditation. And they're right, because each one involves clearing away the mental clutter in your brain and achieving a natural and relaxed trancelike state. However, as effective as meditation has proven to be for reducing pain and certain symptoms, it also has drawbacks.

According to Belleruth Naparstek, MA, LISW, a pioneer in developing guided imagery for cancer patients and author of *Staying Well with Guided Imagery*, one of the drawbacks to meditation is that patients may feel challenged by the learning curve. That's especially true if they're trying to master it on their own instead of in a group. "With guided imagery," Naparstek explains, "there's no learning curve or discipline. You just catch a free ride on the narration and music and so no prep is needed."[9]

Imagery

This is one of the easiest techniques to do on your own, but it's also a popular practice in retreat, therapeutic, and other group settings. Some patient-centered programs combine the practices, or focus on a particular one in order to achieve specific goals, such as pain reduction. It works best in a relaxed, unforced atmosphere. Essentially, you use your imagination to guide yourself to a focused, relaxed state. To get started:

1. **Make yourself comfortable.** You can sit cross-legged, recline in a cozy chair, or even lie down (if you don't think you'll fall asleep).

2. **Close your eyes and begin to take long, slow deep breaths** . . . in and out, in and out until you can feel your panic and anxiety slowly being released. (There's no set time limit for this to happen; take as long as your body needs.)

3. **Begin to daydream, imagining yourself in a relaxed, happy place.** Think about all aspects of that place: what it looks like, how it sounds, what it smells like, how it feels, and even what it tastes like (for example, the salty ocean air at a beautiful beach). Make your vision so vivid that you feel like you could be in that spot right then.

4. **Stay in your happy, relaxed place as long as you need to.** When you're ready to return to reality, count backward from 10. When you reach 1, say out loud, "I am relaxed and peaceful."

That's all there is to it. You can do this anytime, anywhere you can find a comfortable place (even a waiting or treatment room) to help get a handle on your stress.

According to Naparstek, even skeptics have experienced benefits from guided imagery. "I always tell people to try not to get too intense about 'doing it right,'" she says, adding that there are many ways to do it right, but none is necessarily the best. In other words, all ways will lead you to discover that imagery will clear your mind, slow it (and you) down, and calm and strengthen you.[10] Guided imagery is when someone else (or something else, like one of the numerous CDs or podcasts available) is guiding you through this same technique.

Visualization

This relaxation technique is very similar to imagery, but is less formal. You can do it anywhere–in the bath, lying in bed at night, waiting to see your doctor, while you're having treatments. It's as simple as visualizing what you want: to be healthy, to be happy, to be free of cancer. Whatever you want to happen, vividly see it in your mind. Do this technique for at least 5 minutes, and if you can, do it every day.

imagery, visualization, and hypnosis resources

To use imagery or visualization for stress reduction, check with your friends, relatives, local breast center, or public library for recordings that you can borrow. If you'd like to learn to do self-hypnosis at home, we recommend that you start by learning it from a qualified professional certified by the American Society of Clinical Hypnosis (go to asch.net to find a professional in your area).

A particularly good guided imagery resource you may want to check out: *Healing and Transformation through Self-Guided Imagery,* a book by Leslie Davenport, MS, MFT, an integrative psychotherapist in practice at Smith Integrative Oncology in San Francisco. There are also CDs, recordings, and podcasts you can listen to or download online.

- **Health Journeys Meditations to Relieve Stress** by Belleruth Naparstek is available 24/7 at tinyurl.com/nsu3pob

- **Anxiety Relief,** a guided imagery app by Martin Rossman, MD (for iPhone, iPod Touch, and iPad; available on iTunes)

- **"Guided Imagery and Harp Meditation,"** a free MP3 by Leslie Davenport at lesliedavenport.com/invitation.mp3

- **"Guided Imagery and Relaxation for Surgery Patients,"** a free MP3 by California Pacific Medical Center at tinyurl.com/qhr6z2w

- *Self-Healing with Guided Imagery,* an audio CD by Andrew Weil, MD, and Dr. Rossman, author of *Fighting Cancer from Within* (thehealingmind.org)

- **"Taking a Walk,"** a free MP3 from the University of Michigan's Comprehensive Cancer Center (tinyurl.com/celaqy); you can also find other free guided imagery MP3s on this site

Hypnosis

Similar to imagery, hypnosis (and self-hypnosis) involves finding a quiet place and deep breathing until you find yourself relaxing. But with hypnosis, you prepare positive statements, called affirmations, beforehand. Some examples are: "I am healthy. I am strong. I will fight this cancer" or "I am relaxed and comfortable. With every breath, I am becoming more relaxed." And then, once you're in a relaxed state, you say these affirmations out loud over and over until you get into a trancelike state. Most people do self-hypnosis for 15 to 25 minutes.

MEDITATION

Did you know that meditation has a lot in common with the words *medicine*, *medical*, and *medicate*? All are rooted in the Latin *mederi*, which means to heal or cure. Know that meditation isn't always about sitting crossed-legged on a pillow on the floor while chanting for long periods of time. There are many ways people can meditate (a walking meditation, for example), any of which can be done alone in a quiet, calm place, with a partner or teacher, or in a group setting.

Meditation goes by many names and styles: Some popular ones include insight meditation, Transcendental Meditation, Zen, and Kirtan Kriya, a meditation chant exercise originating from yoga that uses finger poses (*mudras*). There's also mindfulness meditation (we'll be showing you how to do this, in this section). Certain forms of chanting (mantras like "Om") and drumming can be meditative, too. And almost every religious and spiritual path worldwide incorporates meditation-like contemplative practices in the form of prayer, rituals, and chanting to help participants focus inwardly. All these practices are rooted in emptying our minds in order to leave the busyness of the world and our thinking mind behind. This allows us to go into a deeper state of self-awareness. The benefits of meditation are that it can:

- Boost your immune function
- Reduce stress and anxiety
- Lower heart rate, blood pressure, and respiratory rate
- Improve your mood and reduce feelings of anger

The proof it works: Probably the best news about the stress-relieving benefits of meditation is that medical professionals and researchers agree that there are plenty of benefits. While there are many different types of meditation, one particular form called mindfulness-based stress reduction (MBSR) has been used in hospitals since the 1990s. It's a nonsectarian, research-based form of meditation derived from a 2,500-year-old Buddhist practice called Vipassana or insight meditation.[11] It's designed to develop the skill of paying attention to our inner and outer experiences with acceptance, compassion, and patience.

In one 8-week MBSR study of two groups of women diagnosed and treated for early-stage breast cancer, all the participants practiced breathing exercises, gentle yoga, body awareness, and meditation together. Nineteen women in the MBSR group also agreed to practice meditation for an additional 45 minutes daily on their own (though not all followed through). Seventeen women in the other group did not do the additional practice. When tested, the MBSR group had lowered their heart rate, blood pressure, and respiratory rates and experienced less stress than the other group.[12]

In another controlled study of 90 cancer patients who did mindfulness meditation for 7 weeks, 31 percent had fewer symptoms of stress and 65 percent had fewer episodes of mood disturbance than those who did not meditate.[13] Some studies have also suggested that more meditation improves the chance of an even more positive outcome.

Another study, conducted by MD Anderson Cancer Center's Integrative Medicine Program, found that a form of meditation called Tibetan sound meditation (a practice that integrates breathing and visualization with ancient Tibetan sounds) helped to improve memory problems and foggy thinking, as well as mental health and spirituality in breast cancer patients undergoing chemotherapy.[14]

How to do it: One of the hardest things for us is to stop being a human *doing* and become a human *being*–to just be present to ourselves from one moment to the next. Practicing mindfulness meditation is a way to do that because in the present moment we can purposefully and nonjudgmentally pay attention to whatever arises inwardly and outwardly from a place of self-compassion.[15]

Bestselling author Jon Kabat-Zinn, PhD, brought the concept of mindfulness into the mainstream of medicine and society in the 1970s.

He reminds us that traditional sitting poses are only one way to cultivate this practice. We can also, he says, nurture nonjudgmental awareness of the present moment while standing, walking, and even eating. In fact, mindfulness can be done in any position or situation because, he says, "The real meditation is your life, and how you inhabit it moment-by-moment."[16] Dr. Kabat-Zinn recommends that beginners start practicing mindfulness meditation by focusing on one of our most constant companions—our breath. Here's one way of doing that, based on Dr. Kabat-Zinn's work, in just a few minutes.

1. **Focus on your breath in bed for a few moments after you wake up or before falling asleep.** Close your eyes, and take deep breaths in and out, in and out. Visualize in your mind that these breaths are waves, ebbing and flowing along the shore. Locate where the breath sensations are most vivid—in your belly, at your nostrils, wherever. Take a moment to continue breathing and just being aware of where you feel these sensations.

2. **Expand this awareness of your breath** until it includes a sense of your whole body lying in your bed breathing. Again, continue breathing and slowly become aware of your breath, your body, and how your body is feeling at the moment.

3. **Become aware of the various sensations fluxing in the body,** including the breath sensations. Continue deep breathing in and out.

4. **Just rest in the awareness of lying here breathing,** outside of time, even if it is only for a minute or two. You'll notice that the mind has a life of its own as it wanders away, thinking about other things. Keep in mind that's what minds do, so you have no need to judge it. Note what is on your mind, and let that be part of your awareness for the moment.

5. **Slowly bring your awareness back to your breath once again,** and make the breath and the body center stage in your mind. Continue deep breathing in and out, in and out.

6. **Embrace how you're feeling right now,** while still focusing on your breath. It's very easy to fall into the thought stream of worrying about and planning for the future, as well as looking back at the past with its remembering and blaming. There's no need to stop this from happening. Instead, just bring openhearted, accepting awareness to these feelings.[17]

7. **Slowly bring your focus back to the present.** Continue breathing in and out, while opening your eyes and taking a moment to appreciate everything you are.

meditation resources

Breast cancer centers and support groups are some of the best places to get feedback about local meditation resources, instructors, books, and educational CDs. Also talk to family members, friends, and coworkers who meditate. Most importantly, seek out the advice of other breast cancer survivors who practiced meditation while they were patients–they may still be doing it as part of a healthy lifestyle. Here are some great places to start.

- *A Meditation to Help You Fight Cancer,* an audio CD or MP3 download by Belleruth Naparstek; there's also *A Meditation to Help You with Chemotherapy* and *A Meditation to Help You with Radiation Therapy* by Naparstek (healthyjourneys.com)

- *Guided Meditations for Difficult Times,* an audio CD by Jack Kornfield (jackkornfield.com)

- **"Loving Kindness Meditation,"** a free guided meditation from the Mindful Awareness Research Center at UCLA; they have six others–all free (tinyurl.com/crh56nd), as well as 13 free mindful awareness exercises available through iTunes

- **Meditation Oasis** (meditationoasis.com), a Web site where you can find meditation how-to's, podcasts, smartphone apps (including Simply Being), and more

- **Mindfulness Meditation** by Mental Workout, a guided meditation app (for iPhone, iPad, and iPod Touch)

- *Wherever You Go, There You Are,* the bestselling book by Jon Kabat-Zinn; the *Guided Mindfulness Meditation* series are audio CDs, also by Dr. Kabat-Zinn (mindfulnesscds.com)

You don't have to do this in bed. You can do this practice anytime, anywhere: on the beach or in a park, in your office, in your backyard, in your treatment center, while you're waiting at your doctor's office. Remember: What happens *inside* your inner space is more important than the space around you.

BIOFEEDBACK

Whenever you're confronted with a stressor in your life—like hearing those words "you have cancer," undergoing treatment, waiting for surgery, and even coping with the fallout in your life from having cancer—your body puts into motion the fight-or-flight response that we talked about earlier in this chapter. Your heart rate increases, your muscles tense up, your mind races, your breathing becomes shallow and panicked, and you start to sweat. This is a result of the surge of cortisol and neurotransmitters into your bloodstream. While we can't control the bodily processes that are happening, we *can* control our response to them. And that's where biofeedback comes in.

How it works: A biofeedback technician attaches electrodes or sensors (similar to the ones used for an electrocardiogram, or EKG) to various locations on your body—typically the shoulders, chest, abdomen, fingers, back, and head. These sensors are connected to a biofeedback computer program or other equipment. They measure your basic bodily functions like heart rate, brain waves, muscle activity, skin temperature, perspiration rate, and breath.

As you think different stressful thoughts, you're able to observe the changes happening to your body on a computer screen—or via auditory tones that get higher or lower, depending on your levels of stress. The goal is to get you to figure out what you have to do—taking a deep breath, counting to 10, changing your negative thought process, whatever—to change the way your body responds so it's less stressed. Then, over time, you'll learn how to do these things to change your stress response in the real world. Biofeedback gives you control over your body—and that, say experts, is ultimately why biofeedback has such an impact on our health and overall well-being.

While this popular form of mind-body therapy has no demonstrated effect on cancer cells, it does have many other benefits.

- It reduces stress and anxiety.

- It can help patients better cope with the pain associated with surgery and other treatments, as well as the sleeplessness and fatigue that often accompany radiation and chemotherapy.

- It can help to lower stress-triggered high blood pressure.

- It gives you concrete, practical ways to manage your stress long term.

The proof it works: Biofeedback has a proven track record of being safe, free of side effects, and beneficial. (You do have to be cautious, though, if you have a serious heart condition or an implanted pacemaker or other implanted electronic device, because the electrical impulses used to monitor your reactions and progress could interfere with the pacemaker's operation. Get your doctor's okay first.)

According to research conducted at the University of California San Diego Moores Cancer Center, biofeedback not only helps relieve the symptoms and side effects of surgery, it's also proven useful in retraining, reconditioning, and strengthening muscles after surgery, and restoring loss of control due to pain or nerve damage.[18]

A small pilot study, conducted at the Applied Brain Research Foundation of Ohio, also found that neurofeedback, a form of biofeedback that concentrates specifically on brain wave readings via sensors attached to the scalp, can improve the cognitive impairment that often results from chemotherapy (also called "chemo brain" because of the thinking and memory problems that can occur posttreatment) and can help reduce fatigue, sleep disturbances (and use of sleep medications), as well as the overall psychological distress (including depression) of breast cancer patients 6 months to 5 years after chemotherapy. Four weeks after the study ended, follow-up testing showed that the survivors were maintaining their improvements.[19]

Additionally, a study from the College of Nursing at Seoul National University in Korea determined that biofeedback can help improve quality of life after a mastectomy–thanks to a reduction in blood cortisol levels and overall anxiety–making it an important intervention for those living with cancer.[20]

How to do it: If you're a "seeing is believing" type of person, then biofeedback may be an interesting, and even fun, way to untie stressful knots, stay healthier, and improve your quality of life while you're being

biofeedback resources

Meeting with a biofeedback therapist to understand how biofeedback works and how you can control your stress response is recommended over trying one of the many home devices, or apps, available today.

The Association for Applied Psychophysiology and Biofeedback (aapb.org) offers a locator to find an expert in your area. On their Web site, you can also find information about biofeedback and how it works.

The Biofeedback Certification International Alliance (bcia.org) is the nonprofit international certifying body for biofeedback experts. They can help point you to additional resources about biofeedback.

But if the option of meeting with a certified therapist isn't available to you (particularly because insurance may not always cover the series of treatments necessary) or you've already met with one and want to continue managing your stress on your own at home, then these options may be worth a try.

BioZen is an Android app from the Department of Defense's National Center for Telehealth and Technology. Geared toward members of the military suffering from post-traumatic stress disorder, this biofeedback app can also be used to mitigate the stress response. It uses Bluetooth-coupled sensors to show the user how her body is responding to certain stressors and tracks the user's progress over time. While the app is free, you do need to purchase medical sensors (which cost between $75 to $150) to attach to your skin and read your body's stress response. For more information, go to tinyurl.com/mnjujhu.

EmWave is a biofeedback-like device available from HeartMath. You collect pulse data from your finger through a handheld device, which can be connected to your computer and translated into visual graphs so you can see how to control your breathing and thoughts to reduce your stress response. Versions that connect to your iPad or iPhone are also available. For more information, go to heartmath.com.

treated for your breast cancer—and even long afterward. The advantage of working with someone who can teach you biofeedback is . . . the feedback. In other words, you can talk to them about the things that are causing you anxiety, and they'll talk you through how to diminish your stress response, and then they'll monitor your results. If you decide to go that route, you need to work with a certified biofeedback therapist who may be a psychologist, psychiatrist, or some other kind of health-care or trained professional possibly affiliated with your cancer treatment center.

Sessions run 30 to 60 minutes; you'll need at least a few to get the hang of it and learn how to practice on your own. It's daily practice at home, at work, at your treatment center that will bring you the best, long-term results. (Practicing on your own will also reduce the number of in-office sessions you need, which is important to consider financially because not all insurance companies cover biofeedback, and Medicare does not. Each visit can cost up to $150.)

You can, however, also purchase and use biofeedback equipment at home. These typically require you to attach a device to three fingers to measure your pulse. Sometimes you have to use deep breathing and calming thoughts to open doors on the computer screen or to make balloons float up, down, or stay steady. Some are even video-style games that teach you relaxation and meditation techniques, and then have you practice biofeedback to monitor your thoughts, feelings, breath, and awareness.

Ultimately, whether you work with a therapist or use a home computer program, your goal isn't to be wired with sensors or to be glued to a monitor forever. Instead, it's to train your mind and body to make beneficial, incremental changes that can reduce stress without anyone—or anything—but you.

EXPRESSIVE/CREATIVE ARTS THERAPY

You've probably heard the expression, "Music has charms to soothe a savage breast." As a survivor, you know there's truth in those words. Music is a powerful ally in the fight against breast cancer because it helps to soothe the stress you've been feeling since you got your diagnosis.

Often survivors find that some of the most interesting, creative, enjoyable, and helpful stress-busting techniques are therapies that use music, art, creative writing and journaling, and dance. All these psychotherapeutic healing paths hold that your mind and body function together as part of your whole being. Nationwide, medical and breast cancer centers are offering patients this safe form of healing therapy during, and after, their treatments.

The best way to try these stress busters is in a group setting. All professional expressive arts associations require that credentialed therapists have extensive training.[21] However, books and other media can help you to understand the benefits and provide step-by-step guidelines, too.

Whatever creative media you choose to pursue, though, know that the goal is the same: to allow you to find a creative way—through self-exploration and self-expression—of dealing with the physical and emotional stress you're experiencing. It's also to:

- Relax your mind
- Lessen pain and other side effects of treatments and surgery
- Improve energy levels
- Reduce anxiety
- Relieve depression and sleeplessness

Art Therapy

Art therapy has been used in hospitals and other health-care settings for years. Breast cancer patients have reported that these creative experiences help to reduce pain and other side effects of their surgery and treatments.

The proof it works: In one 4-month study on the effectiveness of art therapy on cancer patients conducted by Judith Paice, PhD, RN, director of the Cancer Pain Program at Northwestern Memorial Hospital in Chicago, eight of nine of the patients' symptoms improved, including pain, tiredness, depression, anxiety, drowsiness, lack of appetite, well-being, and shortness of breath. Nausea was the only symptom that did not change as a result of the sessions. Moreover, the patients also reported that they found art therapy energizing.[22] According to Dr. Paice, "Art therapy provides a distraction that allows patients to focus on something positive instead of their health for a time, and it also gives patients something they can control."[23]

Another study, conducted by the Jefferson Myrna Brind Center of Integrative Medicine in Philadelphia, found that art therapy, when combined with mindfulness-based stress reduction, can lower anxiety levels in women with breast cancer. The study found that a combination of the two

"draw" a self-portrait

After reading this, close your eyes and begin to imagine that you're in an art therapy class for breast cancer patients and survivors. After being given instructions and reminders that this is expressive art and it's not about making perfect pictures by coloring inside the lines or following all kinds of "rules," you're invited to draw a self-portrait in your journal. What you and others put down on your paper may range from a pretty good pencil sketch to a primitive stick figure or an abstract shape that's an expression of what you look like to yourself right now. Maybe you'll include more than your head in the portrait. Perhaps your breast will be there. Maybe not.

Now imagine yourself looking at your picture to explore what it may be "saying" or revealing to you about how you feel physically and emotionally. If you feel calm or happy, something about the portrait—like a smile—may convey that. However, it may also reveal deep-seated sadness, anger, loss, or grief that you don't show outwardly or notice in the mirror.

Because you're tapping into the wisdom deep in your body instead of in your head when you do this, don't be surprised if you have "insights" that bring tears. Don't hold them back; they come from a well within that has been waiting to speak to you in some way for a while now.

Art therapy isn't meant to be a onetime experience. If you find it helpful, return to it and try using different media like paint, collage, pastels, and anything else you may be attracted to. For example, many survivors find that working with clay or even Play-Doh is a revealing, satisfying, and, at times, cathartic experience.

stress-relief therapies actually showed changes in brain activity associated with lower stress and anxiety after the 8-week program.[24]

How to do it: During a typical session, participants use assorted media, images, and the creative process as a way to help resolve emotional conflicts, foster self-awareness, build confidence, manage behavior, and reduce stress and anxiety. For example, some breast cancer patients might be encouraged to make beaded bracelets, where each bead is selected to somehow signify a part of their journey. Others might be encouraged to draw self-portraits. Some hospitals, like Memorial Sloan-Kettering Cancer Center in New York, even offer art therapy sessions for breast cancer patients and their children to allow them to learn creative ways to enhance communication together.

Music Therapy

Like art therapy, music therapy can help cancer patients physically, emotionally, and spiritually. In fact, many hospitals have music therapists on their staff.

The proof it works: One study of 40 patients who suffered from anticipatory nausea and vomiting while receiving chemotherapy were given a combination of music therapy and guided imagery. Researchers found that the two therapies together lowered the patients' anxiety. Moreover, by the time these patients went for their third round of chemotherapy, the music therapy and imagery had also reduced the severity and duration of the nausea and vomiting significantly.[25]

Music therapy also seems to help improve mood; lower heart rate, blood pressure, and breathing rate; relieve depression and sleeplessness; reduce muscle tension; and provide an overall feeling of relaxation.

How to do it: Depending on the setting and your needs, a therapist may use singing, listening, instrumental music, composition, creative movement, and even music combined with guided imagery to augment your medical treatments. One great advantage of music therapy for breast cancer patients is you can really do it anywhere, and while lying down, sitting, or standing.

Dance Therapy

Also called dance movement therapy, this technique uses movement and dance to help you to feel more physically and emotionally balanced and whole. Like other expressive arts therapists, dance therapists believe that the mind, body, and spirit are interconnected. Dance therapy has been offered in therapeutic settings across the country for more than 50 years. Clinical reports suggest that dance therapy helps patients to not only reduce stress and anxiety but also develop a positive body image, improve self-esteem, decrease the sense of social isolation, and encourage an overall sense of well-being.[26] The Lebed method of dance therapy (also called Healthy Steps), in particular, is one that's recommended by the National Cancer Institute and is widely used to help breast cancer patients and survivors suffering from the chronic and progressive swelling that comes from lymphedema (see page 197).

The proof it works: In one of the few studies on dance therapy to date, the efficacy of Healthy Steps was evaluated on participants ranging in age from 38 to 82 years. Researchers found that, after about 7 months, the women with breast cancer who did dance therapy had significant improvements in their quality of life, improving body image and shoulder range of motion.[27]

How to do it: A typical session includes a warmup with deep breathing and stretches done to percussive music. Core exercises follow, with upper- and lower-body movements done to music and imagery. Next is dance movement designed to address challenges such as body image, sexuality, sense of control, grief, and loss. The moves are simple and designed for all women, including those who have no dance experience, poor balance, or low self-confidence. The moves come from a variety of musical traditions, including American, jazz, Celtic, Afro-Cuban, reggae, Middle Eastern, and Cajun. Dance therapy also uses props such as stretch bands and long pieces of silk that help provide an external focus and decrease anxiety. As a session draws to a close, a seated ritual typically takes place, which includes gentle stretching, meditative movements, and focused breathing to soothing music. Afterward, the therapist checks in with participants and gives them time to share their thoughts, feelings, and experiences.[28]

MASSAGE

Today, it's common for hospitals and breast care centers to offer their patients massage therapy (with some insurance covering it) because

expressive/creative arts therapy resources

There are plenty of ways to incorporate creative arts on your own–thanks to the numerous CDs, DVDs, and even Web sites you can use at home.

Art therapy: To find an art therapist near you, go to arttherapy .org, the Web site of the American Art Therapy Association. If you want to be inspired–and possibly even inspire other women with breast cancer–go to pinterest.com and sign up. You have to wait to be "accepted," but don't worry, you will be. And once you're on, search for "art therapy" from other women. You may even want to post pictures of some of your own healing art there.

Music therapy: Healing music and sound therapy CDs and DVDs are available from online bookstores. Many use instrumental music corresponding to a rhythmic beat to help promote sleep and help reduce pain, depression, and other side effects of breast cancer. Others use drumming or indigenous instruments (such as the Australian didgeridoo, a wooden trumpet) to create the desired effect. Ones to try include:

- *Music for Sound Healing* by Steven Halpern, a relaxing mix of piano, electric piano, flute, and harp (innerpeacemusic.com)

- *Musical Rapture: A Healing Gift to Humanity*, celestial music from various artists; a free MP3 download is available at fredericdelarue.com

- *The Healing Journey* by Tami Briggs, which uses harp music for healing (available digitally through iTunes and as a CD from dailyom.com)

Dance therapy: You can read about dance therapy's ability to heal at the American Dance Therapy Association's Web site, adta.org. Another resource for you to use at home:

- *Thriving after Breast Cancer* (book and two DVDs) by Sherry Lebed Davis (cofounder of the Lebed method) and Stephanie Gunning; these include essential healing exercises for the body and mind (gohealthysteps.com) this healing touch has been shown to relieve muscle tension, reduce stress and anxiety, improve circulation, and boost your immune system.

The proof it works: Studies of massage for cancer patients suggest massage can decrease stress, anxiety, depression, pain, and fatigue.[29] In one study, conducted at the Touch Research Institute at the University of Miami Miller School of Medicine, 34 women with stage I or II breast cancer were randomly assigned to a massage therapy group or to a control group after their surgery. The women in the first group received 30-minute massages three times per week for 5 weeks. By the end of the study, they had reduced their anxiety, depressed mood, and anger and boosted their immune system as well as the functioning of their neuroendocrine system (which essentially regulates your entire body's response to stress).[30]

Another study of 230 cancer patients found that those who received one 45-minute therapeutic massage session per week for a month felt less pain and took about eight fewer doses of pain medication than those in the control group.[31] Another study found that therapeutic massage reduced cancer pain perception, decreased anxiety, and enhanced relaxation.[32]

How to do it: To experience the benefits of massage, all you have to do is to lie down or sit in a chair, relax, and allow the therapist to take over. Therapists can also come to you at the hospital, while you're in bed or on a bedside chair. (Be sure to talk to your doctor before getting a massage to make sure it's okay.) A simple foot massage may only take 10 minutes and a full-body massage, an hour.

There are many different styles of massage–from aromatherapy (using scented essential oils) to Swedish (essentially a relaxing, full-body massage)–but the underlying principle is the same. A licensed massage therapist manipulates your muscles and soft tissue, stimulating nerves, increasing blood flow, and relaxing your muscles. Many therapists are trained in more than one style of massage and can combine them depending upon a client's needs. But no matter what style of massage your therapist uses, it should never hurt; if it does, tell your therapist immediately. Also, keep in mind these precautions (you may want to bring this book and have your massage therapist read these precautions before getting started).

1. **Lie on your back, if you've just had breast surgery.** It may not be safe to lie on your stomach until your doctor gives you the okay.

2. **Tell your therapist *not* to use strong pressure, if you're undergoing chemotherapy and radiation.** People undergoing chemotherapy and radiation may have a decrease in red and white blood cells and platelets, so with strong pressure, there's more of a risk of developing bruises. Also, if you have any cuts or incisions, make sure your therapist doesn't manipulate those areas because of concern about infection.[33] Lastly, make sure your massage therapist doesn't touch skin that's sensitive or irritated because of radiation treatments (it can make the area feel much worse).

3. **Have your therapist be extremely cautious around the underarm areas** if you've had your lymph nodes removed. This area will be particularly sensitive. Plus, if you've developed arm lymphedema (swelling caused by the accumulation of lymph fluid), your massage therapist should avoid that area altogether as it could worsen the swelling. Arm lymphedema can, however, be treated by a type of massage called manual lymphatic drainage.

massage resources

You can find a licensed massage therapist (LMT) or licensed massage practitioner (LMP) by going to the Web site of the American Massage Therapy Association (amtamassage.org), but make sure he or she has experience with breast cancer patients. Getting recommendations from your doctor, hospital, and/or treatment center may be your best bet. (*Note:* Some states don't offer licensing for massage therapists; if your state is one of them, look instead for a certified massage therapist or CMT.)

If you're suffering from arm lymphedema (a side effect of breast cancer treatment, which can affect lymph node drainage), you can find a certified therapist in this massage technique from the National Lymphedema Network (lymphnet.org) or the Lymphology Association of North America (clt-lana.org). Your doctor or treatment center may also have recommendations.

YOGA, QIGONG, AND TAI CHI

Like many of the forms of stress reduction that focus on the mind, body, and particularly the breath, these ancient practices migrated to our shores from the East. Today, they're popular forms of exercise that are taught in studios, community centers, senior centers, and even daycare centers. Because they're so mainstream and generally believed to be safe, they've become an integral part of breast cancer recovery programs in hospitals and support groups nationwide. They've also become integral because they can bring a sense of inner peace and well-being, improve self-esteem, improve range of motion in areas like the shoulder, fight fatigue, lessen anxiety and stress, reduce depression, and boost immune function.

Yoga

Yoga, which means "to yoke" in the Sanskrit language of India, joins the mind, body, and breath as one unit. It originated in India, and its underlying philosophy is holistic: If the mind is disturbed, the breath and body are affected, too. By doing *asanas* (yogic poses), the mind, body, and breath work together for the sake of inner peace and well-being.

The proof it works: In the first study to compare yoga with stretching, women undergoing radiation therapy who did yoga (which incorporated yogic breathing, postures, meditation, and relaxation) experienced improved energy, physical functioning, better general health, and lower levels of the stress hormone cortisol. They also were better able to find meaning in their cancer experience. During the follow-up period, researchers—from the MD Anderson Cancer Center and India's largest yoga research institution, Swami Vivekananda Yoga Anusandhana Samsthana in Bangalore—theorized that yoga offers psychological and physical benefits for cancer patients beyond those derived from stretching exercises alone.[34]

In another small study—conducted by yogis and medical doctors in India—with women who had metastatic breast cancer, the researchers found yoga, when done daily, was resoundingly effective in decreasing the severity of anxiety, depression, and perceived stress. It also helped improve the emotional well-being, cognitive functioning, and overall quality of life.[35] The biological findings were equally impressive. Cortisol levels dropped, and the study participants who did yoga experienced a significant increase in the percentage of cytotoxins, special "killer" cells, shown to play a therapeutic role in the treatment of cancers.[36]

How to do it: Despite popular thinking, yoga is not all about standing on your head and tying yourself into pretzel-like knots. A pose can be as simple as sitting in a chair while doing breath work and holding your hands and fingers in a certain position (see page 260). In fact, hand yoga poses are called *mudras*, a Sanskrit word for "seal."

Practitioners believe that this simple form of yoga stimulates different parts of the body involved with breathing and affects the flow of *prana* (life) in the body. Since many mudras are easy to learn on your own, you might give the basic chin mudra a try. You've probably seen it many times in pictures of hatha yoga practitioners who are meditating while seated, but the chin mudra can actually be done while walking or standing–almost anytime and anywhere.

Chin means consciousness. This pose joins the thumb (universal consciousness) with the index finger (our individual human consciousness). The goal is to quiet your mind by focusing on your breath and the points where your fingertips touch.

Qigong and Tai Chi

Qigong (pronounced chee-gong) and tai chi (pronounced tie chee) are ancient health-promoting practices that release tension and stress and have many other benefits in common. Both originated in China, and there are thousands of forms worldwide that use slow, deliberate movements, mental focus/meditation, and deep breathing.

Today, hospitals nationwide offer qigong and tai chi as part of their complementary or integrative medicine programs because studies show that with practice either can positively affect your mind and body. For example, both have been shown to enhance immune function, bone health, cardiopulmonary fitness, balance, self-confidence, stress, and quality of life.

The proof they work: Depression and stress often go hand-in-hand, which is why many women feel stressed and have symptoms of depression when they're about to begin treatments for breast cancer.

In one study, published in the journal *Cancer*, researchers looked at women with breast cancer experiencing depressive symptoms at the beginning of radiation treatment. After 5 to 6 weeks of doing qigong for five 40-minute classes weekly, they found their symptoms were reduced and their overall quality of life was improved throughout treatment and 3 months later.[37]

And according to a review of 77 scientific studies that looked at both practices, both are viable alternatives to conventional exercise.[38] This can be especially important to survivors who want to do something gentle but who may also need to build their strength, balance, and immune system while standing in one place or sitting in a chair.

How to do them: Qigong, the oldest therapeutic modality in Chinese medicine, is a canopy for all the forms of both practices. Literally, the

try this simple yoga pose

Sit in a straight-backed chair with your feet (barefoot if possible) on the ground. Relax your jaw, and join your thumb and forefinger on both hands to form a zero. Extend the rest of your fingers. Now place your hands on your thighs. When your fingers point down to Earth, the chin mudra (or hand yoga pose) grounds you. If they point up to Heaven, they are in a position to receive qi (energy) from the universe. (Point them in whichever direction is comfortable for you.)

Try to always stay focused on your breath. It activates the diaphragm, which allows for deep "stomach breathing." This means as you inhale, your diaphragm pushes your internal organs out instead of sucking them in. Begin by doing it as long as you can comfortably. After some practice, try doing it for 15 minutes (or longer) with your eyes open or closed.

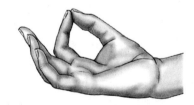

word *qigong* means cultivating your life force or qi; practitioners believe that the gentle movements bring the energy and flow of qi into all parts of your body. Perhaps that's why some studies have shown that tai chi can have a positive effect on lymphedema.

Tai chi, an important branch of qigong, is considered a "soft" martial art and is based on the movements of five animals–the tiger, dragon, leopard, snake, and crane. Each move in tai chi flows into the next one so

yoga, qigong, and tai chi resources

While most hospitals and breast cancer treatment centers can give you lists of yoga, qigong, and tai chi practitioners (and may even offer classes on-site), you can also track down experts through these national organizations: the Qigong Institute (qigonginstitute.org), the National Qigong Association (nqa.org), and the American Tai Chi and Qigong Association (americantaichi.org). If you want to try these Eastern practices on your own, DVDs are a good way to start. There are plenty, taught by top experts, available. Here are a few, tailored to beginners.

- *Qigong Beginning Practice* with Francesco and Daisy Lee-Garripoli is a 2-DVD set that includes moving meditations to ease ailments and boost resilience, loosen joints, increase core strength, and stretch and strengthen the legs (gaiam.com).

- *Sunrise Tai Chi* by Ramel Rones is split into three sections–demonstration, instruction, and workout–and is set to flute and harp music (ramelrones.com).

- *Thriving Yoga: Yoga for Breast Cancer* incorporates poses to increase flexibility, bring healing energy to the areas in breast cancer patients that need it most, and relax the mind and body (yogaforcancer.com).

- *Yoga for Cancer Recovery* with Claire Petretti (a breast cancer survivor) is a gentle yoga program specifically designed for someone going through treatment or recovery (oceansoulyoga.com).

your body is in a state of constant yet gradual motion (think karate in slow motion). It's this gentle movement that's said to help restore a sense of peace and serenity to your mind and body.

Although both ancient practices have only gained popularity in the United States over the last 3 decades, today more than 100 million people practice qigong worldwide and millions of others practice tai chi. Essentially, both are meditation in motion, although most people find qigong is the easier of the two to learn because tai chi is more structured.

Which to choose? If you're wondering whether to take a class in tai chi or qigong, we believe that either can be a beneficial and health-enhancing exercise you can do now—and for a lifetime.

WHAT'S NEXT?

By now we're sure that you are looking at how stress may be impacting your breast cancer journey and wondering what else you can do to manage and reduce it. One step is to join a breast cancer support group as a way to gather support and learn how to manage stress better. In the next chapter, we'll explore several options for finding support groups of all kinds that can offer you many kinds of helpful and healing resources.

New Direction

When she was diagnosed in 2010 with ductal carcinoma in situ–a condition in which cancer cells are present inside a milk duct in the breast–Kimberly Simanca was determined to beat it. "My husband had fought his own battle with a carcinoid tumor in his liver and was now doing fine. I wasn't going to let breast cancer take me," she says.

Kimberly's cancer was caught early, before it had spread to other parts of the breast. Because there was no actual lump, her options included excising the calcifications and receiving radiation. Instead, she chose a much more aggressive and definitive course–to completely remove the breast.

"To me it wasn't a big deal to have a mastectomy; I didn't attach a lot of meaning to my breast," Kimberly says. "What mattered was being completely free of cancer."

Kimberly, 53, continued to work during the months-long reconstruction, but she and her husband decided to take early retirement when "the breast stuff," as she calls it, was finished. "We felt it was time to put ourselves before work."

After a cancer diagnosis, self-reflection can be difficult. Kimberly allowed herself a few pity parties but mostly stayed positive. "Soon after my diagnosis, I learned I'd be a grandma for the first time. That gave me something else to focus on," she says.

She's learned to go with the flow. "I really don't worry anymore about what I can't control," Kimberly says. She takes yearly trips and has started reading again. "Reading sounds so small, but it's something I hadn't done when I was busy working and raising a family," she says.

Because of her choice to have a mastectomy, the chances for recurrence are very low. "It's always in the back of my head," she says, "but that doesn't stop me from enjoying myself."

She'd like women who've been diagnosed to know . . . *try not to be afraid, and don't worry too much about saving your breasts.*

Breast cancer is . . . *scary.*

Tomorrow will . . . *bring new hope.*

"What do we live for,
if it is not to make life less
difficult for each other."

—GEORGE ELIOT

CHAPTER 12

JOINING A
SUPPORT GROUP

Want to reduce the three major stressors—loneliness, loss of control, and hopelessness[1]—that impact breast cancer patients the most? Interested in optimizing your outlook on the future? If so, consider hanging out with other survivors in a face-to-face (or virtual) support group. Along with a healthy diet, exercise, and other life-affirming choices, studies show that a supportive network can improve your quality of life and possibly help you to live longer, too.

For example, in one study from Ohio State University, women with breast cancer were evaluated after their surgery and before starting other treatments. They were randomly assigned to either small groups led by a psychologist or to a control group without psychological intervention. The small groups met for 26 biweekly sessions over the course of a year.

The goal of the meetings was to reduce distress (and stress), improve quality of life, encourage better health behaviors (diet, exercise, smoking cessation), and facilitate cancer treatment compliance and medical follow-up. The long list of strategies used ranged from progressive relaxation techniques to using assertive communication to get medical needs met.

When the study ended, researchers found that the psychologist-led group benefited across the board from the intervention. Moreover, having a group they could discuss things with and get advice from also seemed to strengthen their immune systems. But what may have been the most striking finding came when patients were followed up 7 to 13 years later. Those who had participated in the small groups had a better chance of survival and less chance of recurrence than the control group.

The researchers theorized that when cancer patients get psychological help early, they not only improve their health (both mental and physical) and treatment-relevant behaviors but possibly their biological outcomes, too. If so, the researchers concluded, support groups offer the potential for improved survivorship and survival for cancer patients.[2]

Additional findings from international studies about the benefits of support groups are compelling, too. This research has found that:

Support groups can reduce distress–and pain–as well as trauma symptoms in breast cancer patients, according to research conducted on professionally led support groups at the University of Alberta in Canada.[3]

Support groups can reduce social isolation and enhance ability to cope, according to an Irish study published in the journal *Cancer Nursing*. Investigators reported that peer support for women with breast cancer also provided additional access to information.[4]

Support groups can help women with breast cancer overcome feelings of powerlessness–and increase their sense of control, according to Vestfold University College in Norway. In the study, participants in three professionally led support groups learned about empowerment through weekly discussions that focused on raising awareness, acquiring knowledge, learning from others' experiences, and discovering new perspectives on life–and on themselves. Interviews conducted during, and after, the support groups concluded that the self-help sessions made a valuable contribution to the patients' recovery. Participants also strongly recommended the groups to others.[5]

Support groups can improve memory, feelings of fatigue, and body image. A long-term Swedish study divided women with breast cancer into two groups. One group attended a support group for a week, and the control group did not. The researchers followed up with the women 2 months later and again about 6.5 years later.

The researchers found that the women who attended the support group showed significantly greater improvements, not only in cognitive function, feelings of fatigue, and body image but also in their outlooks on the future.[6]

Even after reading those studies about the benefits of support groups, you may still be saying, "No thanks–that's not for me." Many women feel this way, mainly because they're not interested in sharing their private experience with a group. But before skipping this chapter entirely and moving on to the next, take a look at all options for group support that we discuss. Not all fit the face-to-face profile you may expect. Instead, there are "on demand" groups available 24/7 by phone and in cyberspace that may just be a perfect fit for you.

SUPPORT GROUPS THEN—AND NOW

When you ask people for a successful example of a peer support group, invariably the words "Alcoholics Anonymous" roll off their tongues. And that's not surprising. Alcoholics Anonymous developed what is now called a 12-step program; and, for 75 years, it has served as an exemplary model of mutual holistic support for people of all ages, races, and socioeconomic backgrounds.

But what we call a "support group" today is broader than just this one iconic illustration. In the jargon of the 21st century, it also makes sense for patients, survivors, and their families to think of these multifaceted groups in terms of social networks and connections.

A social network is defined as an interconnected group of cooperating significant others, who may or may not be related, with whom a person interacts.[7] People in these networks are just as likely to live on another continent as they are in your neighborhood, city, or country.

It doesn't matter, though, what you call your group–it could be anything from a social network to a self-help meeting to a book club. And it matters even less how big or small your group is. What counts are the positive benefits of interacting closely with others, as this one study from Kaiser Permanente found.

When a team of scientists looked at the impact of social networks on survival, they found that "socially isolated women were 34 percent more likely to die from breast cancer or other causes than socially integrated women." Moreover, their study of 2,264 women diagnosed with early-stage invasive breast cancer determined that the real benefits were not related to the size of the patient's social circle but to the strength of bonds formed in individual relationships.[8]

Women whose networks were small but offered high levels of support were better off than women who had small networks and low levels of support, according to Candyce H. Kroenke, ScD, MPH, lead researcher of the study. And those who were not well integrated socially were at a greater risk of dying. In fact, women with small social networks and less support were 61 percent more likely to die from breast cancer and other causes.[9]

A GUIDE TO GROUPS

Use this guide to help you find the group that's right for you.

Face-to-Face Support Groups

There are two types of face-to-face groups that can offer emotional, physical, psychological, social, and informational support: "open" and "closed." Open groups are those in which new members are welcome to join pretty much at any time. It may also mean that your family members or friends can join with you as well. In closed groups, people are only allowed to join the group at certain times (for example, at the beginning of the year) or under certain circumstances.

Patients in closed groups may have characteristics in common, such as gender, age, or those that are cancer specific. Under some circumstances, you may need a referral from a doctor, therapist, or other professional to join.

Self-Help/Peer Support Groups

These are classic and newer versions of the face-to-face local support groups. Most are organized and run by their members and meet in community centers, churches and synagogues, and even members' homes. Sometimes a leader has professional credentials, but not always. There's typically no cost to join these groups.

Group Therapy

Because it's easy for many people to confuse self-help groups with group therapy, it's important to know how they're different.

Unlike self-help/peer groups run by members, group therapy is psychotherapy. That means the sessions are run by qualified psychologists, psychiatrists, social workers, or other licensed therapists. For some survivors, these groups are a more affordable alternative or an adjunct to private therapy.

Unless a social service agency, hospital, or health-care organization is covering the cost of group therapy, the charges vary. Whether or not the fees are on a sliding scale depends on who sponsors the group. Most likely you'll need a referral, and the costs may or may not be covered by your health-insurance plan, so be sure to check first. If it's confusing, ask your health provider, your patient navigator (if you have one), or a financial representative at the therapist's office for help and more information.

Organization-Based Support Groups

These groups gather under the banners of national, statewide, or local cancer organizations. The Virginia Breast Cancer Foundation (vbcf.org), for example, is an organization that provides downloadable information about organization-sponsored support groups statewide. Another example is the Beautiful Gate Cancer Support and Resource Center (thebeautifulgate.net), which has four locations in the greater Miami area. Each offers African American women a wide range of breast cancer services, including monthly support group meetings. And in San Francisco, there's BAYS, the Bay Area Young Survivors (baysnet.org), a support and action group that sponsors everything from monthly support group meetings to community-building events–all for young women living with breast cancer.

On a larger scale, the Cancer Support Community is an international nonprofit group offering personalized services and education to support people affected by cancer. It's an initiative that got started after two well-known organizations–the Wellness Community and Gilda's Club–joined together to provide support through a network of 50 local affiliates, more than 100 satellite locations, and online services. The local centers offer free support group meetings for patients, their families, and other caregivers that are run by mental health and other professional volunteers. For a list of centers or information about online groups, go to cancersupportcommunity.org. Here, too, are a few organizations that may be able to steer you to support groups in your area. They also offer one-on-one support by phone, e-mail, or online chat.

- **American Cancer Society** maintains a list of organizations offering support groups. Call 800-227-2345 for information or to talk to a cancer specialist.

- **Cancer*Care*** is a national nonprofit organization providing free professional counseling, educational programs, practical help, and financial assistance to cancer patients. No matter where you live, you can speak with an oncology social worker or join a 12-week telephone group for women with breast cancer who are stage IV and currently receiving active treatment; 800-813-4673, cancercare.org.

- **National Cancer Institute's Support Services Locator** has links to more than 100 organizations nationwide that provide emotional, practical, and financial support for people with cancer and their families; supportorgs.cancer.gov.

- **National Lymphedema Network** organized the first lymphoma support group in the United States, providing education and guidance to women with lymphedema; they can also help you start a support group if one isn't available in your area; 800-541-3259, lymphnet.org.

- **Planet Cancer** is a Livestrong Foundation initiative for young adults with cancer ages 18 to 40; 855-220-7777, myplanet.planetcancer.org.

- **Reach to Recovery** is an American Cancer Society program in which volunteers offer understanding, support, and hope because they themselves have survived breast cancer; tinyurl.com/l792nbn.

- **Sharsheret,** Hebrew for "chain," is a national organization supporting young Jewish women and families facing breast and ovarian cancer. A peer support network connects women newly diagnosed or at high risk of developing breast or ovarian cancer with others sharing similar diagnoses and experiences; 866-474-2774, sharsheret.org.

Special Needs Support Groups

These may be peer groups or ones facilitated by medical, mental health, and other health-care professionals such as nutritionists. Trained, volunteer survivors who represent national breast cancer organizations may also organize and moderate them. Examples are groups that help women deal with postsurgery pain, self-esteem, sexual or childbearing issues, lymphedema, self-empowerment, relationships, and other conditions and concerns. Overall, these support groups may offer short-term follow-up and/or ongoing resources for patients, survivors, and their families. These groups are usually free.

"support groups just aren't right for me"

Are you like many women who hear the words *support group* and immediately think, "Not for me." If so, know this: The decision to join is very personal, and it's not wrong to feel this way. Indeed, there are many valid reasons breast cancer patients and survivors make this choice.

Reason #1: Lack of Communication

Sometimes busy doctors and health-care professionals don't take the time to talk to all of their patients about the benefits of a support group. This can limit or influence their patients' perceptions and decisions about the value and importance of these groups.

This was the conclusion of a study, conducted at the University of Cologne, Germany, which found that patients are given different information about self-help groups depending on which hospital they're being treated at. Additionally, they're also given different levels of contact with the groups based on their age and education. For example, the odds of being informed about self-help groups were significantly lower when breast cancer patients were treated at a teaching hospital. Also, patients ages 40 to 59 were significantly more informed about these support groups than those ages 60 to 69. Moreover, women with the highest education often reported that they were not only informed about the groups, but that they had contact with them, too.[10]

Reason #2: Personality Issues

You may be shy and/or introverted or find it difficult to talk to strangers about feelings, personal problems, and body parts like your breasts. That's okay; if you feel this way, you don't have to join a support group, but read this chapter anyway. You may be surprised to discover a group that works for you.

Reason #3: Learning Styles

Maybe you'd rather get information or support from a licensed counselor or clergy person. Or maybe you're already attending group therapy sessions facilitated by a licensed professional.

Reason #4: Alternate Approaches

You may find other ways of making social connections—through religious and spiritual communities and/or other types of therapeutic groups such as for art, music, drama, poetry, or dance. These groups allow you to express your concerns, questions, and emotions without having to join a formal breast cancer support group.

Reason #5: Logistics

You may find that your schedule is so tightly packed that there's no room for one more thing. Or perhaps you live in a rural area without the means to get to a meeting.

Reason #6: Misperceptions

Maybe you've gotten negative feedback and information about a group from someone else and that discourages you. Perhaps you're worried that you'll have to make uncomfortable revelations in front of strangers (you won't).

Reason #7: Sheer Exhaustion

Women often find it difficult to make choices due to fatigue, stress, depression, and the side effects of their treatment. Or you may simply be tired of talking about or trying to deal with breast cancer. You would rather do something else with your precious and rare free time.

If these reasons and others have contributed to your decision not to consider group support as a viable resource, we encourage you to read about all the options in this chapter before making your final decision.

Online Support Groups

This category covers a range of services that offer peer support and information, medical information and education, professional support, inspirational support, opportunities to read and tell stories, and other services, such as online conferences and newsletters.

In fact, according to a 2011 Pew Research Center Internet and American Life Project survey, one in four Internet users living with cancer or some other chronic ailment say they've gone online to find others with health concerns similar to theirs.[11] Whether people are searching for a quick answer or seeking to gain a deeper understanding of a new treatment option or prescription, the survey concluded that the Internet can be a valuable tool.[12]

THE POWER OF A VIRTUAL COMMUNITY

Since the explosion of social networks on the Internet, research shows that women with breast cancer now use them to meet their psychological, informational, and emotional needs prior to diagnosis and during and after treatment. The results of these studies are not only affirming the need for this resource, but they also offer a new lens for medical and social service professionals to better understand what their patients want and need. For example, researchers have found that:

Information online should be tailored to patients' different interests and needs. In a University of North Carolina study of breast cancer, diabetes, and fibromyalgia online discussion forums, researchers categorized the forums for each of the illnesses into clusters—generic, support, patient-centered, experiential knowledge, treatments/procedures, medications, and condition management. They concluded that narrowing the focus of the forums was indeed helpful because doing so provided the specific information that patients needed at various points during their illness.[13]

Women feel empowered after participating in virtual support groups. A study at the Institute for Behavioural Research at the University of Twente in the Netherlands looked at 528 women with breast cancer, arthritis, and fibromyalgia who participated in online support groups. The women felt empowered from "being better informed" and experienced "enhanced social well-being." The practical implication for

do I need a face-to-face support group?

Having a hard time trying to figure out whether or not a local, face-to-face support group will meet your needs and expectations? First, try journaling about why you're considering or *not* considering doing this. Then make a list in your journal of the pros and cons of joining one. (Plan to come back to these thoughts and ideas after you do the exercise below—and then again, after you read this chapter.)

Here are some suggestions on getting started.

Divide a page into two columns. Mark one column *Upsides*. Mark the other *Downsides*.

List every reason or thought that comes to mind in each column. No idea is off-limits.

Finally, add up the number of reasons in each column. If there are lots of upsides, now is the time to join. If there are too many down-sides, respect what your mind, body, and spirit are saying.

Begin exploring your options if you're ready to look for a group. Use this chapter as a guide.

If you're not going to join a local group, read about alternative ways to get "group" support in this chapter. In your journal, write about your decision—and your decision process. If you *do* decide to join one, however, be sure to use your journal to jot down notes and thoughts about the group—and what you're learning from it.

health-care providers: It's important to inform patients about online support groups and the benefits they offer.[14]

Women don't feel comfortable discussing everything in online sup-port groups. Psychologists at Felician College in Lodi, New Jersey, were the first to look at the perceived benefits of online support groups for women with metastatic breast cancer. Women with this type of cancer participated in online peer support groups. Most reported benefiting in some way from the cohesiveness of the group, the information exchanged, the hope offered, the universality of the members, and the feelings of catharsis. However, although most women said they could discuss many of their concerns freely, researchers found they had difficulty discussing death and dying, critical issues for women with metastatic breast cancer.[15]

Finding Online Support

Here are some of the most popular types of sites that breast cancer patients and their families go to for group, informational, and one-on-one support. Think of them as starting places. Also check with other survivors to see what they recommend.

Cancer and health-care organizations: These include not just the big recognizable names in cancer causes, but smaller national and local ones, too. Many also provide support group opportunities to patients, survivors, and their families. In most instances, you can blog, chat, get expert one-on-one advice, be part of a conference call with breast cancer survivors of all ages, read posts, and post on discussion boards. Here are some examples.

- **Cancer Support Community** (cancersupportcommunity.org) offers the Living Room, an online community where patients and survivors can connect with others 24/7 to discuss concerns, questions, or just speak to someone else going through the same thing. They also schedule real-time support groups that meet online in a chat room–facilitated by professionals trained in running online cancer support groups–for 90 minutes each week. Groups are also available for caregivers and those dealing with bereavement.

- **Cancer Survivors Network** (csn.cancer.org) is an online American Cancer Society community by, and for, people with cancer and their families. It has a member search to find and connect with others as well as discussion boards, chat rooms, and private e-mail. You can also create your own personal space to write about your experience, share photos and audio, start a blog, talk about resources, and more. (You can also do live chats; 877-333-4673.)

- **Living Beyond Breast Cancer** (lbbc.org) is committed to empowering all women affected by breast cancer to live as long as possible with the best quality of life. The organization offers a Survivors' Helpline for those times when you have questions, need someone to listen, or don't know where to turn. Women who have experienced breast cancer answer the calls; 888-753-5222.

Living Beyond Breast Cancer also has opportunities for you to ask questions during free webinars (seminars conducted on the Internet) that discuss medical findings from leading breast cancer conferences, give detailed information on new treatments and clinical trials, and explore emotional issues. Their online first-person videos and stories are another way to "connect" with survivors whose experiences may resonate with yours.

- **National Breast Cancer Foundation** (nationalbreastcancer.org) offers MyNBCF, a support community for breast cancer patients, survivors, and their loved ones.

making sure a group is right for you

Whether a group is open or closed, formal or informal, has half a dozen members or a hundred, when you attend for the first time, just observe, talk to other people in the group, and get a gut sense of whether or not it's a safe place for you and other women with breast cancer to gather. Then, observe how mutually and respectfully the women in the group are able to:

- Talk about their experiences, interests, and stories—and listen to the stories of others
- Experience nonjudgmental acceptance
- Seek others' support for their desire to be well
- Discuss common concerns and problems
- Get information and ask questions
- Become inspired to remain hopeful
- Get the support they need to overcome stumbling blocks

- **Triple Negative Breast Cancer Foundation** (tnbcfoundation.org) is in partnership with Cancer*Care*, a national nonprofit organization; it offers online support groups moderated by an oncology social worker for those diagnosed with triple negative breast cancer.

- **WhatNext** (whatnext.com) is a social network developed in part with the American Cancer Society to help cancer patients, survivors, and caregivers gain firsthand insight into living with cancer (including what cancer treatments are like) and connect with others facing a similar diagnosis. WhatNext also links you to American Cancer Society resources.

Hospital and hospice Web sites: If you're interested in finding out what support groups are available in your area, you'll usually find answers and/or links on hospital or hospice home pages. If not, call the organization directly. If the person answering doesn't have the information you need, ask to be put in touch with a patient navigator or the person managing the Web site. Either should be able to answer your questions.

Social media: Today when someone hears "social media," Facebook, Pinterest, and Twitter—as well as blogs, chat rooms, and discussion boards—usually come to mind. All offer ways to get support and practical information from peers, organizations, and professionals. All also offer these additional benefits, according to one survey: friendships, empathy, humor, freedom to be one's self, diversity, convenience, nonjudgmental atmosphere, relative anonymity, reassurance that others are there for you, and reassurance that there are survivors of the disease. [16]

If you're not already on these social interaction sites, here's a guide to using them. In each case, you'll have to register and create a profile before you can move beyond the home page and have a "voice."

- **Facebook** is the site where you can add different types of personal information and photos—and join breast cancer pages and groups. Facebook is also a place where you can create your own page dedicated to your breast cancer journey and get "Likes" and other feedback from friends. To get started, go to facebook.com.

- **Twitter** members "tweet" each other and their followers through short messages up to 140 characters long. Your tweets are always posted on your browser's Twitter page, but most often, they usually go to your "followers" on their mobile and other devices. To get started, go to twitter.com.

Once you're logged on, test Twitter's style of support by tweeting #BCSM (breast cancer social media) and taking it for a trial run. This Twitter and online community/network is dedicated *exclusively* to women and men affected by breast cancer. Its mission is to help support, empower, and inform their followers about issues related to breast cancer and help them out of the isolation treatment can create. #BCSM on Twitter hosts real-time conversations on Monday evenings at 9:00 p.m. ET/8:00 p.m. CT/6:00 p.m. PT. The moderating team includes a board-certified breast surgeon. Recaps of clinical conferences are part of the schedule. For more information, go to bcsmcommunity.org.

- **Pinterest** focuses on images using "pinboards," which can contain thoughts, pictures, artwork, inspiring quotes, and other information that can then be "repinned" by others with the same interests. You have to sign up for Pinterest and wait a few days to be "accepted." Once you're in, you can get an idea of what Pinterest is like by going to the Living with Breast Cancer board at is.gd/soy53s; it's just one example of a dedicated breast cancer board.

Blogs: These are also called online journals, diaries, and weblogs. They all have one thing in common–they're a Web site containing the writer's or group of writers' own experiences, observations, and opinions. They range from very serious musings to humorous ones. Often they have images and links to other Web sites, too. Thousands of breast cancer patients and survivors have blogs, and a few have been running for 10 or more years. Because they're insightful, inspirational, and informational, many survivors read them daily.

Most of the national breast cancer organizations and many hospitals and cancer centers have their own blogs, too. These are trustworthy places where patients, survivors, and their families can ask questions, tell stories, or just comment on the words of others going through similar experiences.

Here's a sample of a few highly rated breast cancer blogs to explore.[17] Before you find yourself reading the posts, you may want to click the "About" link to get information about the blogger and what compelled her to make such deeply personal information public.

- **Living Beyond Breast Cancer** (livingbeyondbc.wordpress.com) explains the purpose of their blog by saying: "Every woman deserves to live beyond her cancer, to achieve her dreams and goals despite a terrible setback. With this group ready and waiting in the wings, that happy outcome will be a whole lot more doable for women across the country."

- **I Survived Damn Near Everything** (isurviveddamnneareverything .com) is by Carole Sanek, who says, "Life is not about just surviving, we all do that in some form. It is about how we thrive after we survive that matters."

- **ChemoBrain–In the Fog** (chemo-brain.blogspot.com) is written by AnneMarie Ciccarella, an award-winning blogger with a family history of breast cancer. She explains why she started her blog: "There are, for all intents and purposes, five diagnoses of breast cancer among my mom, my sisters, and me. Four of those were premenopausal."

- **Miracle Survivors–Inspiration & Information for Cancer Thrivers** (tamiboehmer.com) is by Tami Boehmer, who explains her blog's purpose: "Since being diagnosed in 2002, and especially since my stage IV diagnosis (2007), my passion is serving other breast cancer survivors."

- **Bumpy Boobs** (facingcancer.ca/bumpyboobs/) is by Catherine Brunelle, a Canadian survivor who went through treatment when she was 28 years old. She explains her blog this way: "I was diagnosed with breast cancer a few days after my 1-year wedding anniversary. That was a shocker. Since then I had a mastectomy, chemotherapy, radiotherapy, and am now 3 years NED [no evidence of disease]. With international relocations, job search drama, fighting off apartment vermin, falling deeply in love, and now navigating fertility, the impact of a cancer diagnosis has been far reaching."

Chat rooms: These are, quite simply, places on the Internet where people can type on their keyboards to "talk" to one another in real time. Many breast cancer organizations sponsor chat rooms that are "open" 24/7. The chat room at Breastcancer.org is a good place to begin to get a feel for this type of group support. All you have to do is register on the site. From that point on, you may find that chat rooms are a great way to get and share information on breast cancer.

Discussion boards: These are places for you to post comments and questions about your breast cancer and get feedback from other patients, survivors, and their families. Discussion boards are typically organized into "forums" where participants discuss specific topics.

Discussion boards are usually easy to follow and are a great way to get support from people worldwide. When someone posts a question, thought, or concern on a board and others respond, they create "threads." On many discussion boards, you can also send and receive private messages.

Once again, we recommend getting the hang of discussion boards by first registering for one sponsored by a respected national breast cancer organization. Breastcancer.org, for example, has very active ones. In 2013, the site's discussion boards had more than 134,000 members in 73 forums discussing more than 106,000 different topics.

Additionally, moderators on this site recommend following these helpful tips for keeping the community safe–and protecting your privacy and security.

- **All posts and screen names are searchable** using Google and other search engines, as well as by using the Breastcancer.org forums search function. Though a private message will not show up in a search, *everything* you post on public discussion boards can be read by others.

- **For your posting ID, never use your real name,** a recognizable nickname, address, phone number, workplace or school, names of kids or pets, or any other details that can specifically identify you to a searcher. If you originally registered using your real name, you can change it any time. Go to the "My Profile" link at the top of the page. From there, go to the "Settings" tab and then the "Edit" link beside your name.

- **Only use the "Private Message" function if you want to share personal information** with members you know and trust.

- **Protect your privacy** by using an avatar–an image that represents you–instead of a real picture of you. Popular avatars are pictures of flowers, animals, mythological creatures, or any other image that says, "This is me"–but in disguise.[18]

caution: browse safely!

Because this is such a vulnerable time for you, use this step-by-step guide to be sure your experience looking for breast cancer information and support on the Internet is safe.

Step 1: Be Sure Your Computer Is Hacker-Proof

First, look at the list of browsers below. If you're not using one of them to get on the Internet, it's time to switch. While no browser is completely foolproof and secure from hackers, these are among the safest ways to get onto the Internet.

- **Firefox:** firefox.com
- **Chrome:** google.com/intl/en/chrome/
- **Internet Explorer:** windows.microsoft.com/en-us/ internet-explorer/download-ie/ (for PCs only)
- **Safari:** apple.com/safari/
- **Opera:** opera.com

Next go to Web of Trust, at mywot.com, and download and install the software for your browser. (If you're not tech savvy, ask a knowledgeable and trustworthy partner, friend, or relative to help you through this process.) When you click on a site, Web of Trust instantly goes into action, identifying whether that site has a proven safety record–and giving you the option to click off and go to another site.

Once Web of Trust is working, it's time for you (or your helper) to get security in place. Many excellent programs have free versions, so you don't have to pay for one with unnecessary bells and whistles. Just search for "best free antivirus software for Mac (or for PC)." Next, read the reviews of those that come up, and opt for the best. Remember, Web of Trust will warn you if the site reviewing the software is "shady." Once you see software that looks like it will do the job, double-check that it finds malicious programs. These harmful programs are called malware. If the software looks comprehensive, download it.

With these safeguards in place, there are just two more things to keep in mind: Almost everything on the Internet is public, so be careful what you type–even if you're in a closed virtual group. And when you go to a site that asks for your information, see if there's a lock by its address or if it reads "https://" instead of just "http://." The s in "https" stands for secure, but either one indicates that your personal information will be safe.

Step 2: Begin Surfing

Now that you've got safeguards in place, here's how to navigate the information you find.

Narrow your search. If you search "breast cancer" on Google, you get a list of about 500 million sites. The top breast cancer sites come up first, and almost all of the ones on the first few pages have a green dot (for "go ahead and check out this page") from Web of Trust. Most of these sites have information about support groups, and many link you to local resources.

Use your browser's bookmark feature. This marks the sites you like so you can quickly access them later.

Don't pay attention to breast cancer–related ads on the side of your search results page. They're distractions, and they may contain viruses. Instead, if you're looking for a specific product or organization, search for it separately.

Keep track of time. The amount of information can be mesmerizing, but spending a lot of time on the Web can cause fatigue, something you definitely don't need right now.

Personal pages: Many hospitals and cancer treatment centers offer patients these services via CarePages (carepages.com), CaringBridge (caringbridge.org), or MyLifeLine.org (mylifeline.org). These sites allow cancer patients and other patients to set up a personal, secure, and free Web site in order to share news, stories, pictures, and other information with their families and friends. The goal is to help you create your own social health network. Like blogs, discussion boards, and Facebook pages, there are places for people to comment on the posts. If you want, they can even make donations to help out with medical bills and other financial concerns. According to CaringBridge, over half a million people connect through their site every day.

In closing, keep in mind that if a support group isn't a part of your road map at this time, it may be in the future. In the next section, we'll talk about moving beyond breast cancer. Because life always puts challenges in our paths, we hope this chapter can always be a place to revisit to find resources for working through them.

New Beginnings

On 9/11, Meryl Marshall faced a horrible challenge when she lost her husband, Robert Mayo, in the World Trade Center attacks. She started coping with her loss and rebuilding a life with her son, who was 11. On the path to healing, she met widower Craig Marshall and married him in 2004, becoming a stepmother to his sons, who were then 8 and 12.

But just 6 months after walking down the aisle, Meryl, then 46, was diagnosed with stage I breast cancer. "One day as I sat down with my coffee, I watched some morning show hosts discuss a new technique for doing breast self-checks. I decided to try it, and sure enough, almost immediately I found a lump the size of a pea."

Meryl's doctor wasn't worried. Her breast exam just a month earlier and the previous year's mammogram had been clean. But she went for another mammogram, an ultrasound, and ultimately a needle biopsy. "When I got the diagnosis, all I could think was, *Why?*" says Meryl, now 54. "I finally had a chance at being happy, and here was another very large staircase to climb."

A lumpectomy, six rounds of chemotherapy, and 5 weeks of radiation took its toll on her body. "It's a daily battle to regain strength," says Meryl. "Going through something like 9/11, and then through breast cancer . . . those challenges really shape you."

After treatment, Meryl started exercising, revamped her diet, and switched to nontoxic products for her home. She and her husband now own a chemical-free makeup line.

Meryl cherishes simple moments. "I don't need an outrageous vacation, but I do need to meet my friends or my sons for lunch. I want to provide memories for them and enjoy special life moments for myself."

She'd like women who've been diagnosed to know . . . *to learn to relax; being stressed won't help you.*

Breast cancer is . . . *a hurdle.*

Tomorrow will . . . *be there.*

*"It is more important to know what sort
of person has a disease than to know
what sort of disease a person has."*

—HIPPOCRATES

CHAPTER 13

COMPLEMENTARY AND ALTERNATIVE MEDICINE

When one part of your body isn't working well–your breasts, for example–the mental, emotional, and spiritual side of you is out of balance as well. Chances are you've already felt and experienced this phenomenon. It's the foundation of thought behind complementary medicine. Complementary medicine encompasses the use of healing therapies, such as acupuncture and reflexology, used along with conventional (sometimes called Western or allopathic, or conventional) medicine. Complementary medicine is also known as integrative or holistic medicine because it integrates mind-body-spirit therapies with–in the case of breast cancer–mainstream scientifically proven medical treatments such as surgery, chemotherapy, and radiation. The idea is to treat the *whole* person (hence the word *holistic*), inside and out, so the body can get back into balance and help heal itself. And just as chemotherapy or radiation is tailored to your body and the breast cancer you have, so too is complementary medicine tailored to the individual. The thinking: The therapies that are right for *you* might not necessarily be right for the woman with breast cancer who's sitting next to you in the waiting room. Health care, say complementary medicine practitioners, must be personalized to what *your* body, mind, *and* spirit need.

Perhaps you've been wanting to try complementary medicine since you got your diagnosis, or perhaps you're already using it. You're not alone. Today, up to 80 percent of all women use some form of complementary and alternative medicine, and 57 percent of those with early-stage breast cancer will try at least one over the course of their illness[1] to reduce symptoms and the side effects of treatments, to gain some semblance of control over their health and their recovery, to help treat or cure their breast cancer, and to maintain a positive outlook.

In fact, you may have already experienced complementary medicine without realizing it. Meditating to reduce stress, sipping herbal tea to sleep better, having acupuncture treatments to help reduce pain, practicing tai chi to stimulate your immune system, or visualizing the best possible outcome are all forms of this type of medicine. Even taking nutritional supplements is one. In fact, supplementation is the number-one form of complementary medicine used in North America by both cancer patients and the general population.[2] And for more than 20 years, complementary medicine has also included spiritual practices, such as prayer and other spiritually based rituals and healing practices. Even cancer support groups have been classified as complementary medicine in several recent studies that looked at their efficacy.

THE 5 CATEGORIES OF COMPLEMENTARY AND ALTERNATIVE MEDICINE

According to the National Cancer Institute, experts use these five categories to describe complementary and alternative medicine.

1. **Biologically based practices** include "treatments" based on plants and animals found in nature. This includes vitamins, herbs, foods, special diets, and aromatherapy.

2. **Manipulative and body-based practices** work with one or more parts of the body by manipulating or adjusting them. This includes massage, acupressure, and reflexology.

3. **Mind-body medicine** is treatment based on the belief that your mind and body are an interactive system, and one can affect the other. Included are meditation, biofeedback, hypnosis, imagery, yoga, and creative or expressive arts.

4. **Energy medicine** involves the belief that the body has energy fields that can be used for healing and wellness. Included are tai chi, qigong, reiki, therapeutic touch, and healing touch.

5. **Whole medical systems** are complete, unconventional healing systems and beliefs that have evolved in different cultures and different parts of the world. Ayurvedic (eye-yur-VAY-dik) medicine is a system from India emphasizing balance among body, mind, and spirit. Chinese medicine is based on the belief that health is influenced by a balance in the body of two forces called yin and yang. Homeopathy uses very small doses of substances to trigger the body to heal itself.

WHAT DOES *YOUR* DOCTOR THINK OF COMPLEMENTARY MEDICINE?

While there's no scientific evidence that complementary medicine can prevent or cure breast cancer, don't be surprised if your oncologist or health-care team suggests trying some form of complementary medicine over the course of your treatment and recovery.

Just 25 years ago, this type of recommendation from a mainstream doctor was unheard of. At that time, most of these traditional doctors resisted learning about complementary and alternative medicine and rarely recommended it. Back then, it was untested and commonly considered unsafe, even quackery, in the broad medical community. Today, however, many doctors give their patients a green light to use acupuncture, mindfulness meditation, breath work, guided imagery, and other forms of alternative medicine that have a proven track record of safely helping people.

Why the attitude adjustment? First, more and more people are using it, so doctors can't ignore it anymore. In fact, studies show that use of complementary and alternative medicine increases following any kind of cancer diagnosis, with breast cancer survivors being the heaviest users among all survivors.[3] Plus, a growing number of top medical schools and cancer centers, including Harvard, Yale, Johns Hopkins, the University of Massachusetts, Duke University, Georgetown University, Columbia University, the University of Texas MD Anderson Cancer Center, and Memorial Sloan-Kettering Cancer Center, are embracing it as well. To date, 50 of the 141 accredited American medical schools[4] have established integrative medicine departments and programs.

So if you're planning on using (or already are using) alternative therapies, don't be afraid to talk to your oncologist about it. Mainstream medical doctors want to have open communication with their patients about complementary and alternative medicine to advise them about what may be helpful and what could be harmful (for example, any form of therapy that recommends discontinuing conventional medical treatments and/or guarantees a cancer cure). We cannot stress this enough: You should *never* discontinue a medication or treatment in favor of an alternative medicine without discussing it with your doctor first, because it could interfere with your healing, recovery, and even your long-term prognosis.

IT'S ABOUT QUALITY OF LIFE

Conventional medical treatments such as surgery, chemotherapy, and radiation can improve your health, but their primary focus is on treating the disease and not necessarily on improving your quality of life. Quality of life takes into account:

- How well you feel, physically and mentally
- How well you do everyday activities, such as eating, bathing, and dressing
- How content and/or stressed you are
- How rewarding your relationships with family, friends, and others are

As you read through this list, spend some time pondering how your diagnosis and treatments may be impacting one, a few, or all of those factors. Most likely you can name at least one. And if that's true, then it may be just enough reason for you to begin using complementary medicine because *these* are the things that complementary medicine has had the most success treating.

Even the National Institutes of Health, which funds complementary and alternative medicine studies, categorizes therapies that improve a breast cancer patient's quality of life as a priority. Other government and private agencies that financially support investigative complementary and alternative studies agree, too. For example, the Department of Defense funded a Michigan State University College of Nursing study to analyze which complementary and alternative therapies, such as massage, supplements, and reflexology, are used the most, and why.

The study enrolled 220 women with breast cancer who were tracked to determine their use of complementary and alternative therapies. The research showed that the sickest women enrolled in the study were more likely to use multiple therapies. Biological-based therapies were the most

BETWEEN THE LINES

complementary and alternative medicine in a nutshell

While many of the names for complementary and alternative medicine are used interchangeably, they have slightly different meanings. Here's a quick rundown.

Alternative medicine refers to healing practices that replace conventional medicine and are not part of standard care. For example, using homeopathy in place of mainstream medicine, or replacing chemotherapy with Chinese herbs and other dietary supplements, is considered alternative medicine.

Complementary medicine refers to medical systems, therapies, and practices that are used as an adjunct to conventional medicine. For example, using acupuncture in addition to mainstream medical care to help lessen pain or other symptoms is considered complementary medicine.

Holistic medicine looks at, and treats, the body as a whole and can be used along with conventional medical treatments for breast cancer, like chemotherapy, radiation, and surgery. For example, holistic practitioners may treat cancer by changing the diet and adding support groups and counseling. Holistic practitioners also typically recommend healthy lifestyle habits, such as exercising, eating a nutritious diet, getting enough sleep, and working toward inner peace.

Integrative medicine is a total mind, body, and spirit approach to patient care that combines treatments from conventional medicine and alternative medicine and for which there is some high-quality evidence of safety and effectiveness.[5] It's also called integrated medicine and integrated health care.

popular, followed by mind-body therapies using audiotapes, video, and music therapy.[6] Lead researcher Gwen Wyatt, PhD, RN, concluded that: "Patients link symptoms to quality of life; if you have to live with breast cancer, then let's have the highest quality of life we can during the process and make it as humane as possible."[7]

But don't expect any form of complementary or alternative medicine to be a quick fix. For example, if you're not sleeping well and hope that complementary medicine can cure that problem right away, set that expectation aside. Even if numerous studies found that hypnosis and/or guided imagery (see Chapter 11 for more on these) are highly effective, you still won't cure insomnia overnight. It usually takes time and sustained daily practice for your z's to improve, and the same is true for most complementary and alternative therapies and whatever problem you're looking to them for solutions.

CONSIDERING COMPLEMENTARY MEDICINE?

There are risks associated with any medical treatment you receive for breast cancer. Complementary and alternative medicine is no different. In fact, because these therapies don't fall under the same rigorous scrutiny as traditional medicine, many are not regulated, making them even more risky. So if you choose to use complementary and alternative medicine, we strongly advise taking some precautions.

Research

Read through this chapter and the stress management chapter to learn about a particular practice or therapy that may interest you. If you have health-care insurance, find out if the treatments are covered. If so, ask how many are included and what your co-pay will be. For example, some plans now cover acupuncture, biofeedback, and massage, but only when your doctor prescribes them.

Communicate

Even if your hospital or medical center offers these therapies free to breast cancer patients, still talk to your health-care team first. Why? As we mentioned in Chapter 9, some nutritional supplements, for example, may interact negatively with your medications and/or with other supplements, or they can contain harmful ingredients not listed on the label. By giving your health-care team a comprehensive picture of how you're managing all aspects of your healing journey, you're taking an important step to ensure that your self-care and your medical care are always coordinated, beneficial, and safe.

Don't Neglect Your Doctor's Treatment Plan

Although you may assume your doctor will automatically say "no" to using a complementary therapy exclusively, that may not be the case. It will depend on what therapy you're planning to use, and your reason for discontinuing a medication. For example, let's say you've talked to your doctor about using complementary and alternative medicine therapies because you both agree that your insomnia medication may not be helpful, perhaps due to side effects or perhaps because it's just not working. So instead of prescribing another medication, your doctor may give you the go-ahead to try hypnosis, imagery, or acupuncture as a path to a good night's sleep.

Learn about Practitioners

Begin by asking your health-care team and other survivors for recommendations for practitioners. Then, just as you did to select your medical team, book an informational interview to meet with a potential provider. If practitioners tell you to stop conventional treatments to use their "medicine," call it quits right then. Otherwise, begin by asking lots of questions such as:

- Why did you choose to practice this form of medicine?
- What is your philosophy of health and healing?
- How much experience do you have working with women who have breast cancer?
- In what ways has your treatment helped other breast cancer patients?
- Are there studies that can help me better understand why your treatment may help me?
- Does this treatment have any side effects, and will it affect my daily routine at all?
- What reasons would you give to your mother, sister, or partner for using your treatment? What reasons would you give them for *not* using your treatment?

Ask Questions

For example, if your insurance plan covers acupuncture, but the provider you want to use doesn't accept yours (this is not uncommon), you'll be responsible for filing a claim and paying additional out-of-network fees. Find out how many treatments you'll need, what your initial appointment will cost, what subsequent treatments will cost, and the provider's cancellation policy if you can't keep an appointment or choose to stop treatments.

Be Flexible

If there isn't a qualified practitioner in your area for the therapy you want to try, see if someone nearby specializes in a similar practice. For example, if you want to do tai chi, but no one teaches it, see if a qigong instructor is available instead.

CHOOSING THE RIGHT THERAPY FOR *YOU*

To help you figure out what's best for you, we recommend that you consider all the information we're giving you in this chapter and the next as maps with decision-making guideposts. The samplings of therapies we include here are recommended by the medical community and are considered helpful with a safe track record. Discuss them with your doctor and/or medical team, and consider selecting one (or two) therapies to try.

Acupuncture

Acupuncture is the most practiced component of traditional Chinese medicine. It's been in use for more than 4,000 years. Today, it's still used to diagnose, treat, and prevent disease in countries worldwide, including the United States.

Acupuncture teaches that we each have a life force energy known as *chi* or *qi* within our bodies. This energy travels along pathways called *meridians*. The places where the meridians come to the surface of the body via the skin are called *acupoints*. We have more than 2,000 acupoints throughout our body.

Traditional Chinese medicine holds that whenever our chi becomes unbalanced, we're at risk of becoming ill—physically and/or spiritually. Reasons for imbalances include having too much chi, not enough chi, or a blocked meridian. That's where acupuncture comes in.

To rebalance your chi, an acupuncturist will insert disposable, sterile stainless steel needles of varying lengths into your skin to stimulate the acupoints. The goal is to direct blocked chi into healthier patterns.

Does it work? Though there's no definitive scientific explanation of how acupuncture works, one Western school of thought contends that

take a deep breath . . . and relax

Intrigued by complementary and alternative medicine, but don't know where to begin? Try breathing; that is, taking *deep* breaths in and out . . . in and out. . . . Most of us don't actually breathe correctly: We engage in something called chest breathing (where we're only breathing with the top part of our lungs), when we should be doing something called diaphragmatic breathing (also called abdominal breathing or belly breathing), which is essentially breathing with our entire lungs. By getting more oxygen into your lungs and then into your bloodstream, your muscles will have more fuel and your heart won't have to beat as quickly and use so much effort, ultimately slowing down your body's levels of stress.

Today, diaphragmatic breathing is one of the most popular complementary mind-body medicine techniques. That's because it's easy to do (essentially it's just breathing to engage the diaphragm muscle, which is located beneath your lungs) and it gets results.

Once you get the hang of this method of breathing, you can use it anytime—to pause in the midst of a stressful day, before treatment, before surgery—to slow down your heart rate and possibly even lower your blood pressure. Here's how to get started.[8]

Begin by sitting with your back straight (to open up your chest), feet flat on the floor, and your head, neck, and shoulders relaxed. (If you need to do this while lying down, you can.)

acupuncture stimulates points that trigger chemicals that influence our hormones and glands (endocrine system). These chemicals include pain-killing endorphins and brain-altering neurotransmitters and neuropep-tides, which affect our moods, energy, and immune systems.[9] Thus, in response to receiving acupuncture, cancer patients may be better able to

Close your eyes, relax, and breathe as you typically do. Then begin slowly to breathe in through your nose, and out through your mouth, continuing to take normal breaths.

Place one hand on your upper chest. Place the other hand on your abdomen. Continue to breathe normally, and notice how your hands move when you breathe. (You want to breathe so your chest hand doesn't move and your belly hand does. This is a sign you're engaging in diaphragmatic breathing.)

Breathe in again, counting slowly to four. If you need to, count *one one-thousand, two one-thousand, three one-thousand, four one-thousand* to really slow down your counting. (If you start to feel light-headed, hold your breath for one or two counts before exhaling.)

Now exhale slowly, and gently, out of your mouth (pursing your lips), counting to six. Try to sigh slightly to provide extra tension relief. (You always want your exhale to be longer than your inhale.)

Hold your breath for up to four counts when you reach the end of this cycle.

Begin another cycle. Note that you may have to repeat this exercise a few times to get into a calming rhythm because it takes practice to slow down our unnaturally rapid way of breathing. And it's only with practice that diaphragmatic breathing can become automatic.

manage stress, reduce fatigue, sleep better, control hot flashes, and decrease nausea and pain.

One study, from the University of the Saarland in Homburg, Germany, determined that acupuncture could help breast cancer patients manage postoperative pain related to arm movement. Forty-eight women received acupuncture on the third, fifth, and seventh days after surgery to remove lymph nodes. They also had a treatment on the day they were discharged. A control group of 32 postsurgery women did not receive the acupuncture. After each treatment and upon being discharged, the acupuncture group reported significant pain relief. During the postoperative period, their range of arm motion in the affected arm also increased significantly when compared with the control group.[10]

In another small study of acupuncture, conducted by the British government's Complementary Health Service, breast cancer patients received acupuncture treatments for 6 weeks. All the patients were suffering from chemotherapy-induced peripheral neuropathy, which causes a loss of sensation, and pain or mobility problems in their arms and legs. After 6 weeks of treatment, 82 percent reported an improvement in symptoms. Some reported additional benefits that included using fewer painkillers and sleeping better.[11]

What to expect: As you might have already guessed, acupuncture is not a do-it-yourself treatment, although acupressure–a first cousin of acupuncture that doesn't use needles–can be (see page 296). When you go for your first visit, expect to spend a couple of hours if a treatment is included. Remember, this is a holistic health practice, so your acupuncturist will want to do an in-depth interview with you to know what's going on physically, mentally, emotionally, and spiritually. If you have medical records, mammograms, and other medical information, plan to bring them along. This will be an ideal time for both you and the practitioner to ask and answer lots of questions, so don't be shy.

Most of your treatments will take place on a massage table; you will be fully clothed or semiclothed and covered with a sheet. After determining which acupoints to use, your acupuncturist will insert the appropriate number of needles. Unlike the hollow hypodermic needles used for injections, acupuncture needles are very sharp and hair thin, and most (but not all) are barely felt upon injection. Make sure that you check with your doctor and health-care team about the use of these needles, particularly if you have had recent surgery or are on active treatment (receiving chemotherapy and/or radiation).

Don't be surprised by the location of the needles. Because chi travels along the meridians, or channels, acupoints addressing a particular condition may not be where you feel pain or other symptoms. For example, needles in your ear may help to relieve pain in your armpit. If you're curious about how, and why, it's done that way, use your time on the table to ask questions. If not, talk about something else, or just rest (some people find acupuncture so relaxing, they fall into a deep sleep while having a treatment).

When the needles are in place, your acupuncturist may move them up and down and/or twirl or vibrate them to influence the flow of your chi. He or she may then leave the needles in place for $\frac{1}{2}$ hour or more to give your body a chance to integrate the treatment. Sometimes the needles will also be stimulated by heat, pressure, cold, or newer techniques that add electrical and other forms of stimulation.

Reflexology

Reflexology, an ancient, noninvasive healing practice, is often used to help manage pain, nausea, and stress. Practitioners—called reflexologists—believe that finger pressure applied to specific areas of the feet and hands eliminates blocked chi that affects organs and systems throughout the body and promotes an overall sense of relaxation.

Does it work? Although reflexology is being offered to breast cancer patients in a growing number of hospitals, there is no consensus about its overall efficacy. Some studies have shown benefits, however. One study showed that patients with breast or lung cancer experienced a significant decrease in anxiety after receiving 30 minutes of foot reflexology from a certified reflexologist. The breast cancer patients also experienced a significant decrease in pain.[12]

Another study found that after reflexology, patients experienced 100 percent improvement in the quality-of-life categories of appetite, breathing, communication (with doctors, family, nurses), concentration, constipation/diarrhea, fear of future, mobility, mood, nausea, pain, and sleep.[13]

Other evidence comes from a recent pilot study at Johns Hopkins University, where a research team compared the effectiveness of 20 minutes of Swedish massage and reflexology on nursing home residents ages 75 or older (an age group rarely studied) who had been diagnosed with cancer up to 5 years earlier and had already finished their treatments. The study concluded that both massage and reflexology resulted in significant declines in stress and pain, and it improved overall mood, too.[14]

Finally, a much larger study looked at the effectiveness of reflexology on women with advanced-stage breast cancer. At the time of the study, all the participants were receiving chemotherapy and/or hormone therapy.

PERSONAL PRACTICE

do-it-yourself acupressure

Have you ever bought a wristband with a hard plastic stud to help overcome motion sickness or nausea from chemotherapy? If so, you've already discovered the benefits of applying acupressure to the pericardium meridian (P6 or PC6). In traditional Chinese medicine, this is also known as the Nei-Guan or "inner gate" acupoint.

Acupressure is older than acupuncture and it, too, originated in China. (Shiatsu is the Japanese variation.) Like acupuncture, this therapy uses the same (or similar) acupoints, but without needles. Instead, the acupressurist stimulates your chi by using his or her fingers or hands to apply pressure to specific acupoints. Because you can also do acupressure on your own or buy the over-the-counter wristbands for nausea, this therapy is a practical, portable, and cost-effective form of complementary medicine.

Studies show that using acupressure after chemotherapy can help reduce and/or control its side effects, which include nausea and/or vomiting. For example, in a randomized controlled trial in England, women wore acupressure wristbands for 5 days after their chemotherapy treatments. The results showed that the pressure on the P6 acupoint significantly reduced the patients' distress from nausea and vomiting.[15]

The women who received reflexology had significant improvement in their physical functioning. Afterward, the research team recommended that reflexology be added to support care because it is effective and generally considered to be safe.[16] Note that reflexology is *not* recommended for people with diabetes or those with conditions that affect the feet, legs, and circulatory system, such as deep vein thrombosis.[17]

What to expect: If treatments are not offered at your hospital, be sure to get recommendations for practitioners from your doctor and from

Acupressure can address other symptoms, too. In a preliminary study of acupressure at the University of Michigan that focused on breast cancer survivors with persistent cancer-related fatigue, the research team reported that acupressure had been shown to decrease fatigue levels by as much as 70 percent in cancer survivors.[18]

How to do it: If you want to try using acupressure to help control nausea, follow the instructions given here. The theory: Because the chi in the digestive system is supposed to flow downward, you can suffer from nausea whenever the chi moves in the opposite direction. Traditional Chinese medicine holds that, by gently massaging P6, you help to reverse this disruptive flow.

1. **Turn your palm up,** and place the middle three fingers from your opposite hand on the inside of your wrist.

2. **Make sure the edge of your top finger is at the top of your wrist crease.** Directly beneath the lower third finger is your P6 point; it's located between the tendons there.

3. **Stimulate it by gently applying pressure** and lightly massaging it for about 30 seconds. You can repeat this three to five times.[19] Do as often as necessary.

other survivors. Because reflexology is not regulated in the United States, practitioners are not licensed, so anyone can hang out a shingle offering those services.

A reflexology session typically begins with the practitioner asking you questions about your health. This is the time to bring up your breast cancer and any side effects you've been experiencing from treatments, such as pain or nausea, or quality-of-life issues, like feelings of

do-it-yourself reflexology

As an alternative to going to a reflexologist for treatments, a growing number of patients are doing reflexology on themselves. Like acupressure, it's even taught in some hospitals. (If you want to learn even more about how to use reflexology, contact the American Reflexology Certification Board, arcb.net, to find courses, as well as practitioners, in your area.) But know that your symptoms determine what spots on your feet to apply pressure to. The step-by-step guide that follows is for general pain and discomfort you might be experiencing from your breast cancer and/or your treatments. You can also find a reflexology foot map—a chart mapping out which areas of the foot correspond to which areas of the body—online (for example, you can find one at reflexologyfootmap.net).

How to do it: Before beginning any home reflexology session, remove your shoes and socks and sit cross-legged on the floor or your bed, if that's more comfortable for you. Then, cradle one foot in your lap (do one foot at a time, then switch) to get started.

1. **Start with the toes.** Apply pressure to the entire surface area and then to the joints of your toes, using both thumbs and forefingers. Apply pressure to all points for about 10 seconds at a time.

depression, poor self-esteem, and fatigue. Having a specific condition in mind allows the reflexologist to carefully work the area corresponding to the presenting problem.

Then you'll lie or sit down, remaining fully clothed except for your shoes and socks. The practitioner may wash your feet and soak them in warm water, then position them at his or her chest level. He or she will then apply gentle pressure to specific points on the foot, starting at the

2. **Move to the ball of the foot.** Apply pressure with the thumbs of both hands across the ball of the foot, concentrating on any areas that feel pain or discomfort (these, say reflexologists, correspond to areas of the body that are out of balance). Again, apply pressure for 10 seconds before moving on to the next area.

3. **Apply pressure to the instep,** which is the non-weight-bearing area on the inside of your foot. (*Note:* This is also the area you work on if you are feeling gut-wrenching emotions.)

4. **Apply pressure to the outer edges of your foot,** working your way down the foot.

5. **Cover all areas of the foot** and finish by applying pressure to the heel.

6. **Return to any painful points,** and gently apply pressure to these areas until you no longer feel the discomfort.

Remember: This process is meant to be relaxing. Don't rush through it, and be sure to take time to breathe deeply while you're doing each point on each foot.

toes and working down the foot. (He or she may also apply pressure to your hands–and even to your ears–depending on what symptoms you're seeking relief from.) Each session typically lasts from 30 minutes to 1 hour. You can rest, talk, or fall asleep during the session.

Aromatherapy

Do you wash your sheets in lavender-scented detergent because you believe that fragrance helps you relax and fall asleep? Do other scents you smell during the day seem to stimulate you and make you feel sharp and on top of your game? If so, you already know the power of smell to affect your mind and body.

Aromatherapy is one of several sensory therapies that use smell, taste, sight, sound, touch, and the body's energy to enhance and balance your mind, body, and spirit.[20] It's been used for therapeutic purposes for nearly 6,000 years. It involves inhaling or massaging the skin with specific preparations of highly concentrated scents, called essential oils, naturally distilled from herbs, flowers, and fruits. The most popular essential oils are lavender, rosemary, eucalyptus, chamomile, marjoram, jasmine, tea tree, peppermint, lemon, geranium, and the oil from the flowers of ylang ylang (an aromatic Asian tree).[21]

Does it work? Aromatherapy is an ancient healing practice that's never been proven to cure anything. However, it *is* believed that aromatherapy can be a beneficial complement to conventional medicine as well as other complementary and alternative medicine therapies. Moreover, studies are under way worldwide to determine which extracts may have anticancer properties.[22]

How does it work? One theory is that the smell receptors in your nose communicate with the parts of your brain (the amygdala and hippocampus) that regulate mood and emotions.[23] This, in turn, not only affects your moods but also your metabolism, stress levels, and libido.[24] When used topically, some oils have been shown to have antiseptic (tea tree oil), anti-inflammatory (rosemary), anesthetic (clove leaf oil), and analgesic (black pepper) effects.[25]

Although credible controlled studies and professional articles on the benefits of aromatherapy are in short supply, there are a few that specifically focus on its efficacy for breast cancer patients. For example, one article published in the journal *Professional Nurse* concluded that aromatherapy massage benefited breast cancer survivors with

at-home aromatherapy: is it safe?

Generally, aromatherapy is considered safe, but it's not regulated, so there can be risks associated with using it. Don't try it on your own at home before checking with your oncologist or a qualified aromatherapist who works with cancer patients.

If you are already using aromatherapy, it's still important to get professional advice *now* to find out if the essential oils you're using could have a negative effect on your breast cancer or interact with any of your treatments, including medications.

Some oils can interact with certain medications and affect the strength and effectiveness of others. Finally, if you have preexisting conditions and sensitivities, some oils can cause rashes or allergic or asthmatic reactions. Plus, it's important to keep in mind the following:

Essential oils are volatile oils. They evaporate very quickly, so a tiny bit goes a long way. (It's easy to overuse them because they evaporate quickly.)

Essential oils should always be of high quality and diluted in a "carrier," such as almond or coconut oil. (If used directly on the skin, they could cause irritation or a rash.)

Each essential oil has a different chemical composition that affects its smell, the ways in which it's absorbed, and how the body uses it.

***Never* take any essential oil internally,** because many are irritants and some are highly toxic.

Aromatherapists don't need to be licensed, so getting word-of-mouth recommendations from your oncologist, treatment center, or other survivors is the best way to find a qualified expert. One of the governing bodies for national educational standards, the National Association for Holistic Aromatherapy (naha.org), *is* currently attempting to standardize aromatherapy certification in the United States, which should make finding a qualified aromatherapist easier.[33]

lymphedema because it helped them to relax and feel more comfortable.[26]

And in a study of British oncology patients who inhaled aromasticks (essentially aromatherapy-infused sticks), 65 percent reported feeling more relaxed and 51 percent felt less stress. Of those with nausea, 47 percent felt better using aromatherapy, as did 55 percent of those with sleep disturbances.[27]

What to expect: As with other complementary therapies, you begin an aromatherapy session by talking to the practitioner about your health and your health history. This is the time to bring up any concerns you have and what problems you're there to treat. From there, the aromatherapist will tailor the rest of your visit to your individual needs. Many aromatherapists are also massage therapists and will give you a massage using scented massage oils. But there are other ways to experience aromatherapy, too. For example, your therapist might use steam inhalations, vaporizers, sprays, and/or compresses (typically a warm washcloth or towel soaked in essential oils). Your first session should last 45 minutes to 1 hour. [28]

Energy Healing: Therapeutic Touch, Healing Touch, and Reiki

Therapeutic touch, healing touch, and reiki are considered energy medicine, or energy-healing therapies, that originated with ancient religious laying-on-of-hands techniques. These healing therapies share common roots grounded in one theory: All living things have a vital energy field that extends throughout and also beyond the body. This is also referred to as an *aura*. The thinking is that when channels in this field become blocked, we become unbalanced and ill. A practitioner attempts to rebalance and harmonize a patient by transferring energy through his or her hands into the patient's body in order to open these gateways. Ultimately, the goal is to jump-start the patient's self-healing processes.

Therapeutic touch, healing touch, and reiki are popular forms of complementary and alternative medicine used by nurses and other health-care professionals in hospitals and breast centers. And because of the growing number of integrative medicine programs nationwide, doctors and osteopaths are learning these practices, too. In a survey of hospitals offering complementary and alternative medicine, the American Hospital Association reported in 2006 that 15 percent, or more than 800 American hospitals, offered reiki among their patient services.[29]

Reiki (pronounced *ray-key*) is a Japanese holistic healing therapy that means universal (*re*) + life force (*ki*), or universal life force. In practice, it's a vibrational or subtle energy therapy with a spiritual component that's intended to promote higher consciousness. (Although it's spiritual in nature, it's *not* a religion.) A physicist describing what is happening might say that reiki acts at an atomic level by causing molecules throughout the body to vibrate with higher intensity. This, in turn, dissolves energy blockages that lead to disharmony and disease.[30]

The basic principles of reiki, according to its founder Usui Mikao, are healthy guidelines for anyone to follow daily:

> *The secret art of inviting happiness*
> *The miraculous medicine of all diseases*
> *Just for today, do not anger*
> *Do not worry and be filled with gratitude*
> *Devote yourself to your work. Be kind to people.*
> *Every morning and evening, join your hands in prayer.*
> *Pray these words to your heart*
> *and chant these words with your mouth.*

—Usui Mikao[31]

Does it work? Unfortunately, there is no significant body of scientific studies that have looked at the effect of energy-healing therapies like reiki on illnesses like breast cancer. But in one pilot research study conducted at Hartford Hospital in Connecticut, researchers found that reiki improved patient sleep by 86 percent, reduced pain by 78 percent, reduced nausea by 80 percent, and reduced anxiety by 94 percent.[32]

What to expect: Treatment sessions are about 1 hour long. If you decide to have one, you'll lie, fully clothed, on a table while the practitioner places his or her hands lightly on or above you. He or she will use 12 different hand positions to transmit life force and dissolve blockages in the energy centers known as chakras that result in disharmony and disease.

Therapeutic touch and healing touch are the same in many ways. The differences between them have to do with the practitioner's training and the techniques used. Therapeutic touch, taught in many nursing schools nationally and internationally, is a standardized energy technique that was cofounded in the 1970s by Delores Krieger, PhD, RN, professor emeritus of nursing at New York University, and Dora Kunz, an energy healer. Healing touch, on the other hand, incorporates a collection of practices from well-known healers along with concepts borrowed from ancient shamanic and aboriginal healing traditions. The techniques used by practitioners today were developed and compiled in the 1980s by Janet Mentgen, RN.

 BETWEEN THE LINES

ayurvedic and traditional Chinese medicine

Ayurveda and traditional Chinese medicine are ancient medical systems with shared roots and philosophies. They focus more on the patient than the disease by taking a holistic body, mind, and spirit approach to treating illnesses. Whenever a patient uses either one *instead* of Western medicine, it is considered *alternative* medicine.

But when ayurvedic or TCM dietary, herbal, and other practices, such as acupuncture, massage, hatha yoga, qigong, or meditation, are used *alongside* conventional Western medical treatment, they are considered *complementary* medicine.

Because these are complex and individualized medical systems, discuss them carefully with your physician to ensure that dietary changes or prescribed remedies don't interfere with your treatments or cause drug interactions.

Ayurveda (*Ayur* = life, *Veda* = science or knowledge) is the traditional medicine of India, dating back to 1200 BC. Its guiding principle: Optimal health consists of physical, mental, and spiritual harmony, and the pathway depends on the individual's principal *dosha*, or constitution.

It's founded on the principle that the universe is made up of combinations of the five elements: *akasha* (ether), *vayu* (air), *teja* (fire), *aap* (water), and *prithvi* (earth), which are coded into three

Does it work? Patients also give these energy-healing therapies high ratings for helping them deal with wide-ranging symptoms and side effects.[34] For example, breast cancer patients report that after having had therapeutic or healing touch, they have reduced pain following surgery, faster wound healing, and relief from lymphatic disorders and fatigue as well as headaches and other stress-related conditions.

doshas (*kapha*, *pitta*, and *vata*), which govern all life processes. Each is composed of one or two elements; collectively, they regulate each of our physiological and psychological processes. When the doshas are in harmony, they create balance and health. Imbalance shows up as symptoms of disease.[35]

Diet plays an important role in achieving balance, especially ayurvedic diets and herbs. When qualified practitioners make dietary recommendations, they are always dependent on the patient's diagnosis, and their recommendations change seasonally.

Ayurvedic treatments may include dietary modification, herbal preparations, massage, yoga, meditation, and *pranayama* (breathing) exercises.

Traditional Chinese medicine is also based on principles of harmony and balance. Practitioners believe that the unobstructed flow of chi prevents illness and promotes wellness. TCM also incorporates the concept of yin and yang—that the opposites like male and female, hot and cold, dry and moist are interrelated and interdependent. Because yin and yang are relative and each rises and falls, practitioners focus on acheiving balance and harmony to help patients heal and prevent illness.

TCM uses diet, exercise (tai chi and qigong), herbs, acupuncture, and massage as primary paths for managing and treating patients.

In one review of 66 clinical studies, done to see if energy-healing therapies were helpful, investigators found strong evidence supporting the use of energy therapies to reduce pain for a variety of illnesses. Investigators also noted that therapeutic touch, healing touch, and reiki helped breast cancer patients reduce their fatigue and enhance their quality of life.[36]

Other studies have shown that when energy-healing therapies are used in conjunction with guided imagery, massage, music therapy, and other complementary medicine modalities, some patients report even better results.

What to expect: Both therapeutic and healing touch sessions can last for as little as 5 minutes or as long as 1 hour. Usually the practitioner has you lie down, fully clothed, on a table, but these therapies can also be done while you're sitting. Because they're calming and meditative experiences, many patients fall asleep during their treatments.

At the beginning of the first session, the practitioner will ask you about your health, symptoms, expectations, and goals. He or she will then:

- **Focus inwardly** to be in the present moment and concentrate his or her attention on your highest good. This is called *centering*. In healing touch, centering is followed by an *attuning*. During these few moments, the practitioner sets an *intention* (goals) for your highest good.

- **Assess your energy field** by doing a scan above you with his or her hands. The purpose of the scan is to determine where there may be blockages. Practitioners report they feel different sensations that can include heat, coolness, heaviness, pressure, and/or tingling.

- **Clear and mobilize your energy field** with hands-off sweeping strokes and then direct energy to balance and harmonize it.

- **Do another scan to reassess your energy field** and then close the treatment.

- **Request feedback** about your experience and answer your questions.

CONTINUING THE CONVERSATION

This chapter introduced you to complementary and alternative medicine therapies that are currently available. However, data on the effectiveness of these therapies is not robust. It is very important that you discuss these strategies with your health-care team to ensure the safety of pursuing these strategies as you travel through your treatment of breast cancer and beyond.

Fishing for Fun

Patricia Huxta has one reply when asked how she is: "I'm fishing for fun.

"Breast cancer is life changing for the whole family," says the 63-year-old survivor. "I learned to flip my priorities. Today, fun comes first for me—work is something I do, but it no longer dictates my days."

When Patricia's doctor found a lump on her left breast and explained what she could expect with stage I breast cancer, she recalls that she felt as if she were looking at him through a telescope. "It was so unbelievable; cancer is a scary word," says the mother of four. "The first thing I thought was that I wasn't going to get to be a grandma."

Patricia had a lumpectomy and surgery to remove her lymph nodes. Several rounds of chemotherapy, 3 months of radiation treatments, and a 5-year course of tamoxifen were followed by an aromatase inhibitor to block estrogen production and prevent cancer recurrence.

Patricia's ability to find humor in her situation helped her through the toughest parts. In charge of a large class at a child care center, she says, "I didn't really take time off work, and I remember the kids and me laughing whenever the wind would whip up and blow my hair away.

"I dealt with my diagnosis by picturing my life as two separate roads: the medical road and the life road," she explains. "I'm not someone who needs all the information in the world. I didn't want to know about all the science stuff; I trusted my doctors and let them steer me along my medical road. For the life road, I'd go to work and be with my family and not think about cancer. Compartmentalizing really helped me."

When she finished radiation in 2005, Patricia went to Paris. She also made time for favorite activities. Then, in 2009, a mammogram showed what turned out to be a benign spot. "If I knew how to do flips, I would've done them after that second scare," she says.

"Fun comes first now; that's my thing," Patricia says.

She'd like women who've been diagnosed to know . . . *you deserve to have fun, so look for opportunities to smile and laugh.*

Breast cancer is . . . *life changing, for you and your family.*

Tomorrow will . . . *be great.*

PART FIVE

THRIVING—
Not Just
SURVIVING

Congratulations! You've made it through one of the toughest ordeals you've probably ever faced. The long months from diagnosis through treatment are over, and it's time to make the transition from patient to survivor. Chances are you've learned a lot about yourself along the way and discovered reserves of courage and strength you never knew you had. As you begin your new postcancer life, here's your guide to follow-up care that can help reduce your chances of recurrence and keep you healthy. You'll find tips for sharing your experience and your hard-won wisdom with other women and for creatively moving on to the next phase of your life. Bon voyage!

*"There is no medicine like hope,
no incentive so great, and no tonic so powerful
as expectation of something tomorrow."*

—ORISON SWETT MARDEN

CHAPTER 14

FOLLOW-UP CARE

Congratulations on completing your primary breast cancer treatment! Whatever the exact path that brought you here, going on from this point brings some responsibilities along with relief. Follow-up care will certainly be less involved than primary treatment, but no less important. It's natural to look for a "finish line" in your cancer journey, and you've certainly earned the right to celebrate. Still, it's important to remember that follow-up care is an essential part of your fight to get and stay healthy.

REGULAR EXAMS

You're no doubt tired of doctor appointments by now, and fortunately you'll have far fewer of them moving forward. For the first 3 years after primary therapy (that is, your original breast cancer treatment), you'll need an exam every 3 to 6 months; for the next 2 years, every 6 to 12 months; and annually thereafter.[1]

Many women prefer to have these appointments with their primary care provider rather than with an oncologist; it just feels less frightening to be examined by your regular doctor. According to the latest recommendations from the American Society of Clinical Oncology, patients with stage I or II breast cancer may transfer their care to a primary care physician 1 year after diagnosis.[2] It's important, though, that your primary care physician is experienced in cancer surveillance and breast examination, including the examination of irradiated breasts if you've had radiation therapy.

If you do choose to use a primary care physician for your follow-up care, make sure that you, your doctor, your oncologist(s), and any other members of your medical team coordinate your care and maintain good communication. You may be referred back to an oncologist for reassessment, especially if you're receiving adjuvant endocrine therapy. Keep in mind that a referral for further oncology assessment doesn't mean that your cancer has returned; it just means that your doctor is being careful with your health and prefers to have a specialist weigh in on anything questionable.

Alternatively, you may feel more comfortable continuing to see your oncologist for follow-up exams. After all, you and your oncologist have been through a lot together, and you've ideally developed a good relationship based on trust and mutual respect. This also avoids the potentially alarming situation of being referred to an oncologist in the situation described above. Really, it comes down to your personal preference; statistically, outcomes are the same regardless of whether or not you receive your follow-up care from a specialist.[3]

In addition to breast exams, you'll need an annual pelvic exam. This is especially important if you're receiving tamoxifen therapy because it puts you at increased risk for endometrial cancer. Longer intervals between pelvic exams, and especially Pap tests, may be recommended if you've had a total hysterectomy and oophorectomy. However, breast cancer survivors should consult their primary care physician or gynecologist for the latest recommendations.

TESTS

A mammogram is the most common test following breast cancer treatment. Women who've had breast-conserving surgery should expect to have a mammogram 1 year after the initial mammogram and usually 6 months after completion of radiation therapy.[4] After that, you may be able to have a mammogram annually.

It's possible that your doctor will recommend periodic breast MRIs as well. These are not routinely prescribed for everyone who's had breast cancer but may be a good idea depending on your family history and the density of your breasts. Breasts that contain more connective and glandular tissue than fat are considered dense. Mammograms of dense breasts don't always yield clear results, and 40 percent of women have dense breasts.[5] You can't tell how dense your breasts are by look or feel, but in the course of your diagnosis and treatment, someone probably mentioned whether your breasts appear dense on your mammograms. If they didn't, be sure to ask. If you have dense breasts, another option is to have a screening bilateral ultrasound at the time of your routine mammogram.

If you're prescribed an aromatase inhibitor, talk to your doctor about whether or not you should have a bone density test. In some women, aromatase inhibitors have been shown to reduce bone density, which could lead to fractures and other problems. This can also happen with tamoxifen, but it's less common.

Based on the latest guidelines from the American Society for Oncology, blood tests such as CBC (complete blood count), automated chemistry studies, and tumor marker tests are not currently recommended for routine follow-up care. Also not recommended are imaging studies like chest x-rays, bone scans, CT scans, and liver ultrasounds.[6] Keep in mind that your doctor may want you to undergo one or more of these tests anyway, based on your particular situation and his or her own experience and preferences. As always, if you don't understand your doctor's reasoning in recommending a test or course of treatment, ask for an explanation.

Genetic Testing

Patients at high risk for familial breast cancer syndromes are often referred for counseling to discuss the option of undergoing genetic testing for one of the BRCA genetic mutations. Different hospitals and treatment centers define "high risk" differently, but it may include any of the following criteria:

- You're of Ashkenazi Jewish heritage.
- You've had ovarian cancer.
- You have a first- or second-degree relative (first-degree relatives are parents, siblings, and children, while second-degree relatives are aunts and uncles, nephews and nieces, grandparents, half-siblings, and first cousins) who has had ovarian cancer.
- You have a first-degree relative who was diagnosed with breast cancer before the age of 50.

- You have two or more first- or second-degree relatives who were diagnosed with breast cancer at any age.

- You or a relative have had a diagnosis of bilateral breast cancer (tumors in both breasts).

- You had breast cancer diagnosed before menopause and have a relative who was diagnosed with either premenopausal breast cancer or ovarian cancer at any age.

- You have a male relative who has had breast cancer.

- You are male.

- You have a relative who has a BRCA1 or BRCA2 mutation.

It may seem redundant to undergo this sort of testing after you've already had breast cancer, but determining whether you have a genetic mutation may impact your follow-up treatment regimen. In addition, women who have an altered BRCA1 gene have a 40 to 60 percent risk of developing ovarian cancer by age 85, and women with an altered BRCA2 gene have a 16 to 27 percent risk.[7] Still, whether or not to have this test is a personal choice and one that you should make based on your own situation after talking with a genetic counselor.[8]

HORMONAL THERAPY

After completion of your primary breast cancer treatment, your doctor may recommend hormonal therapy if you had estrogen receptor positive (ER+) tumors. These types of tumors are "fed" by estrogen, and hormonal therapy works to reduce or eliminate any remaining cancer cells by cutting off their supply of estrogen. Estrogen receptor negative (ER-) cancers—about 20 percent of breast cancers—are not affected by hormonal therapy, so it's not prescribed for patients with this type of tumor.

Tamoxifen

For premenopausal and some postmenopausal women, your hormonal therapy will likely be in the form of tamoxifen, also known by the brand names Nolvadex (tablets) and Soltamox (liquid). It's believed that tamoxifen works by binding with the estrogen receptors on breast cancer cells, thereby blocking them from estrogen. Without estrogen, the cancer cells can't grow or multiply.[9]

The standard duration of tamoxifen therapy is 5 years, although there's new evidence that extending the treatment to 10 years offers significant benefit, cutting the rate of breast cancer deaths in the second decade after diagnosis in half.[10] Unfortunately, extending the treatment may extend the side effects, so discuss with your doctor whether this is a reasonable option for you.

Benefits of tamoxifen therapy include the following:

- **Tamoxifen reduces the risk of breast cancer recurrence** by 40 to 50 percent in postmenopausal women and by 30 to 50 percent in premenopausal women.

- **Tamoxifen reduces the risk of a new cancer developing in the other breast by about 50 percent.**[11]

Because tamoxifen mimics some of the actions of estrogen in the body, it can offer additional health benefits besides treating breast cancer. For example, in some women, it's been shown to lower cholesterol, help stop bone density loss, and improve cardiac health.[12]

Unfortunately, tamoxifen does carry with it the risk of side effects, most of which are minor. These include the sorts of symptoms you can expect to (or did) experience in menopause, such as weight gain, hot flashes, loss of bone density, vaginal dryness, nausea, and mood swings. Tamoxifen can cause either vaginal dryness or increased vaginal lubrication and bone density loss or an improvement in bone density. Every woman is different, and there's no way to predict which side effects you'll experience. You may experience none at all. There are a couple of more serious, although uncommon, side effects to be aware of.

Endometrial Cancer

This is a type of uterine cancer. While the prospect of an additional cancer diagnosis is daunting, keep in mind that this type of cancer is fairly rare. The average woman's risk of endometrial cancer in her lifetime is 2.6 percent,[13] and tamoxifen therapy increases that risk by 1 to 2 percent.[14] If this type of cancer does occur, it is most often treatable with surgery, which includes a hysterectomy (surgical removal of the uterus).

Another thing to know about endometrial cancer is that it almost always announces itself by causing vaginal bleeding. As tamoxifen may suppress menstruation, this provides a helpful warning sign. Keep in

your role in follow-up care

Taking an active role in your posttreatment care keeps you in control and on track to continue moving forward on your healing journey.

Step 1: Make—and keep—all the appointments your doctor recommends. If your primary care provider suggests that you see an oncologist, do it. If your surgeon wants to see you again in 2 months, put it on your calendar. It may seem obvious, but many people who've had a major health scare procrastinate when it comes to follow-up appointments.

Step 2: Once you and your medical team have decided on a long-term treatment plan, make sure to follow it. It will be significantly less effort and discomfort than the primary treatment you endured, but it still requires daily attention. Tamoxifen therapy, for example, is usually administered in one or two pills a day for 5 years. While this sounds like a small commitment compared with, say, chemotherapy, it still requires that you think about your breast cancer every single day for years, which may be difficult when you just want to forget about it.

Step 3: Have good breast self-awareness. It's important to be aware of any new change to either breast. Even if you've had a mastectomy with or without reconstruction, it's impossible for every bit of breast tissue to have been removed during surgery. So any change in feel or appearance of your chest or reconstructed breast should be brought to the attention of your doctor.

mind that not all or even most vaginal bleeding while on hormonal therapy indicates endometrial cancer; this is just something to watch for and report to your doctor. Pelvic pain or pressure is another possible

Step 4: Take care of yourself. Continue to eat well, exercise, and manage your stress. In addition to potentially reducing your risk of recurrence, these actions may help you to avoid other serious illnesses, including heart disease, diabetes, and other forms of cancer.

Step 5: Pay attention to your body. Another benefit of good diet, exercise, and stress reduction is that it makes you more attuned to your physical self. Stretch, look in the mirror, run your hands over your skin, breathe deeply, and listen to what your body is telling you.

Step 6: Consider following the 2-week rule. If you notice a possible symptom that's worrisome but not particularly alarming or painful, do the following:

- **Write down the date you first noticed something wrong,** along with any information that could explain the cause (overdoing it at the gym, an allergy attack when the pollen count was high, and so on).
- **Mark a date on the calendar 2 weeks later.**
- **Try to put it out of your mind for those 2 weeks, as long as you don't feel worse or notice additional symptoms.**
- **Make an appointment with your doctor** if the symptom is still there on the date you marked.

Step 7: Reevaluate your treatment plan from time to time. Talk with your doctor about the results of any tests you've had and any new studies or therapies you may have heard about. Then ask if your current plan still represents the best possible course for you.

symptom. If you experience either or both of these, your doctor may suggest a transvaginal ultrasound and/or an endometrial biopsy to rule out endometrial cancer.

Blood Clots

Taking tamoxifen can increase your risk of developing a blood clot (thrombosis), which could travel to your lung (where it's called a pulmonary embolism). It's not a common side effect, but it is a serious one and it can be fatal. Signs of pulmonary embolism include shortness of breath and chest pain. Clots usually form in the leg, thigh, or pelvis, where they're called deep vein thrombosis. They're usually accompanied by redness, swelling, or pain. If you experience any of these things while on tamoxifen, seek medical care right away.

Aromatase Inhibitors

Like tamoxifen, aromatase inhibitors work to keep estrogen from contributing to the growth of estrogen receptor positive (ER+) tumors. Aromatase inhibitors work differently than tamoxifen, though. Rather than blocking the ability of the tumor to bind with estrogen, aromatase inhibitors suppress estrogen production. Because aromatase inhibitors can't suppress the quantity of estrogen produced by active ovaries, they're reserved for treatment of postmenopausal women, who still produce estrogen through other tissues but in smaller amounts. Some postmenopausal women are prescribed an aromatase inhibitor after tamoxifen therapy, usually for a total treatment regimen of 5 years.

There are three aromatase inhibitors currently in use for cancer treatment: anastrozole (known by the brand name Arimidex), exemestane (known by the brand name Aromasin), and letrozole (known by the brand name Femara).

Some advantages of aromatase inhibitor therapy over tamoxifen for postmenopausal women include the following:

- **Aromatase inhibitors have fewer side effects than tamoxifen.**
- **Aromatase inhibitors have less serious side effects.**
- **Aromatase inhibitors result in a 3 percent *lower* cancer recurrence 6 to 8 years after diagnosis than with taking tamoxifen alone.**[15]

Also, aromatase inhibitor therapy following tamoxifen therapy has additional benefits:

- **Switching to an aromatase inhibitor** after taking tamoxifen for 2 to 3 years (for a total of 5 years of hormonal therapy) offers more benefits than 5 years of tamoxifen alone.[16]

- **Taking an aromatase inhibitor for 5 years** after taking tamoxifen for 5 years continues to reduce risk recurrence, compared to no treatment after tamoxifen.[17]

As with tamoxifen, you may experience some menopausal symptoms while on aromatase inhibitor therapy, but the most common complaint among women taking it is joint pain and stiffness. There's also a chance that you'll experience cardiovascular problems or loss of bone density. This is because estrogen provides some protection against these problems. Tamoxifen, as we discussed earlier, does not work to eliminate estrogen from your body, so it's less likely to cause these issues.

As medical research continues to evolve, treatment recommendations may change (even during your own treatment course) regarding type of treatment and length of treatment recommended. Be sure to discuss with your doctors whether any new research developments have occurred that may change your course of treatment.

RECURRENCE

Everyone fears recurrence of their breast cancer. No one can predict with certainty whether or not you'll experience a recurrence, but your doctor can give you an idea of the odds for someone in your situation based on the stage of the cancer you had, the pathologic type, and the specific gene signature of your tumor. Other issues, such as your age, your family history, the type of treatment you had and how your cancer responded to that treatment, and how long it's been since you finished your treatment, may be considered as well.

There are Web sites and tables that medical professionals use to aid them in determining your odds of recurrence and even your odds of survival. We recommend that you don't use these tools to make predictions on your own. Even though you have no doubt educated yourself quite a bit about your cancer, you may fail to take some aspects of your situation into account or enter the data incorrectly. If you come up with a "good" number and your doctor tells you that your odds of recurrence are actually higher, you'll feel let down. Conversely, you could cause yourself unnecessary panic by calculating a number that's erroneously high. Even if you do manage to calculate a risk assessment that matches your doctor's it's better not to find out "your number" while sitting alone in the dark staring at your computer. Your doctor will be able to frame your odds of recurrence within the context of a plan for follow-up care, answer any questions you have, and provide perspective.

Recurrence is different from progression, which is a spreading or worsening of the original cancer. It's sometimes difficult to know whether the presence of cancer in someone who was previously declared cancer-free is a recurrence or a progression, because it's not possible to be completely certain that the cancer is truly gone at the end of treatment. Most doctors would say that a return of the cancer after less than 3 months probably indicates that the cancer has progressed rather than recurred.[18]

It's also possible to have breast cancer a second time that is not a recurrence of the original cancer. If the tumor is located in the other breast or a different area of the same breast, it's likely a new cancer, called a second primary cancer. In about one-third of cases when localized breast cancer is discovered a second time, it's a second primary cancer.[19] By examining the cancer cells under a microscope, a pathologist can determine if you have a local recurrence or a second primary cancer. It may sound frighteningly unfair to realize that you could have a whole new breast cancer to deal with, but these cancers are usually easier to treat than recurrences.

If you do have a recurrence, and you were not satisfied with your care during your last bout with cancer, you may want to consider looking for a second opinion about your condition and course of treatment. However, if you were happy with your oncologist, and especially if you have grown to trust your provider, don't feel obligated to do so. The delay taken in order to see other providers could change your prognosis.

There are three different types of recurrence.

1. Local recurrence. This means the cancer has come back in the breast or, in the case of mastectomy, the chest wall or skin on the chest. Local recurrence comes with symptoms isolated to the breast where the cancer first occurred.

If you've had a lumpectomy, the symptom might be:

- A new lump in your breast or an irregular area of firmness
- A new thickening or "orange peel" texture of the skin
- A new pulling back of the skin or dimpling at the lumpectomy site

- Skin inflammation or redness, sometimes accompanied by warmth
- Open sores or a "velvety" rash
- Changes in your nipple, such as flattening or indentation

If you've had a mastectomy, the symptom might be:

- One or more painless bumps or nodules on or under the skin of your chest wall
- A new area of thickening at or near the mastectomy scar

Most of the time these symptoms turn out to be indicative of something other than cancer recurrence, something harmless. A new lump could be a suture granuloma, that is, a bit of scar tissue that forms around a surgical suture. Swelling in the entire breast, especially if the breast is warm and sore, may be an infection that can be treated with antibiotics. Fat necrosis is a benign condition in which fatty tissue dies and turns into scar tissue or liquid, which can present as lumps (this can be caused by any type of breast surgery, including biopsy). A rash is very likely eczema or psoriasis. So pay attention to your body and follow up with your doctor, but don't panic if you notice something new.

Even if you *do* have a local recurrence following lumpectomy, there's about an 80 percent chance that it's still isolated to the breast and has not moved on to other areas of the body.[20] Your recommended treatment will depend on what sort of treatment you had the first time around. If you had breast-conserving surgery, your doctor will probably recommend a mastectomy. If the first treatment was a mastectomy, you'll probably have surgery to remove the new tumor. Radiation will likely follow if you didn't have it the first time; radiation isn't usually done in the same spot more than once. Chemotherapy, hormonal therapy, or both may be suggested.

2. Regional recurrence. This means the cancer has come back in the lymph nodes near the breast, perhaps in the armpit or collarbone area. Regional recurrences of breast cancer are fairly rare. Still, you should watch for the following symptoms on the side of your body in which you had the cancer:

- A lump or swelling in the lymph nodes under your arm, between your ribs, or above your collarbone
- Swelling of your arm

- Persistent pain in your arm and shoulder
- Rarely, loss of sensation in your arm and hand

Regional recurrence is treated by surgical removal of the affected lymph nodes, sometimes combined with chemotherapy and/or hormonal therapy. When the cancer comes back in both the breast and the nearby lymph nodes, it is called local-regional recurrence, and the treatment is a combination of those two regimens.

3. Distant recurrence or metastatic disease. This means the cancer has come back in another part of the body, such as the liver, lungs, bone marrow, or brain. Distant recurrence tends to be accompanied by more systemic symptoms than local or regional recurrence. These include:

- Persistent headache
- Chronic coughing, chest pain, or difficulty breathing
- Bone pain or fractures
- Abdominal pain
- Jaundice
- Extreme fatigue
- Weight loss or decreased appetite
- Vision changes
- Confusion
- Uneven gait or balance problems
- Seizures

Because these symptoms cover so many systems of the body, it can be easy to interpret every tension headache or chest cold as a sign of cancer. Again, remember that the odds are that your symptom is merely a temporary discomfort. If what you're experiencing isn't particularly severe or uncomfortable, consider following the 2-week rule (page 317). On the other hand, if you find that you can't relax until you get checked out, by all means call your doctor right away. Sometimes, not knowing what's going on is just unbearable, and your doctor will understand that.

As you might expect, the prognosis is better for locally or regionally recurring cancers than for distant ones. It's generally accepted that local and regional recurrences may be curable, but distant recurrences, while

resources for follow-up care

If you want additional information about follow-up care, here are some resources to check out.

- The American Society of Clinical Oncology Recommendations for Follow-Up Care are written for an audience of medical professionals, but if you'd like to read them, you can find them at tinyurl.com/q8ap3w8.

- *When Cancer Comes Back: Cancer Recurrence* by the American Cancer Society offers straightforward, easy-to-understand information. It's available for download at tinyurl.com/odlmkdv.

- *A Survivor's Guide to Life After Breast Cancer Treatment* (New York: Bantam, 2006) by Hester Hill Schnipper, an oncology social worker and two-time breast cancer survivor, is a very personal yet informative guide to follow-up care and beyond.

- *Breast Cancer Recurrence and Advanced Disease* by Barbara Gordon, Heather Shaw, David Kroll, and Brooke Daniel (Durham, NC: Duke University Press, 2010) is packed with expert information about this difficult topic. Everything from minimizing your chance of recurrence to planning for end-of-life care is covered in a way that's clear and frank without being harsh.

- *After Breast Cancer: All the Questions You're Afraid to Ask* by Musa Mayer (Sebastopol, CA: O'Reilly and Assoc., 2003) provides solid facts, statistics, and answers in a way that's reassuring but never condescending.

often treatable, cannot be cured. Even so, many women with distantly recurring or metastatic breast cancer are able to have good quality of life for years, even decades. Many oncologists encourage patients to think about this sort of cancer as a chronic condition, like diabetes or heart disease. While it's true that some people die of diabetes and heart disease every year, many others are doing quite well.

Sadly, some cancers cannot be controlled with any treatment available today. This is a frightening prospect, but it is important to remember that no doctor can predict your outcome with 100 percent certainty. Remember that new therapies are being researched every minute of every day by teams of scientists who want nothing more than to make breast cancer a thing of the past. Where there is life, there is hope, and quality of life should be an important consideration for you in this stage of disease.

· · · · · · · · · · · ·

It's important to fight the natural superstition that engaging in follow-up care somehow increases the likelihood of the cancer coming back. After months spent in the care of physicians, it is certainly tempting to put the entire experience behind you and try to reenter your life unencumbered by thoughts of your illness. You may have a strong aversion to the settings and experiences associated with cancer and its treatment. You may subconsciously blame those entrusted with your care for the difficulties you have endured. This is entirely understandable, but you must not allow those feelings to get in the way of following through with your responsibilities to yourself and those who love you.

Conversely, you shouldn't believe that you can prevent a recurrence through constant vigilance. Your quality of life is dependent on moving on and letting yourself take pleasure in the people and things you care about, without fear. Life is a gift, and we all have a limited amount of time to enjoy it. In the next chapter, we'll talk about how to find peace with your status as a breast cancer survivor.

A Fresh Start

In 2008, Summer Bondurant's life seemed perfect. Working part-time in compensation and benefits, she was able to balance her workload and spend lots of time with her sons, then 3 and 7, plus train for charity running races.

Then one day she looked at the breast self-exam instruction card she'd recently been given. "It was the first self-exam I'd ever done," she says, "and I felt something in one breast that wasn't in the other."

Her gynecologist sent her for a mammogram, which confirmed something suspicious. "The biopsy was very painful," she says. "And the technician told me that if the biopsy is painful, it's usually cancer." In fact, it was invasive ductal carcinoma.

Summer says her first thought was *I've got to preserve this great life I have for my sons.* So instead of opting for a lumpectomy, she chose an aggressive course and had a double mastectomy with TRAM flap reconstruction (see page 105) and four rounds of chemotherapy.

"Treatment was very painful, but believe it or not, it was also a happy time," says Summer, now 37. "I threw a birthday party for my son. I threw a big birthday party for myself. I kept busy at work, and I went out whenever I could. I was just focused on living."

In hindsight, Summer says she put many of her emotions into a box; when treatment ended, she "crashed." That's when she looked inward and says, "I realized I had an opportunity to see my life fresh." Big changes followed: She left her corporate job and founded a consulting firm. "I've never been a risk taker or a thrill seeker. I never would have had the courage to leave a steady job before breast cancer," she says. And she's committed to helping others: "I was lucky that a woman gave me a plastic sheet that told me how to do a breast exam."

Summer says, "I made changes in my life because I knew in my heart it was the right thing to do."

She'd like women who've been diagnosed to know . . . *it's okay to accept help.*

Breast cancer is . . . *rough, but it's not the end of the world.*

Tomorrow will . . . *not be worth all the worry.*

*"In three words I can sum up everything
I've learned about life: It goes on."*

—ROBERT FROST

CHAPTER 15

MOVING ON

You've completed your treatment and been declared cancer-free. Now what?

You may tell yourself that you should feel relieved, even euphoric. You've looked forward to this date for so long, endured so many moments of pain and fear, and now here you are, ready to put your cancer diagnosis firmly in the past. So why doesn't it seem so easy? Why do you sometimes still feel sick, scared, or confused?

First, keep in mind that this sort of response is normal. All sorts of complicated emotions—which you've probably been too physically drained to consciously deal with—are beginning to come to the surface. Your joy and gratitude may be mixed with anger, self-pity, or dread. You're likely experiencing physical aftereffects of your primary treatment or side effects from ongoing adjuvant therapy. You may find that your ability to communicate with your spouse or partner is weakened, even if he or she was extremely supportive during your treatment. You may find that your children, coworkers, or friends seem less patient with you now that the cancer is "behind you." You may wonder if your self-image or your libido will ever improve or if you'll ever be as physically and mentally capable as you were before. Above all, you may wonder if you'll ever stop feeling afraid.

In this chapter, we're going to look at some of the challenges that you may face going forward and help you find ways to make your recovery easier on yourself and those you care about.

RECOVERING PHYSICALLY

Late effects are essentially side effects that show up or linger after treatment is completed. While there's no way to predict which effects you'll experience (and maybe you won't experience any), we'll discuss a few of the more common ones and what you can do to help yourself get through them.

Chemo Brain

Chemo brain and *chemo fog* are terms sometimes used to describe the memory, concentration, or other cognitive problems that can follow cancer treatment. Complaints include difficulty multitasking, having a short attention span, being especially disorganized or forgetful, or a general feeling of mental fogginess. Of course, these are things that can also be brought on by the fear and distraction of fighting a serious illness, so it can be difficult to separate the symptoms brought on by treatment from those brought on by circumstances. It's not even clear whether chemotherapy is the sole cause of mental fuzziness after cancer treatment; it may be caused by other cancer treatments (such as radiation or hormone therapy), the side effects of cancer treatments (such as anemia or insomnia), or even the medications used to treat the side effects of these treatments (such as painkillers or sleep aids).

It's clear, though, that chemo brain is a real syndrome. In a study completed in 2012 at Rutgers University,[1] scientists found evidence of postchemotherapy disruptions to the hippocampus, the part of the brain responsible for transferring information from short-term memory to long-term memory. Tracey Shors, PhD, the neuroscientist who headed the study, said, "Chemotherapy is an especially difficult time as patients are learning how to manage their treatment options while still engaging in and appreciating life. The disruptions in brain rhythms and neurogenesis during treatment may explain some of the cognitive problems that can occur during this time. The good news is that these effects are probably not long-lasting."[2] In fact, while most chemotherapy patients *do* experience some degree of mental fogginess during and after treatment, for roughly 85 percent, these symptoms are temporary.[3]

Knowing that your mental fog will likely clear over time is helpful, but it can still be frustrating to not feel as sharp as you used to. There are things you can do in the short term to help improve your cognitive function and make your life flow more smoothly.

- **Get plenty of sleep.** Adequate sleep is crucial to proper brain function.
- **Exercise regularly.** Increasing the flow of oxygen to the brain has been shown to help improve cognitive function.[4]
- **Keep your mind active.** Mental challenges like math problems, crossword puzzles, or memory games can help.
- **Eat well.** Healthful foods, such as blueberries, salmon, avocados, and whole grains, may support brain function.[5]
- **Make lists and keep a calendar** to help you remember tasks and appointments.
- **Keep a journal**, and reread it from time to time; this will help transfer events from short-term to long-term memory.
- **Ask for help.** Request that the people you live with help you keep track of things. Simple things such as always putting back household items like keys where they belong and writing down phone messages rather than giving them to you verbally can relieve a lot of frustration. If you live alone, try to be careful about putting things away after you use them, and leave notes for yourself where you'll see them.
- **Focus on a single task** rather than trying to do too many things at once.
- **Be patient with yourself.** Stress and panic over feeling that your mind is failing can make it harder to remember or process things. Try to relax and give it time.

Weight Gain

It does seem horribly unfair on top of everything you've been through, but weight gain can be a side effect or late effect of chemotherapy and hormonal treatment, or the medications that accompany these therapies. Fortunately, the amount of gain is usually minimal (5 to 10 pounds).[6] It's difficult to know, of course, the exact causes of weight gain, because cancer treatment is often accompanied by stress, reduced activity, and insomnia, all of which can contribute to weight gain. In addition, going through menopause (either naturally or as a result of the treatment) plays a part, as does the normal aging process.

Regardless of the causes, though, the treatment for any kind of weight gain is the same.

Eat well. We're sure that by this point in this guide, you're probably growing tired of being told, but a healthy, balanced diet is one of the best things you can do for your health and well-being. Refer to Chapter 9 if you need to renew your commitment to eating well.

Exercise. See Chapter 10 if you need to get back into a gentle exercise plan. If you're already exercising, talk to your doctor about ways to safely step up your workout and set new goals for yourself.

Get enough sleep. In one recent study, subjects who were restricted to 5 hours of sleep a night gained an average of *2 pounds* in a single week.[7] If you're having trouble sleeping, talk to your doctor about lifestyle changes or medications that can help.

Don't sit for too long. Even if you're getting regular exercise, long periods of sitting can lead to weight gain and a host of other health problems.[8] Anything that gets you out of your chair will help. If you work at a desk, set a timer on your computer to remind you to get up and stretch or walk around your office for a couple of minutes every half hour. If you're watching TV, stand up during the commercials and do a few jumping jacks, gentle stretches, or a few of the exercises mentioned in Chapter 10. (Just don't use this as an excuse to head to the kitchen for a snack.)

Fatigue

If you're tired of feeling tired, you're not alone: Fatigue is one of the most common complaints among those recovering from breast cancer. In most cases, this is temporary, but it can be frustrating to be unable to keep the schedule you once did. If you were an especially busy, high-energy person, it's a big adjustment to have to admit that you can't do it all. Here are some tips to get you through the fatigue until you feel more like yourself.

Schedule naps. Yes, it feels like kindergarten, but you'll find it easier to cope if you give yourself a break. At first, you may have difficulty falling asleep during the day if it isn't something you're used to, but after a week or so the habit will feel more natural. Try for 20 minutes as a starting point, but adjust to longer or shorter naps based on what your body asks for. If you work, let your family know that the first hour after you get home is your rest time. Try to avoid long naps late in the day, though; it can lead to insomnia at night.

Look carefully at your schedule. When you were first diagnosed and going through treatment, a lot of commitments probably got pushed off the calendar: volunteer work, community or parents' association meetings, church obligations, and so on. Maybe you even took medical leave from your job. People may now be asking when you can pick up where you left off. Consider each obligation carefully before taking it on again. You'll want to prioritize your activities so the ones that are most important to you get your energy and the ones that aren't so vital wait until a few months down the road. You may even find that your time was being expended on some things that you don't miss very much.

Get used to saying "no." When someone asks you to do something that you don't feel up to, don't let guilt force you into it. Friends, family, and coworkers may assume that they're being kind by including you in activities or asking you for help. For them, it sends the message that they don't see you as less fun or less capable since your illness. You, on the other hand, may feel that since they supported you when you were sick, you "owe" them now. If you're worried about making them feel bad for asking, try keeping your response light: "I'm sorry, Barb, but chemo kicked my butt, and if I don't get my 14 hours of beauty sleep, I'll need to lie down while I'm taking a shower."

Consider using caffeine—judiciously. Coffee and tea haven't been shown to increase breast cancer risk, and there is evidence that they may even reduce it slightly.[9] (If you're unsure about your particular situation, though, ask your doctor.) A cup of black or green tea or coffee can give you enough of a boost to get you through times when you'd love a nap but just can't manage one. Stop at one, though, and avoid getting your caffeine fix from soda, which is full of sugar (and the diet ones have zero nutritional value plus chemical sweeteners). Also, go easy on the sweets; sugar might make you feel more energetic for a brief time, but the inevitable crash will make you feel worse than before.

Menopausal Symptoms

The combination of the cancer and your treatment has wreaked havoc with your hormones. (Refer to "Hormonal Therapy" on page 314 for more on this.) If you were premenopausal before your diagnosis, you'll likely find that your periods have stopped either temporarily or permanently. (This depends on a variety of factors, including your age, the type of treatments you had, and the form and duration of adjuvant therapy you're receiving now.) If you've been through menopause already, you may experience some of the same symptoms again.

Hot flashes and night sweats are among the most common complaints. Here are some ways to cope.

Tailor your sleeping conditions. If you share a bed with someone whose internal thermostat doesn't match yours, consider a dual-control electric blanket or a blanket on only your partner's side of the bed. Some companies even make custom comforters with more down filling on one side than the other so that sleeping partners can each have their own level of warmth.

Use cotton or modal sheets; they're more absorbent than synthetic fabrics. (Modal is a fiber made from beech trees.) This will help you feel less sweaty during the night.

Carry water everywhere. Invest in an insulated BPA-free water bottle, or buy a set of refillable ones and keep the fridge stocked with them. You might even consider putting one of those small dorm fridges in your bedroom.

Use ice packs or damp washcloths liberally. Applying one to your forehead and one to the back of your neck can do a lot to make you feel cooler fast. You can find small, flexible, gel-filled ice packs in the first-aid section of most pharmacies. Again, a small fridge next to the bed would be helpful for preparing for middle-of-the-night discomfort.

Dress in layers. There's a special kind of frustration in having a hot flash at work and realizing that you have to keep your turtleneck sweater on for the rest of the day because it's all you have.

See an acupuncturist. Recent studies indicate that acupuncture may relieve hot flashes as well as other symptoms of menopause. Talk to your doctor about including this complementary therapy in your regimen. You can read more about acupuncture on page 291.

Lymphedema

This is fluid retention caused by removal of the lymph nodes. In breast cancer survivors, this usually shows up as swelling in the arm on the same side of the body where the mastectomy and/or radiation was performed. Besides the swelling, you may notice in the same area some tightness or restricted movement, a sense of heaviness or aching, or thickening of the skin.

These symptoms can show up any time after breast cancer treatment, even years later. If you notice any of them, tell your doctor right away because lymphedema can lead to infection. While lymphedema is not curable, there are a number of things you can do to manage it and minimize your discomfort.

Avoid straining that arm. For instance, don't carry heavy suitcases or bags in that hand.

Avoid cuts, scratches, and burns on that hand or arm as much as possible. Consider using an electric razor to shave your armpit, use insect repellent, wear thick gloves while doing household chores or gardening, and don't cut the cuticles on that hand. Also, if you need to have blood drawn or get an IV, ask the phlebotomist or nurse to use the other arm, if possible. To avoid burns, use long oven mitts that go well up your arm, and don't forget sunscreen.

If you do get a wound on that hand or arm, clean and treat it carefully, then be alert for any sign of infection. Call your doctor right away if you notice pus, warmth, or redness or if you have a fever or chills.

Consider massage or gentle exercise; both help to move fluid out of the arm. Exercises that focus on gently contracting and releasing the muscles are often prescribed; your doctor may suggest that you see a physical therapist to learn how to do them properly.

Ask your doctor if a compression bandage or sleeve is a good idea for you. These work to keep fluid from building up in the arm by exerting pressure. Even if you don't use one regularly, you may be advised to wear one in certain situations that can make lymphedema worse.

Don't wear tight cuffs or bracelets on that arm or carry hair elastics or rubber bands around your wrist.

Rest and elevate your arm above your heart when you notice swelling or achiness. This can be done by lying down and propping two or three pillows under your arm.

Most breast cancer centers have a lymphedema specialist, so make sure to discuss with your doctor whether you should see one.

RECOVERING EMOTIONALLY

Cancer treatment, no matter how physically unpleasant it is, can be psychologically helpful in that it gives a sense of purpose and direction to your life. It can even help to make you feel safer as you and your medical team are actively fighting the disease. Experts have been closely monitoring your condition, giving you instructions, supporting you, and reminding you that while you are at the center of this battle, you are far from alone. Now that the fight is over, you may find yourself feeling scared and adrift.

Fear

Many women say that the worst aftereffects of breast cancer aren't the hot flashes or the chemo brain–it's the fear. While we all know that we're mortal, most of us do a pretty good job of forgetting about it most of the time. A diagnosis of breast cancer, even if it comes with a good prognosis, is a stark reminder of our mortality.

You've no doubt spent a great deal of time contemplating the possibility that your cancer could return. You probably know the recurrence and survival rates for your particular kind of cancer like you know your phone number. It's fine to educate yourself about the risks and face the reality of your situation, but moving on with your life means getting yourself out of the health-crisis mind-set. It's not easy, but there are ways to get out from under the shadow of constant worry.

Don't go it alone. Breast cancer support groups aren't just for patients currently in therapy; having people to talk to who understand your fears can be a huge help. As the old adage goes, a worry shared is a worry halved. If you feel more comfortable getting in touch online rather than in person, there are safe message boards at sites like Breastcancer.org.

Consider seeing a psychologist or therapist, if you haven't already. He or she can work through your emotions with you and help you to move past the fear.

Remember that for every year your cancer doesn't return, your odds of recurrence go down. Before you go to sleep, try saying to yourself, "I should be a little less afraid tonight than I was last night."

Remind yourself that statistics can't predict whether or not your cancer will return. Odds are all about large numbers, not about individual outcomes.

Keep up with the coping strategies that got you through diagnosis and treatment. If meditation or journaling helped to calm you down, keep those practices going.

Do a postcancer purge. It's likely that your home contains items that you don't need any longer now that your primary therapy is over. If you have any medications left over from your treatment, contact your pharmacist for information about how to dispose of (or donate) them properly. If you find that you're too superstitious to permanently get rid of breast cancer books or head scarves, put them in a box in the guest room closet or attic. The point is to not have reminders everywhere you look unless they're part of your spiritual or emotional healing process.

If you find yourself fretting about all the things you'll never get to do if your cancer returns, start doing them. Train for a marathon, visit Europe, write a book. Try to see your fear as a galvanizing force rather than a paralyzing one.

Anger

Even if you've never been a "why me?" sort of person, a diagnosis of breast cancer very likely brought that question to your mind. You may find that you're resentful of friends who have good health and have very little patience for their mundane, day-to-day complaints. Maybe you find yourself lashing out at family members with little provocation because they "just don't understand."

Anger is a natural response to an unfair situation, and few things in life are as unfair as cancer. Here are some ways to handle your feelings.

Consider joining a support group, in person or online, and/or seeing a therapist. You need to have a place to vent your anger other than on your family and friends.

Don't confront people you're angry with just yet. If you find that you're carrying a grudge toward a particular person for a particular grievance, give it some time before you have a confrontation. If you can't get past how your sister failed to come visit you after your surgery or how your best friend didn't call often enough while you were sick, it may be a good idea to bring it up with them. But keep in mind that you were in a very raw state emotionally during your diagnosis and treatment, and that means that small slights from that time carry extra weight in your memory. Wait until you feel more like yourself before you have a confrontation. If you can't wait, talk to your therapist or another trusted person first, so they can help you frame the complaint in an appropriate way.

If you do lash out, remember that most people will understand. Apologize sincerely, and then try to be more in control in the future. But don't beat yourself up over an occasional outburst–you're still processing a lot of things, including anger.

Try very hard, however, not to blow up at young children. They likely already feel insecure because of your illness and the changes in routine that accompanied it, so it's important that you not give them any reason to feel at fault.

Don't turn your anger inward. You may find yourself questioning whether you brought the cancer on yourself through diet or other lifestyle choices. The truth is, some women do everything right and still get breast cancer.

Get it out physically. Running, kickboxing, Spinning, or any other sport that gets your heart rate up releases endorphins and helps you to relieve your stress and anger. Talk to your doctor first about what exercises are safe for you and what your target heart rate should be.

Poor Body Image

In our society, we're constantly exposed to images of physically and sexually attractive women. It's just about impossible to watch an hour of TV, check the news online, or flip through a magazine without seeing young, fit, healthy, barely dressed women trying to sell something. Before your cancer diagnosis, you may have hardly noticed these images, but when you're feeling insecure about your body, they seem to be everywhere.

Learning to accept and even love your body again is possible, but it takes time and perspective.

The changes that you see in your body will improve after treatment is over. Consider what they say about pregnancy: 9 months up, 9 months down. This is a way of reassuring women that the weight they gain during pregnancy takes at least that much time to lose, but it's a good philosophy for recovering from any major physical endeavor or trauma. Be patient with your body. Scars will fade, hair will grow back, chemotherapy bloat will subside.

Keep in mind that everyone ages. Yes, you've gone through a body-altering experience, but every day, everyone is a little different than they were the day before. Life is change. During the time you were in treatment, your friends may have noticed new freckles, new laugh lines, or new gray hairs. Eventually, you'll go back to noticing these trivial changes about yourself, too. Odds are, though, you'll be able to see them for what they are: glorious signs of a long, full life.

As your energy returns, you'll be more able to pay attention to your physical appearance. You may have had days during your treatment when it felt like an effort just to brush your teeth. Something like painting your toenails or giving yourself a facial at those times seemed impossible. Now you can begin to consider what makes you feel beautiful inside and out, and do those things. Or grab a friend and go to a spa so someone else can do them for you.

Frame your situation in terms of what you can control. You may not be able to say, "I'm going to be a size 4 by Christmas," but you can say, "I'm going to eat at least five servings of fruits or vegetables a day" or "I'm going to go to the gym four times a week."

If you have clothes that don't fit because of weight gain or loss, get them out of your closet and drawers. You don't have to get rid of them, but store them somewhere where you won't have to shove them out of the way when you get dressed every day.

Consider whether the colors that flattered you before your therapy are working for you now. Your skin may have more yellow tones after chemotherapy, and your hair may be growing back in a different color than it was. If you don't know how to choose clothing or makeup colors, get help from a stylish friend, a beauty-savvy daughter, a professional stylist, or your local breast center.

Remind yourself that attractiveness and sexiness are about more than what someone looks like. Everything from your sense of humor to your self-confidence comes into play. All of these things can be affected by your diagnosis and treatment, but you *will* get them back.

Relationship Concerns

Your spouse or partner has probably been with you through this entire process and has had to deal with many of the same kinds of fears and frustrations that you have, combined with the helplessness of watching a loved one suffer. Now that you're both trying to get back to your normal life, your partner has to find a way to put your illness into context. This isn't easy, and everyone handles it differently.

Maybe things are better than ever between you, and this experience has only strengthened your bond and made you each appreciate what you have. If so, congratulations. If not, though, there are ways to help your spouse or partner through this time of transition. Examples of behaviors that you might see are:

- **Avoiding any discussion of the cancer** and becoming upset or quiet when you bring it up
- **Being overprotective** and resisting your attempts to resume your normal routine
- **Getting resentful or frustrated** when you aren't yet able to do all the things you could
- **Being emotionally distant, physically distant, or unaffectionate**
- **Seeming sexually uninterested**
- **Feeling the need to keep up a strong front** at all times or being overly jovial or optimistic

Keep in mind that your spouse or partner is coping as best as he or she can. Sometimes they're called silent victims. During the time of your disease, most of the concern and care has been appropriately directed toward you. Family, friends, and medical professionals were understandably much more concerned with how you were feeling, physically and emotionally, than how your partner was doing. Your partner has also had to shoulder a lot of responsibility and carry around a lot of fear. Now that you're trying to get back to a more normal routine, he or she may be dealing with some complicated emotions, and this can come out in ways that seem unloving or destructive.

Remember, it is always a good idea to seek help if you feel that you need it. Ask your doctor for a referral to a specialist in sexual health. Many centers have these specialists available or can refer you to the appropriate person. Here are some ideas to help get your relationship back on track.

Get your spouse or partner talking. Explain how you're feeling, and encourage your spouse or partner to do the same. Agree that you won't judge each other for having "wrong" or "bad" thoughts, like "Sometimes I feel angry with you for getting sick" or "I hate that the kids depend on you more than me since my cancer." These aren't easy conversations to have, so consider couples therapy if you're worried about how to start them or how to keep them loving and respectful. Or encourage your spouse or partner to see a therapist to work through some of the feelings before bringing them to you.

Give your spouse or partner a break. If he hates talking about the heavy stuff, work out times when you don't discuss it. Maybe you declare weekends to be your days off–no talk about cancer, your relationship, or whatever else causes stress. As long as you set aside time when you *do* talk about the things that are bothering you, it's healthy to forget about them for a while.

Get your spouse or partner a book or two that specifically addresses his or her experience of breast cancer. Marc Silver's *Breast Cancer Husband: How to Help Your Wife (and Yourself) During Diagnosis, Treatment, and Beyond* (Emmaus, PA: Rodale Inc., 2004) is well-written, engaging, and at times refreshingly funny. This is a great resource for spouses, significant others, and even friends or other family members.

Make sure your spouse or partner has some leisure time away from you. It's likely that when you were in treatment, he or she stopped doing some enjoyable activities to be there for you and take on some of your duties around the house. Send your partner out for an afternoon on a bike, to a baseball game with friends, or for a day on the golf course.

Get back to doing the things that you enjoyed as a couple before your illness. If you used to go hiking but aren't physically up for that yet, try a walk at a local park. The point is to bring back the sensation of having fun together that you had before cancer interrupted your lives.

Have sex or talk about why you aren't having sex. Sex releases dopamine and oxytocin into the brain, two chemicals that are responsible for feelings of well-being and affection,[10] which can strengthen your bond with each other and fight depression. If you don't feel physically or emotionally ready after your cancer treatment, talk to your partner about your concerns. You can also talk to your doctor about vaginal dryness, low libido, or difficulty achieving orgasm, all of which can be side effects of hormone therapy.

Don't give up. You've been through a frightening, painful, exhausting ordeal together. Despite myths to the contrary, divorce rates are *not* higher among breast cancer survivors, and couples who have been through breast cancer diagnosis and treatment together report no less marital satisfaction than other couples.[11]

• • • • • • • • • • • • •

Moving on after breast cancer is never easy. You've no doubt lost some things along the way, but you've gained some things, too: an appreciation for the resiliency of your body. A deeper knowledge of the love of your family and friends. A clarity of priorities in the way you spend your time. A reminder of the beauty and fragility of life.

No one ever says, "I'm glad that I had breast cancer." All you can do is find the small gifts, the moments of kindness, of insight, that made your time as a breast cancer patient bearable. Try to hold on to those gifts as you go forward. Try to be kind to others and insightful about yourself and the world around you. The path ahead of you may not be free of obstacles, but no one's path is. The only option is to trust that all will be well, and take the first step.

GETTING INVOLVED—YOUR WAY

About $6 billion a year goes into breast cancer awareness and research campaigns in the United States.[12] You don't have to look far to see a pink ribbon, particularly during National Breast Cancer Awareness Month in October, when they show up on everything from socks to pencils. Some women who have recovered from breast cancer find this comforting and encouraging, a sign that our society cares about them and is constantly working toward a cure. Others may find it becomes nearly impossible to escape reminders of the disease. Only you know how you see yourself fitting into society as a breast cancer survivor.

When you feel up to it, consider giving something of yourself toward this cause or another one that speaks to you. There are few things more empowering than feeling that you're doing something positive in the world. If you choose to get involved with breast cancer issues, here are some ways to make sure that your time or money does the most good.

Consider peer mentoring at your hospital or cancer treatment center. Think about how confused and frightened you were when you received your diagnosis. Talking to another survivor who has been through the same thing can be invaluable to someone in that situation.

reward yourself

Something to mark the end of your treatment can help you internalize the sense of completion and accomplishment that should accompany it. Planning for that reward can also give you something positive and life-affirming to focus on. Cancer diagnosis and treatment involves a lot of waiting, often in stressful situations, which can set your mind to rehashing the worst-case scenarios over and over. Break the cycle by creating a notebook—or a file on your laptop or phone—dedicated to your project, which you can work on during these moments.

Choose something meaningful to you. A trip is a popular choice and gives you a break from the environment of your cancer experience. You may love your home, but you've spent months forming "cancer" associations with everything from your bed to your drinking glasses. Time away can give you fresh perspective and dull some of the frightening memories.

One woman we know spent her time in treatment planning a party for her family and friends. She worked out every detail, from the menu to the live music to the invitations. Every element had meaning and celebrated her life and those she cared about. She called it her INDY (I'm Not Dead Yet) party.

A party or a trip isn't your style? Figure out what calls to you. Perhaps a class in something you've always wanted to learn to do

Participate in a clinical trial for breast cancer survivors. These trials study things like the impact of lifestyle on cancer recurrence or quality of life after treatment. You can search for trials in your area at breastcancertrials.org.

Fund-raise for an organization. If you'd like to coordinate a fund-raiser, or if your friends or family want to make a donation in your honor, or a redecoration of a room in your home. (This can help remove some of those negative associations we mentioned.) The point is to have something to focus on during your treatment that helps you look toward the future. When you need a distraction from all the cancer talk, put your energy into researching hotel deals in Greece or finding the perfect bedspread. With the Internet, you can do these things at home. No Internet access? Just gather catalogs, brochures, or books on the topic to take along to appointments.

Remember, your project doesn't have to be expensive. A potluck dinner keeps costs down and gives your friends a chance to contribute to the celebration. A class at your local library or community college can get you started on a new path. A camping trip is a relatively inexpensive way to vacation, providing time in nature, which can bring a sense of peace and rejuvenation. The important thing is that you mark the end of your treatment in a meaningful way that gives you joy.

One caveat: Don't plan to take your trip or tear out your old carpeting the day after your treatment ends. Depending on your specific treatment and side effects, it will take time for you to feel up to celebrating. Discuss with your doctor what your recovery expectations should be, and wait until you know how the treatments are affecting you before you set a date.

consider one of these well-respected organizations as the recipient. These institutions spend most of their funds on research and treatment.

- Breast Cancer Research Foundation (bcrfcure.org)
- Memorial Sloan-Kettering Cancer Center (mskcc.org)
- University of Texas, MD Anderson Cancer Center (mdanderson.org)

- Dana-Farber Cancer Institute (dana-farber.org)
- The Johns Hopkins Avon Foundation Breast Center (hopkinsmedicine .org/avon_foundation_breast_center)[13]

Remind the people you know that not everything with a pink ribbon supports breast cancer research. Encourage them to find out more about an organization before they buy or donate.

Lobby for increased government support of breast cancer–related issues. Many aspects of public policy–from funding for research to the regulation of industrial chemicals–play a part in the causes, treatments, and cures for breast cancer. Learn more about an issue that gets you fired up, then write your representatives.

GLOSSARY

Acupuncture: A form of holistic healing therapy that falls under the umbrella of complementary medicine and involves the insertion of thin needles at various points of the body to ease pain or other negative conditions.

Adjuvant therapy: Therapy in addition to surgery that is designed to limit the recurrence of breast cancer. Examples include chemotherapy, hormonal therapy, and radiation therapy.

Alternative therapy: Healing practices that replace conventional medicine and are not part of standard care. For example, using homeopathy in place of mainstream medicine, or replacing chemotherapy with Chinese herbs and other dietary supplements is considered alternative medicine.

Anticarcinogen: Any substance that has the capacity to counteract a carcinogen. Examples include various types of plants and foods.

Antioxidant: An agent consumed in food that works to prevent free radicals from damaging your tissues and genes. Because antioxidants can hinder free radicals and prevent disease-causing damage, they're being widely studied for their potential to prevent and eradicate breast cancer.

Apoptosis: The normal life cycle of a cell, in which healthy cells go about their everyday business signaled by directions from DNA and then die a natural death. This process is thought to be mutated by cancers.

Aromatase inhibitors: Agents that work to keep estrogen from contributing to the growth of estrogen receptor positive tumors by suppressing estrogen production. Because they cannot suppress the quantity of estrogen produced by active ovaries, they're reserved for treatment of postmenopausal women, who still produce estrogen through other tissues, but in smaller amounts.

Axilla: The underarm area.

Axillary dissection: Surgical removal of lymph nodes in the underarm area.

Axillary lymph nodes: Lymph nodes located near the underarm area.

Benign: Classification of a tumor meaning it is slow-growing and does not metastasize, or spread to other parts of the body (noncancerous).

Biopsy: The removal of tissue as a means of testing for cancer.

Bone scan: Imaging study that tests for cancer by injecting radioactive material that collects in any abnormal bone areas and can be seen through a scanner. This is not currently recommended as a form of routine follow-up care.

BRCA1/BRCA2 genes (BReast CAncer genes): Tumor-suppressing genes that, if genetically mutated, indicate a disposition to breast and ovarian cancer.

Brachytherapy: Form of radiation therapy (or radiotherapy) that helps eradicate any remaining cancer cells from the body after lumpectomy or mastectomy. This therapy involves placing radioactive pellets in the breast tissue near the location of the excised tumor.

Breast cancer: Condition where out-of-control cell growth and division occurs in the breast, eventually leading to a tumor.

Breast cancer advocacy: Assistance and support offered by groups and individuals to those affected by breast cancer.

Breast density: The measure of connective and glandular tissue in the breasts. Breasts that contain more connective and glandular tissue than fat are considered dense.

Breast reconstruction: Surgical procedure to re-create the appearance of breasts after a full or partial mastectomy.

Breast self-examination: Method that can be used to detect any abnormalities in one's breasts. Not recommended as the only form of cancer screening. Professional screenings are much more detailed and accurate.

Calcifications: Calcium deposits that can form throughout the breast.

Cancer: Abnormal cell processes involving uncontrolled cell growth and division caused by mutations in DNA. There are more than 100 forms of cancer.

Carcinoma in situ: Cancer that has not spread beyond the ducts or lobules. *Situ* means "in place."

Catheter: A tube that goes into the body.

Chemotherapy: A form of cancer treatment administered in cycles to help combat cancer. It involves the administration of one or a combination of drugs designed to stop and destroy cancer cells.

Clinical trials: Scientific means of testing new cancer treatments with volunteers. Often they are performed through hospitals where individuals can choose to take part in the research for the potential benefits.

Complementary therapies (integrative therapies): Forms of therapy, like acupuncture or massage, backed by research and recommended to ease symptoms and side effects, help heal the body, ease the mind, and uplift the spirits. They should not be used alone to treat cancer, but when combined with standard medical care, they can greatly decrease stress and other negative side effects of medication or cancer itself.

Co-payment: The amount of money a patient must directly pay a doctor. It is not covered by insurance.

CT scan: A method of image screening where an x-ray creates a sequence of images through a computerized system. It is not generally recommended for breast cancer screening.

Cyst: A typically benign mass that contains fluid.

Deductible: Amount of money that must be paid by the patient before his or her insurance company will begin to pay compensation.

Diagnosis: Detection of a condition or disease by a licensed professional based on symptoms the patient exhibits.

Diagnostic mammogram: Mammogram performed to determine whether a patient may have breast cancer based on an abnormal screening mammogram. This can also be used to monitor symptoms of already diagnosed cancer. It involves at least two separate breast x-rays.

Disease-free survival rate: The percentage of individuals who are without cancer and alive after a specific increment of time since last treated (for example, 5 years).

Duct: Part of the breast where milk is transported during pregnancy and lactation. Breast cancer can often begin in the ducts.

Ductal carcinoma in situ (DCIS): Generally considered an early stage of cancer, categorized as "stage 0." Highly effective treatments are available, and survival rates for this condition are close to 100 percent.

Early-stage breast cancer: Generally classified as stage I or stage II, when cancer is confined to only the breast and/or underarm lymph node region.

Edema: Swelling that is often painful due to excess fluid in tissue.

Endometrial cancer: Cancer of the uterus, specifically the uterus's lining.

Enzyme: Type of protein that creates other reactions in the body without being destroyed itself.

Epidemiology: The study of diseases. Specifically, what causes diseases and how to prevent disease.

Estrogen: Reproductive hormone that can spur significant growth in cancer cells.

Estrogen receptors: Proteins to which estrogen attaches in cells. Some cancer treatments act by blocking estrogen receptors so that estrogen cannot attach and allow the cancer to grow.

False negative: Test results that incorrectly indicate that an individual is disease-free when he or she has a disease.

False positive: Test results that incorrectly indicate that an individual has a disease when he or she does not have that disease.

Fat necrosis: A benign condition in which fatty tissue dies and turns into scar tissue or liquid, which can appear as lumps. This can be caused by any type of breast surgery, including biopsy.

Fine-needle aspiration (FNA, fine needle biopsy): The suction method of removing a few cells from the breast for examination.

First-degree relative: An individual's father, mother, brother, sister, son, or daughter.

Genes: The area in a cell where DNA is located. Genes are responsible for the transmission of traits and characteristics from parent to child.

General practitioner: A family doctor who may perform mammograms and discover early signs of breast cancer.

Generic: Term for medication unattached to a brand name that instead uses the medication's chemical name.

Genetic: Relating to genes and heredity, the traits and characteristics passed from generation to generation.

HER2/neu (human epidermal growth factor receptor 2, ERBB2): Protein that may be found in some breast cancer cells, which promotes cancer growth but can be inhibited by drug therapy.

Homeopathy (homeopathic medicine): Treatment that uses very small doses of substances to encourage the body to heal itself. Evidence to the safety of this treatment has not been exhaustively proven.

Hormones: Chemicals created by glands and some nerves that control and regulate the functions of different organs and tissues throughout the body.

Hormone receptors: Proteins that accept hormones, which can make cancer grow more aggressively. Some treatments include blocking hormone receptors so they cannot attach to hormones and encourage cancer growth.

Hormone receptor status: Indicates whether your breast cancer is hormone receptor positive or hormone receptor negative, meaning whether or not the cancer needs hormones to grow. If hormone receptor positive, the cancer will require hormones in order to grow, and treatment can be adapted to block hormones from their receptors to discourage cancer growth.

Hormone therapy (endocrine therapy, endocrine manipulation): Therapy that involves blocking hormone receptors from the hormones that would attach to them, and therefore denying the cancer a way to grow.

Hospice: Center dedicated to the special needs of terminal breast cancer patients and their loved ones. They focus on providing comfort, controlling pain and other physical symptoms, and offering emotional support.

Immunotherapy: Therapy that stimulates the immune system to stop the cancer by targeting the biology of the cancer cell.

Implant (breast implant): Silicone material placed in the breast to reconstruct the breast following a mastectomy.

Incidence: The number of new reports of a disease within a certain period of time.

Induction chemotherapy (*see also* Neoadjuvant chemotherapy): Hormone-blocking therapy or chemotherapy prior to surgery. These treatments can shrink a tumor, permitting you to undergo a lumpectomy instead of mastectomy.

Inflammatory breast cancer (IBC): A condition in which the breasts become red and inflamed. It is a particularly aggressive and invasive cancer.

Insurance premium (premium): The amount of money an insurance company charges you in a specific time period.

Intraductal: A classification for breast cancer that has not spread beyond the milk ducts of the breast.

Intravenous (IV): A way of administering treatment or medication through the veins.

Invasive breast cancer: A type of breast cancer where the disease spreads beyond the ducts into other parts of the breast and/or body.

Investigational new drug (new experimental treatment): Drugs that are permitted to be used in clinical trials but are not otherwise available for treatments.

Lesion: Tissue that is pathologically changed.

Lifetime risk: The likelihood of ever developing breast cancer throughout one's lifetime.

Lobular carcinoma in situ (LCIS, lobular neoplasia in situ): Abnormal cells found only in the lobules. Their presence indicates an increased risk for developing breast cancer.

Lobules: Glands that produce milk in the breast.

Local treatment: Breast cancer treatment that involves surgery (with or without radiation) and eliminating the cancer from a specific location in the body.

Localized breast cancer: Cancer that is located only in the breast and currently has not spread anywhere else in the body.

Locally advanced breast cancer (stage III breast cancer): Involves a tumor larger than 5 centimeters that has spread to the lymph nodes under the arm, or a tumor that is any size with cancerous lymph nodes that adhere to one another or to surrounding tissue.

Local recurrence (recurrence): Another case of cancer in the same breast.

Lump: Any mass located on part of the body.

Lumpectomy (breast-conserving surgery): Surgery that removes the tumor and a small amount of normal tissue around it, not the entire breast.

Lymphatic system: Bodily system that plays a role in eliminating waste and is an important first defense against immune intruders, such as bacteria and cancerous cells.

Lymphedema: Painful swelling in the arms due to excess lymph fluid caused by surgery or radiation therapy to the lymph nodes.

Lymph nodes (lymph glands): Clusters of immune cells that are located in different areas throughout the body. Locations include underarms, neck, groin, and so on.

Lymph node status: The indication that cancer cells have traveled to the lymph nodes. If this is the case, systemic therapy is warranted.

Magnetic resonance imaging: *See* MRI.

Malignant: A classification for a tumor that indicates it is cancerous.

Mammary duct: *See* Duct.

Mammary glands: The area of the breast where milk is produced.

Mammogram: A screening technique to detect the presence of breast cancer in an individual. It involves x-ray images of the breast.

Margins: Edges of tissue that once surrounded a removed tumor. When the surgeon excises a tumor, he or she will examine the margins for cancer cells. If none are found, the excision is considered to have "clean" or negative margins, which are a good indication the surgery was successful in removing the cancer. If the edges are positive, it means cancer cells lined the edge of the excised tissue and more surgery is needed.

Mastectomy: Surgery in which part or all of the breast is removed.

Medical oncologist: A doctor who specializes in the treatment of cancer using a variety of therapies.

Menarche: First menstrual period.

Menopausal hormone therapy (postmenopausal hormone use, hormone replacement therapy): Treatment of menopausal symptoms through the use of hormone pills.

Menopause: The gradual process of ending the menstrual cycle for women that usually occurs between the ages of 40 and 59.

Meta-analysis: A study that combines and examines the results of multiple trials.

Microcalcifications: Calcium deposits that can indicate ductal carcinoma in situ.

Modified radical mastectomy: Surgery where the breast and lymph nodes are removed.

Mortality rate: Number of deaths within a specific period of time.

MRI (magnetic resonance imaging): An imaging method that uses radio waves and a powerful magnet linked to a computer to create detailed pictures of the body. It's rarely used as a screening tool.

Mutation (gene mutation): DNA change that can positively or negatively affect the functions of cells.

Naturopathy (naturopathic medicine): School of medical thought founded on the belief that natural elements can be used to achieve health and wellness (for example, massage).

Neoadjuvant chemotherapy (induction chemotherapy, primary chemotherapy, preoperative chemotherapy): Chemotherapy used as a first treatment to shrink tumors, often before a surgery.

Neoadjuvant hormone therapy: Therapy used as a first treatment where hormone receptors are blocked to reduce cancer. This treatment can be used to shrink tumors prior to surgery.

Neoadjuvant therapy (preoperative therapy): Therapy used to shrink tumors prior to a surgery. It is typically the first treatment.

Neoplasm: An abnormal growth of cells.

Nipple-sparing mastectomy: Surgical removal and reconstruction of the breast that removes the cancerous area but does not remove the nipple and areola.

Noninvasive: Breast cancer that currently has not moved past the area where it began. It also refers to a treatment that does not physically enter the body with any instrument (for example, massage).

Normal tissue: Noncancerous cells in the body.

Nuclear medicine imaging of the breast (molecular breast imaging): A way of detecting breast cancer that lights up areas where metabolic activity is going on. Breast cancers are more active than the benign tissue and produce strongly lighted areas. However, this is not a usual cancer screening method.

Observational study: A form of research in which the subjects report their behaviors, such as diet and exercise, to the researchers.

Oncologist: A doctor who specializes in cancer treatment.

Osteoporosis: A condition that involves weakened bones, which breast cancer patients may develop from their treatments and medication.

Overall survival (overall survival rate, survival): The percentage of people still alive after being diagnosed with breast cancer in a specific time period.

Paget disease of the breast (Paget disease of the nipple): A rare form of breast cancer that occurs in the nipple and involves an additional tumor in about half of all cases that may be invasive or noninvasive.

Palliative therapy (palliative care, palliation): A therapy common for those with stage IV breast cancer, which is unlikely to be cured, and therefore the treatment is centered around preventing pain and other uncomfortable symptoms rather than treating the disease itself.

Palpable: A description of a tumor that can be definitively felt in either a self-examination or a clinical examination.

Partial mastectomy: *See* Lumpectomy.

Pathologist: A physician who identifies breast cancer by studying cells and tissues under a microscope.

PET (positron emission tomography): Procedure sometimes used to evaluate the extent of breast cancer. It involves the insertion of short-term radioactive sugar into the body through an IV and looks to see which areas of the body consume the most sugar (cancerous areas usually consume more sugar).

Placebo: A pill that will have no effect on the taker; it is often used in studies to demonstrate the effects of a new medicine. One group in the study typically takes the drug while others are given a placebo, and the varying reactions are recorded.

Pooled analysis: The collection, grouping, and analysis of results and data found from many studies and research.

Positron emission tomography: *See* PET.

Postmenopausal hormone use: *See* Menopausal hormone therapy.

Premenopausal women: Women who regularly menstruate.

Premium (insurance premium): The cost of insurance coverage within a specific time period.

Preoperative chemotherapy: *See* Neoadjuvant chemotherapy.

Prevention: Actions to help diminish the chance of a condition, illness, or disease.

Primary chemotherapy: *See* Neoadjuvant chemotherapy.

Primary tumor: The first tumor to appear in the breast region.

Progesterone: A hormone involved in menstrual cycles, pregnancy, and other body functions. Some cancers feed on progesterone, but hormone therapy addresses this through the use of hormone-blocking drugs.

Progesterone receptor: A receptor to which progesterone will attach itself. This can encourage cancer to grow more aggressively, but hormone therapy and hormone-blocking drugs can be used to block the receptors and stop the cancer from spreading.

Progestin: A natural or synthetic substance that has the same effects as progesterone.

Prognosis: The most likely progress of a disease and the expected outcome.

Progression: The course the cancer takes within the body.

Prosthetic (breast prosthetic, prosthesis): An artificial breast that some choose to wear instead of undergoing full breast reconstruction after mastectomies.

Protocol: The official plan for a treatment process or procedure, experimental or non-experimental.

Quality of life: The assessment of an individual's comfort and happiness in life.

Radiation oncologist: Specialist with additional/advanced training in cancer treatment using radiation therapy.

Radiation therapy (radiotherapy): Treatment that involves using high-energy x-rays to eliminate cancer and/or stop it from growing.

Radiologist: Doctor who specializes in the interpretation of x-rays, mammograms, and diagnostic scans in general, as well as performs needle biopsies and wire localizations.

Radiotherapy: *See* Radiation therapy.

Raloxifene: Drug that can be used by postmenopausal women to lower the chance of breast cancer.

Reconstruction: *See* Breast reconstruction.

Recurrence (relapse): Reappearance of cancer in the body.

Regimen: A plan for the treatment of a disease.

Regional lymph nodes: Clusters of immune cells that are located near the breasts. This includes the axillary lymph nodes, the clavicular lymph nodes, and internal mammary nodes.

Relative survival (relative survival rate): A measurement that demonstrates whether a disease is shortening the lifespan. It compares the survival of individuals who have breast cancer versus those who do not, following treatment.

Remission: The absence of cancer symptoms either permanently or temporarily.

Risk (of disease): Chance that an individual will contract a disease.

Risk factor: Anything that influences the chance of an individual contracting a specific disease.

Schedules: In terms of breast cancer, the times for the administration of chemotherapy or other treatments.

Screening: A method of detecting diseases like cancer in an otherwise healthy person.

Screening mammogram: X-ray test performed to detect breast cancer when a patient has neither symptoms nor palpable lumps. A mammogram finds tumors before they're palpable and still easily treatable and curable.

Selective estrogen-receptor modulator (SERM): Drug designed to bind to breast cancers that have estrogen receptors and block their effects.

Sentinel node biopsy: Removal of tissue from first axillary lymph node to determine if cancer has spread.

Simple mastectomy: *See* Total mastectomy.

Sonogram: *See* Ultrasound.

Stage of cancer (cancer stage): A number corresponding with the size of a tumor and extent of cancer following surgery.

Staging (cancer staging): A way of evaluating the size of a tumor and extent of cancer following surgery.

Standard treatment (standard of care): General means of caring for a condition or disease that is seen as effective and therefore widely practiced.

Surgeon: A doctor who specializes in performing surgical procedures, many times including biopsies.

Survival: *See* Overall survival and Relative survival.

Survivor (breast cancer survivor): An individual who is living and who either has or has had breast cancer in her lifetime.

Survivorship: The well-being and care of someone who is living with breast cancer from diagnosis until the end of her life.

Systemic (adjuvant) treatment: *See* Adjuvant treatment.

Tamoxifen (Nolvadex): Hormone-blocking medication that is taken in pill form to treat hormone receptor positive breast cancers. It blocks estrogen from estrogen receptors and therefore stops the growth of cancer.

Targeted therapy: Cancer treatment that targets specific agents that are contributing to the growth of the cancer.

Therapeutic touch: Form of energy and complementary medicine where the practitioner attempts to rebalance and harmonize a patient by transferring energy through his or her hands into the patient's body in order to open the gateways in the body's energy channels. Ultimately, the goal is to jump-start the patient's own self-healing processes.

Tissue: Collection of cells.

Total mastectomy (simple mastectomy): Surgical removal of the breast and nipple as a way of eliminating breast cancer.

Trastuzumab (Herceptin): Medication that works via the body's immune system to disable the protein HER2.

Triple negative breast cancer: An aggressive form of breast cancer that manifests itself as basal-like tumors. It is estrogen receptor negative, progesterone receptor negative, and HER2/neu negative.

Tumor: An abnormal growth of cells.

Tumor grade: A system used to classify cancer cells in terms of how abnormal they look under a microscope and how quickly the tumor is likely to grow and spread. Many factors are considered, including the structure and growth pattern of the cells.

Tumor marker: A biochemical substance that indicates the presence of a tumor.

Ultrasound (sonogram): Diagnostic test usually used after a screening mammogram shows a mass, to help determine if a mass is solid or cystic (liquid filled). It can also be used for screening in addition to or instead of a mammogram.

Vaginal dryness: Form of discomfort during intercourse that is a symptom of loss of estrogen.

X-ray: The use of radiation to examine a part of the body to detect disease (for example, a chest x-ray).

INDEX

Chia seeds, 188
Children
  communication with, 59–61, 62, 64–67
  insurance coverage for, 136
  patience with, 335
Chinese medicine, 291, 304–5
Chin mudra, 259, 260
Chocolate, dark, 187
Cholesterol, dietary, 191
Cholesterol levels, 166
Cigarette smoking, 81, 105
Citrus fruits, 185
Cleaning for a Reason, 149
Cleaning products, 81
Clergy, 39
Clinical staging. *See* Staging, of cancers/tumors
Clinical trials, 120–21, 340
Clips, 86
Clothing, 336
CMF combination regimen, 124
COBRA, 143
Codes and coding, 145–46
Coffee, 187, 330
Cognitive distortions, 54–55
Cognitive impairment, 123, 248, 327–28
Collagen, 172–73
Colloid carcinoma, 91
Colon cancer, 179
Combination, of therapies, 117–18
Combination regimens, in chemotherapy, 124
Communication
  about death and dying, 19–20
  about diagnosis, 6–8, 48–63, 66
  about financial concerns, 57
  in changing circumstances, 64–67
  with children, 59–61
  of expectations, 67–72
  with medical teams, 15–18, 16, 40–42, 124, 286–87, 290–91, 294
  preparation tips, 63–64, 66
  questions
    about adjuvant therapy, 118–19

about cancer types, 90
from children, 62
communication role, 40–42
for doctors, 17–18
leading, avoiding, 41
for spouses, 57–58
writing down, 41
for yourself, 52
saying "no," 330
with spouse/partner, 55–60, 64–69, 72, 337–39
support group role, 270
Community of supporters, 9–10.
  See also Medical teams; Support groups
Complaints, preparing for, 65
Complementary medicine
  acupuncture, 291–95, 331
  aromatherapy, 256, 300–302, 301
  categories of, 285–86
  vs. conventional medicine, 286–87
  evaluating, 289–91
  overview, 284–85, 288, 304
  practitioners, communication with, 290, 294
  quality of life and, 287–89
  reflexology, 295–300
Compression bandages, for lymphedema, 332
Computer safety, 279, 280–81, 283, 319. *See also* Resources
Connective tissue disease, treatment contraindications, 105
Control
  of message, in discussing diagnosis, 50–54
  sense of, 124, 132, 144, 265, 336
Conventional, vs. complementary medicine, 286–87
Co-payments, 137
Core needle biopsy, 15, 85–86
Corporate Angel Network, 153
Cortisol, 234
Costs, of cancer, generally, 136–37.
  See also Financial concerns
Counseling, 58–59, 338. *See also* Psychotherapy

Coworkers, communication with, 61–63
Creative arts therapy, 250–55
Cross-training, 229
Cruciferous vegetables, 158, 182, 183–84
Cyclophosphamide, 124
Cytotoxic medications. *See* Chemotherapy
Cytoxan, 124

D

Dairy products, 159, 189, 190
Dance therapy, 253–54, 255
Davenport, Leslie, 242
Davis, Sherry Lebed, 255
DCIS (ductal carcinoma in situ), 89–91, 109
Death and dying, 8, 19–20, 25–26, 274. *See also* Life expectancy
Deegan, Donna, 29
Deep vein thrombosis, 318
Denial, 9
Dense breasts, 14, 82, 85, 313
Depression, 58, 181, 233, 260
Detection techniques, 81–85
Diabetes, treatment contraindications, 105
Diagnosis
  coming to terms with, 8–11, 28
  communication about, 6–8, 48–63, 66
  defined, 13
  in pathology reports, 15–16, 39, 43, 86–87, **87**, **88**, 90
  tests used in, 13–15, 24
Diagnostic imaging, 14, 82
Diaphragmatic breathing, 259, 292–93
Diet and nutrition
  appetite loss, 168–69
  checklist for, 190–91
  colorful foods role, 159
  complementary medicine and, 305

healthy eating basics, 162–80
  importance of, 157–58, 328
  mood and, 181
  plant-based diets, 182–89
  for reduced cancer risk, 158–60, 192–93
  as risk factor, 81, 163, 166–67, 173–74
  supplement recommendations, 165, 171
Dietary fat, 159, 165–67, 181, 189
Dip exercise, 214, **214**
Disability insurance, 141
Discussion boards, 279
Distant metastasis, 88
Distant recurrence, 322–24
DNA mutations, 77
Docetaxel, 125
Doctors
  accreditation of, 34
  communication with, 15–18, 40–42, 124, 286–87, 290–91
  rating of, 34
  on second opinions, 44
  selection of, 30–37, 32–33, 39–40, 137, 311–12
Dopamine, 338
"Dose-dense" chemotherapy schedule, 125
Doxorubicin, 124, 125
Drains, surgical, 100, 103
Drugs. *See* Medications
Ductal carcinoma in situ (DCIS), 89–91, 109
Ductal tumors, 89–91, 109, 188

E

Eli Lilly, 151
Emotional health, complementary therapies for, 300. *See also* Quality of life; Stress, management techniques
Employment issues, 61–63, 70–71, 143
EmWave, 249

I

Imagery (mental technique), <u>27</u>, 28
Imaging tests, 14–15, <u>39</u>, 82–85, 139
Immune system
    infection risks, 111, 196, 257, 321,
        332
    stress and, 233
Immunotherapy, <u>129</u>, 130–31
Implants. *See* Breast implants
Individual path, of cancer, 25–26.
    See also Personalized
    treatment
Indoles, <u>183</u>
Infection risks, 111, 196, 257, 321,
    332
Infertility. *See* Fertility issues
Infiltrating cancers, 91
Inflammation, 173, <u>181</u>, 190
Inflammatory breast cancer, 92
Information resources. *See*
    Resources
Insulin growth factor, 81
Insurance card copies, 142
Insurance coverage
    ACA, 135–37
    denial/withdrawal of, 131,
        136–38
    lack of, <u>143</u>
    organization tips, 142–45
    policy copies, <u>141</u>
    resources regarding, 137, 138, 152
    second opinions and, 42
    services covered, 104, 136, 239
Integrative medicine, <u>288</u>. *See also*
    Complementary medicine
Internal radiation, 110–11, 112
Internet. *See* Computer safety;
    Resources
Interval trials, <u>120–21</u>
Interval workouts, 219, <u>219</u>
Intraoperative radiation, 116
Introverts, 49–50
Intuition, listening to, 42
Invasive cancers, 91
Iodine, 176–77
Iron, 177
Isoflavones, 163–64, <u>183</u>

Isolation, 9, 265
Isothiocyanates, <u>183</u>, 184
Ixabepilone, <u>151</u>
Ixempra, <u>151</u>

J

Job discrimination, <u>70–71</u>
Job performance, 61–62
Joint pain, 319
Jolie, Angelina, 80
Journals and journaling
    exercises using, <u>33</u>, <u>45</u>, <u>68–69</u>,
        90, <u>236–37</u>, <u>252</u>
    for exercise tracking, 200, 229
    getting started, <u>6–7</u>
    for help with cognitive
        impairment, 328
    for worry management, 54–55

K

Kabat-Zinn, Jon, 244–45, <u>246</u>
Knee Tuck exercise, 226, **226**
Knowledge, power of, <u>90</u>. *See also*
    Resources

L

Lab tests, cost planning, 139
Language
    age-appropriate, 60
    glossary of terms, 343–54
L-ascorbic acid, 172–73
Latissimus dorsi flap procedure,
    <u>105</u>
Lavender, as estrogen mimic, <u>301</u>
LCIS (lobular carcinoma in situ), 89
Lebed method, of dance therapy,
    254
Legal issues, <u>70–71</u>, 150, 152
Leg Extension exercise, 227, **227**
Leg Slide exercise, 224, **224**
Legumes, 184
Letrozole, 128, 318

National Cancer Institute, 32–33, 269
National Cancer Legal Services Network, 150
National Lymphedema Network, 257, 269
National Patient Travel Center, 153
Nausea
  exercise and, 193, 196
  treatment for
    complementary therapies, 294, 295, 296–97, 301–2, 315
    creative arts therapy, 251, 253
    diet and, 168–69
    medications, 149
    visualization, 239
  as treatment side effect, 57, 121, 131
Needle localization, 99
Negative comments, preparing for, 65
Negative thinking, 55
Neoadjuvant therapy, 83, 110, 117
Neurofeedback, 248
Neuropathy, from chemotherapy, 123
Neurotransmitters, 234–35
NeuVax, 129
Night sweats, 331
Nipples
  cancers in, 91–92
  reconstruction, 106
Nolvadex. See Tamoxifen
Nonmedical costs, planning for, 147
Not Feeling Your Best workout, 224–25
Novartis, 151
Nurses/nurse practitioners, 37
Nutrients, essential, 170–80
Nutrition experts/nutritionists, 39, 160, 161. See also Diet and nutrition
Nuts and seeds, 181, 187

O

Obesity and overweight, 81, 167, 190
Observational trials, 120–21
Olive oil, 191
Omega-3 fatty acids, 164–65, 166–67, 181, 191
Omega-6 fatty acids, 166–67
Oncofertility Consortium, 127
Oncologists, 30–37, 39–40, 312
Oncotype DX, 122–23
One-Arm Row exercise, 206, **206**
Online resources. See Computer safety; Resources
Optimism, 8–9, 55
Oral contraceptives, 80
Organic foods, 189
Organization-based support groups, 268–69
Organization tips, 39, 51, 53, 141, 142–45
Organosulfides, 183
Osteoporosis, 128, 175
Out-of-pocket costs, 43, 136–37, 146
Ovarian ablation, 115
Ovarian cancer, 313, 314
Ovarian suppression, 130
Ovaries, removal of, 115
Overdiagnosis, 109
Overtreatment, 109
Oxidative damage, 186–87
Oxytocin, 338

P

Paclitaxel, 124, 151
Paget's disease, 91–92
Pain
  management approaches, 265, 293–94, 295, 298, 305–6
  phantom, 103
  postoperative, 294
Palliative therapy, 116
PAM50, 123
Paperwork, 39, 43, 141
Papillary cancer, 91
Partial-breast radiation, 116

Progesterone-sensitive/
    progesterone receptor
    positive (PR+) tumors, 92,
    125–26, 160
Prognosis, 18–20, 21, 322–24
Progression, vs. recurrence, of
    cancer, 320
Prostate cancer, 130
Prosthetics, fitting of, 103
Protein, dietary, 162–65, 180, 184,
    191
Protein kinase C, 174
Psychiatrists, 39
Psychologists, 39
Psychotherapeutic healing, 250–54
Psychotherapy, 267–68, 333, 338
PTSD (post-traumatic stress
    disorder), 239
Public policy, 342
Pulmonary embolism, 318
Pushups, 218, **218**

Q

Qi, 291
Qigong, 260–62, 261
Qigong Beginning Practice (DVD),
    261
Quadrantectomy. *See* Lumpectomy
Quality of life
    complementary medicine and,
        287–89, 295
    exercise role, 193–94
    factors in, 6
    stress management for, 248
Questions. *See also*
        Communication
    about adjuvant therapy, 118–19
    about cancer types, 90
    from children, 62
    communication role, 40–42
    for doctors, 17–18
    leading, avoiding, 41
    for spouses, 57–58
    writing down, 41
    for yourself, 52
Quinoa, 188

R

Race, as risk factor, 79, 113
Radiation
    with chemotherapy, 117–18
    cost planning, 139
    for DCIS, 91
    dietary considerations, 187
    exercise and, 196
    intraoperative, 116
    with lumpectomy, 98
    from mammography, 83
    with mastectomy, 106, 111
    overview, 110–12
    partial-breast, 116
    recurrence statistics, 100
    risks of, 109
    scheduling and duration, 107,
        116–17
    stress management for, 257
    in treating recurrence, 321
Radiation oncologists, 37
Radiation physicists, 39
Radiation technologists, 39
Radical mastectomy, 101
Radioactive seed localization,
    99
Radiologists, 37
Radiology reports, interpretation
    of, 43
Raloxifene, 89, 126, 128, 151
Raquel's Wings for Life, 153
Reach to Recovery, 269
Reaction, vs. response, 45
Reconstructive surgery, 57–58,
    103–4, 105
Recover and Rejuvenate workout,
    211–18
Recurrence
    chemotherapy and, 119
    diminished chances of, over
        time, 333
    after lumpectomy, 100
    after mastectomy, 106
    overview, 319–20
    prediction of, 123
    vs. progression, 320
    with tamoxifen, 315

with triple negative cancers, 93
types of, 320–24
Re-excision surgery, 102
Reflexology, 295–300, 298–99
Regional lymph nodes, 88
Regional recurrence, 321–22
Relationship concerns, 58–59,
    64–67, 336–39
Research campaigns, 339
Research studies, evaluating,
    22–23
Resistance training, 196, 197, 201
Resistant starch vegetables, 184
Resources. *See also* Apps
    breast cancer, 73
    clinical trials, 121
    complementary medicine, 298
    counseling, 59
    diet and nutrition, 161, 165
    exercise, 47, 200, 230
    fertility issues, 127
    financial, 148–53
    follow-up care, 323
    fundraising, 341–42
    insurance coverage, 137, 138, 152
    for medical team research, 32–34
    patient navigation services, 38
    patient portals, 35–36
    psychological support, 59
    stress management tools, 242,
        246, 255, 257, 261
    support groups, 272–82
    transportation, 152–53
    treatment options, 119
Response, vs. reaction, 45
Response duration, defined, 118
Retinoids, 170, 172
Rewarding yourself, 340–41
Risk assessment
    chemotherapy, 119
    radiation, 109
Risk factors
    diet, 163, 166–67, 173–74
    existing/previous cancer, 89
    gene mutations, 80, 178, 313–14
    LCIS as, 89
    overview, 78–81
    scanning/imaging, 84

Road to Recovery program, 148–49
Rx Outreach, 150
Rye flour, 188

S

Saline, in vaccines, 129
Salt, 176–77, 190
Saturated fats, 166, 189, 191
Saying "no," 330
Scar tissue, 321
Scribes, 40
Seafood, 164–65, 191
Seated Twist pose, 223, **223**
Seated Workout, 226–28
Second opinions, 42–44, 46, 98,
    115, 320
Second primary cancers, 320
Sedentary lifestyle, 329
Seeds. *See* Nuts and seeds
Segmental mastectomy. *See*
    Lumpectomy
Selective estrogen-receptor
    modulators (SERMs), 126,
    128
Selenium, 176, 177–78
Self-awareness, 52, 252,
    316–17
Self-care, 316–17
Self-education, regarding
    treatment options, 124.
    See also Resources
Self-esteem, 194
Self-exams. *See* Breast exams
"Self-Healing with Guided
    Imagery" (recording), 242
Self-help support groups, 267
Semicircle Crunch exercise, 225,
    225
Senior citizens, insurance coverage,
    138, 161
Sensation
    loss of, 104, 322
    preservation of, 58
Sentinel lymph nodes
    biopsy of, 43, 106, 108–9, **108**
    removal of, 100, 101

SERMs (selective estrogen-receptor modulators), 126, 128
Serotonin, 181
Sex/sexual issues, 58, 67, 337, 338
Sharsheret, 269
Show Me (Gingrich), 94
Side Sweep exercise, 210, **210**
Silver, Marc, 338
Simanca, Kimberly, 263
Simple mastectomy, 101
Skin-saving mastectomy, 102–3
Sleep problems, 233, 235, 289, 328, 329–30
Smokers/smoking, 81, 105
Snack recommendations, 181
Social isolation, 265, 266
Social media, 276–77
Social Security Administration, 152
Social workers, 39
Soda, 190, 330
Sodium, 176–77, 190
Solitude, 50
Soltamox. *See* Tamoxifen
Soy foods, 163–64
Special needs support groups, 269
Speed Skater exercise, 205, **205**
Spices, 187, 191
Spiritual counselors, 39
Spiritual practice, 303
Spouses, communication with, 55–60, 64–69, 72, 336–39
Squat to Raise exercise, 213, **213**
Staging, of cancers/tumors
  in pathology reports, 87, **87**, 88, 89–90
  systems for, 23–24, 26, 43, 86
  treatment selection based on, 97, 115–16, 119
Standing Crunch exercise, 217, **217**
Statistics
  cancer survival, 4, 5
  evaluation of, 19, 22–23
Stereotactic core-needle biopsy, 15, 85–86

Strength training. *See* Resistance training
Stress
  benefits of, 240
  coping strategies, 181
  effects of, 233–35
  management techniques
    biofeedback, 247–50
    exercise, 229, 258–62
    expressive/creative arts therapy, 250–55
    imagery/visualization, 238–39, 241
    massage, 254, 256–57, 295–96, 332
    meditation, 240, 243–47, 246, 262
    overview, 235, 238
    self-assessment, 236–37
Stretching, 196
Sugar, 167, 181, 190, 330
Sulforaphane, 183
Summary Stage system, 26
Sunrise Tai Chi (DVD), 261
Supplements, dietary, 165, 171, 285, 290–91
Support groups. *See also* Community of supporters
  benefits of, 264–66
  resources, 268–69
  role of, 112, 333
  selecting, 275
  self-assessment, 270–71
  vs. twelve-step programs, 266–67
  types of, 267–69, 272
Surgeons, 36–37
Surgery
  body image and, 57–58
  cost planning, 140
  lumpectomy, 98–100, **101**
  mastectomy, 100–104, **101**, 106
  neoadjuvant therapy, 110, 117
  preparation and aftercare, 110
  reconstructive, 57–58, 103–4, 105
  sentinel node biopsy, 43, 106, 108–9, **108**